Fractal and Fractional Analysis in Biomedical Sciences and Engineering

Fractal and Fractional Analysis in Biomedical Sciences and Engineering

Guest Editor

Andjelija Ž. Ilić

Basel • Beijing • Wuhan • Barcelona • Belgrade • Novi Sad • Cluj • Manchester

Guest Editor
Andjelija Ž. Ilić
Institute of Physics Belgrade
University of Belgrade
Belgrade
Serbia

Editorial Office
MDPI AG
Grosspeteranlage 5
4052 Basel, Switzerland

This is a reprint of the Special Issue, published open access by the journal *Fractal and Fractional* (ISSN 2504-3110), freely accessible at: https://www.mdpi.com/journal/fractalfract/special_issues/07796134G7.

For citation purposes, cite each article independently as indicated on the article page online and as indicated below:

Lastname, A.A.; Lastname, B.B. Article Title. *Journal Name* **Year**, *Volume Number*, Page Range.

ISBN 978-3-7258-4847-8 (Hbk)
ISBN 978-3-7258-4848-5 (PDF)
https://doi.org/10.3390/books978-3-7258-4848-5

Cover image courtesy of Radmila Janković

Contents

About the Editor

Andjelija Ž. Ilić

Andjelija Ž. Ilić was born in Belgrade, Serbia. She received the Dipl. Eng., M.Sc., and Ph.D. degrees in Electrical Engineering in 1998, 2004, and 2010, respectively, from the University of Belgrade (Belgrade, Serbia), the University of Massachusetts Dartmouth (MA, USA), and the University of Belgrade (Belgrade, Serbia). She was a Postdoctoral Research Associate with the School of Science and Technology at the University of Westminster, London, UK (2013–2014). She is now a Principal Research Fellow with the Institute of Physics, University of Belgrade. Her research interests span the fields of applied physics and applied electromagnetics, encompassing numerical methods in physics and electromagnetics, microwave components and circuits, accelerator physics and technology, the application of novel materials in electrical engineering, electromagnetic field interactions with biological systems, and biomedical image and signal processing. Dr. Ilić is a Senior Member of IEEE and a Member of Optical Society of Serbia. She was the recipient of the 2006 Young Scientist Award and the 2014 Best Paper ETRAN Award, as well as the "Prof. Aleksandar Marinčić" Award, given annually by the IEEE MTTS Serbia chapter, for the best journal paper in 2016.

Preface

The ten original studies presented in this Special Issue Reprint explore innovative ways of using fractal and fractional models in the life sciences, with the aim of better understanding and quantitatively describing the structure and behavior of the modeled specimens and systems. The subject and scope of the Special Issue were defined in such a way as to allow prospective authors to choose a research topic of their current interest, as long as it concerns the complexity in biological systems. Therefore, the subject considers application of fractal and fractional analysis in any basic or applied scientific investigation in life sciences. The wide scope of this Special Issue resulted in the collection of very interesting studies on diverse research topics, all of which were connected by the methodology employed in the studies. Another factor connecting the authors of these studies is their motivation to apply fractal methodology towards the improvement of objective specimen evaluation, data classification, and understanding of the underlying mechanisms in the studied processes, as well as improvements in diagnostics where the topic is linked to the field of medicine. In summary, the presented works seem to have the potential to contribute to future improvements in science and technology. On the other hand, the studies also have the potential to make students in life science majors more interested in applied mathematics and in discovering how it can help elucidate the causes and developments governing the behavior of biological systems. This Reprint is prepared with the confidence that it will be of interest to researchers, students, and practitioners in the fields of applied mathematics, life sciences, and medicine.

Andjelija Ž. Ilić
Guest Editor

fractal and fractional

MDPI

Editorial

Fractal and Fractional Analysis in Biomedical Sciences and Engineering

Andjelija Ž. Ilić

Institute of Physics Belgrade, University of Belgrade, Pregrevica 118, 11080 Belgrade-Zemun, Serbia; andjelijailic@ieee.org

The visual appearance of fractal patterns in biology has been noted from the early days of research in this field and, henceforth, has been studied for a long time. The typical examples that first come to mind include the branching of the airways in the lungs, the vasculature in the liver, and the shape of cauliflower and broccoli. Then, there are signals —heart signals, brain signals, measured gait patterns, and DNA sequences. The more the research in fractal and fractional phenomena progresses, the more the pronounced fractal behavior of biological systems at every level of organization is noticed. This Special Issue illustrates the breadth of problems, which are being investigated today using the mathematical apparatus of fractal and fractional calculus, by presenting ten papers on very diverse topics in bioscience.

Contribution No. 1 employs fractional calculus in a study of honeybee population dynamics, which is becoming a problem of increasing importance, with honeybee losses being reported in many countries nowadays. The disruption of pollination causes serious additional problems in economics, agriculture, and ecology.

Contribution No. 2 explores the potential of the fractal analysis of intestinal cell nuclei, to serve as an observer-independent histological tool for pediatric ulcerative colitis diagnosis. The investigation was motivated by the noted unfolding of chromatin in the cell nuclei in some diseases, being reflected macroscopically in the altered textures of the nuclei.

A novel unsupervised deep learning approach for characterizing the degree of fractality of dried drop patterns of plant-based homeopathic remedies is proposed in Contribution No. 3. The self- assembled structures formed in evaporating droplets differed for the three mixing procedures that were applied (turbulent, laminar, and diffusion-based mixing).

The corneal geometry of the human eye is studied in Contribution No. 4. The non-integer behavior of the corneal-shaped model is studied using several machine learning models, with the best results achieved through the use of artificial neural network based on the hybrid biogeography-based heterogeneous cuckoo search optimization technique.

The Contribution No. 5 proposes the use of a novel orthogonal matrix decomposition method in combination with the orthogonal generalized Laguerre moments of fractional orders for the analysis of large bio-signals. Due to the highly accurate and stable calculations of higher-order moments, the analysis tested on the arrhythmia dataset is very efficient.

The fractal analysis of immunohistochemical images of invasive cutaneous squamous cell carcinoma is proposed in Contribution No. 6 as the method to potentially inform the development of new diagnostic and therapeutic strategies targeting the tumor microenvironment. Quantitative analysis of the spatial distribution patterns of immune and vascular markers is used for the classification of pre-invasive and invasive lesions.

In Contribution No. 7, fractional electrodamage induced by the electrical stimulation of A549 human lung cancer cells is investigated. Experimentally obtained data is fitted and the order of the fractional derivative is selected to provide the best model of cell elongation during the electrochemical changes. Significant electrocapacitive effects were exhibited by the cells.

The scale-free dynamics of the resting state fMRI is considered in Contributiom No. 8 as a possible multimodal biomarker to study both spatial (brain tissue type and functional networks) and temporal (activation and cognition) brain dynamics. The microstate segmentation method served to obtain topological maps, and the EEG and fMRI data were used simultaneously.

The simulation-based investigation of the tumor growth and chemical diffusion in biological tissues is described in Contribution No. 9, contributing to a deeper understanding of the chemical diffusion mechanisms within tissues and tumor growth under different conditions. Fractional stochastic calculus was used to model these processes.

Finally, in Contribution No. 10, the fractional Fourier transform is combined with the error back-propagation neural network, with an aim of performing advanced image feature extraction and model generalization in tumor diagnostics. The main focus of the prediction model was distinguishing between the benign and malignant cases.

In conclusion, most of the presented articles rely on empirical, real-world data and advanced non-integer models to achieve good agreement between experimental observations and the models aiming to provide deeper insights into the studied phenomena. Numerical models, developed and trained on real-world data, can be valuable tools for the prediction of process progression and, in some cases, treatment monitoring in biomedical sciences. All of the selected papers have the potential to contribute to addressing practical problems. The proposed new methods can be applied in future to diverse sets of problems.

Funding: This research received no external funding.

Acknowledgments: The author acknowledges the funding provided by the Institute of Physics Belgrade, University of Belgrade, through the grants from the Ministry of Science, Technological Development, and Innovations of the Republic of Serbia.

Conflicts of Interest: The author declares no conflicts of interest.

List of Contributions

1. Georgiev, S.; Vulkov, L. Parameters Identification and Numerical Simulation for a Fractional Model of Honeybee Population Dynamics. *Fractal Fract.* **2023**, *7*, 311. https://doi.org/10.3390/fractalfract7040311.
2. Makević, V.; Milovanovich, I.D.; Popovac, N.; Janković, R.; Trajković, J.; Vuković, A.; Milosević, B.; Jevtić, J.; de Luka, S.R.; Ilić, A.Ž. Fractal Parameters as Independent Biomarkers in the Early Diagnosis of Pediatric Onset Inflammatory Bowel Disease. *Fractal Fract.* **2023**, *7*, 619. https://doi.org/10.3390/fractalfract7080619.
3. Acuña, C.; Kokornaczyk, M.O.; Baumgartner, S.; Castelán, M. Unsupervised Deep Learning Approach for Characterizing Fractality in Dried Drop Patterns of Differently Mixed *Viscum album* Preparations. *Fractal Fract.* **2023**, *7*, 733. https://doi.org/10.3390/fractalfract7100733.
4. Waseem; Ullah, A.; Awwad, F.A.; Ismail, E.A.A. Analysis of the Corneal Geometry of the Human Eye with an Artificial Neural Network. *Fractal Fract.* **2023**, *7*, 764. https://doi.org/10.3390/fractalfract7100764.
5. Aldakheel, E.A.; Khafaga, D.S.; Fathi, I.S.; Hosny, K.M.; Hassan, G. Efficient Analysis of Large-Size Bio-Signals Based on Orthogonal Generalized Laguerre Moments of Fractional Orders and Schwarz–Rutishauser Algorithm. *Fractal Fract.* **2023**, *7*, 826. https://doi.org/10.3390/fractalfract7110826.
6. Buruiană, A.; Șerbănescu, M.-S.; Pop, B.; Gheban, B.-A.; Gheban-Roșca, I.-A.; Hendea, R.M.; Georgiu, C.; Crișan, D.; Crișan, M. Fractal Dimension Analysis of the Tumor Microenvironment in Cutaneous Squamous Cell Carcinoma: Insights into Angiogenesis and Immune Cell Infiltration. *Fractal Fract.* **2024**, *8*, 600. https://doi.org/10.3390/fractalfract8100600.

7. Martines-Arano, H.; Arano-Martinez, J.A.; Mosso-Pani, M.A.; Valdivia-Flores, A.; Trejo-Valdez, M.; García-Pérez, B.E.; Torres-Torres, C. Fractional Electrodamage in A549 Human Lung Cancer Cells. *Fractal Fract.* **2025**, *9*, 34. https://doi.org/10.3390/fractalfract9010034.
8. Erbil, N.; Deshpande, G. Scale-Free Dynamics of Resting-State fMRI Microstates. *Fractal Fract.* **2025**, *9*, 112. https://doi.org/10.3390/fractalfract9020112.
9. Ghezal, A.; Attia, N. ϑ-Fractional Stochastic Models for Simulating Tumor Growth and Chemical Diffusion in Biological Tissues. *Fractal Fract.* **2025**, *9*, 258. https://doi.org/10.3390/fractalfract9040258.
10. Liu, X.; Gao, N.; He, S.; Wang, L. Application of Fractional Fourier Transform and BP Neural Network in Prediction of Tumor Benignity and Malignancy. *Fractal Fract.* **2025**, *9*, 267. https://doi.org/10.3390/fractalfract9050267.

fractal and fractional

MDPI

Article

Parameters Identification and Numerical Simulation for a Fractional Model of Honeybee Population Dynamics †

Slavi Georgiev [1,2,*] and Lubin Vulkov [2]

1 Department of Informational Modeling, Institute of Mathematics and Informatics, Bulgarian Academy of Sciences, 1113 Sofia, Bulgaria
2 Department of Applied Mathematics and Statistics, Faculty of Natural Sciences and Education, University of Ruse, 7004 Ruse, Bulgaria; lvalkov@uni-ruse.bg
* Correspondence: sggeorgiev@uni-ruse.bg; Tel.: +359-82-888-725

† This is an extended version of our conference paper "Georgiev, S.G.; Vulkov, L.G. Parameter identification approach for a fractional dynamics model of honeybee population. In Lecture Notes in Computer Science; Springer: Cham, Switzerland, 2022; Volume 13127, pp. 40–48".

Abstract: In order to investigate the honeybee population dynamics, many differential equation models were proposed. Fractional derivatives incorporate the history of the honeybee population dynamics. We numerically study the inverse problem of parameter identification in models with Caputo and Caputo–Fabrizio differential operators. We use a gradient method of minimizing a quadratic cost functional. We analyze and compare results for the integer (classic) and fractional models. The present work also contains discussion on the efficiency of the numerical methods used. Computational tests with realistic data were performed and are discussed.

Keywords: honeybee population dynamics; fractional derivative; parameter estimation; cost function minimization

MSC: 26A33; 34A08; 34A55; 65L09; 92D25

1. Introduction

In recent years, honeybee losses were reported in many countries such as the USA, China, Israel, Turkey, and in European countries, especially, Bulgaria [1]. The disruption of pollination causes serious problems in economics, agriculture and ecology.

The honey bees *Apis mellifera* are the main contributors to pollination, and the global loss of honeybees leads to disruption of pollination, which, thus, causes serious difficulties in *economics, agriculture and ecology* [2,3]. The leading factor for the loss of honeybees has not yet been discovered, but it has been found that an ensemble of stressors cause a colony to collapse. Some of the main reasons are infections by viruses, such as Nosema ceranae, Varroa mite [4], the use of pesticides [5], food shortages [6] and severe weather conditions [7].

Colonies of honeybees have been declining for over a decade [8]. Colony losses are due to a combination of stressors [8,9], but the presence of Varroa mites is considered one of the most important factors [10].

Mathematical models have been widely used to examine and predict the dynamics of honeybee population. The paper [11] presents a review of recent progress in mathematical modeling of honeybee colony population dynamics, since the review in [12]. In the latter, models, studying different stress factors which lead to further colony collapse were reviewed. In a recent paper [11], though, the models were divided on the basis of age structure, nutritional effects, pathogens, etc. The common trait between the existing models is that they were derived on the base of the classical (integer) derivative. Their potential to identify different factors causing colony losses are discussed.

On the other hand, fractional-order models have been recognized as a powerful mathematical tool to study anomalous behavior observed in many physical processes with prominent memory and hereditary properties. Thanks to the memory effect, which represents an advantage of the fractional derivative compared to the ordinary derivative, the theory and the application of fractional calculus have been widely used to model dynamic processes in the fields of science, engineering and many others. The last decades, especially, have seen a rapid development, both in theory and applications, of fractional ordinary differential equations, as in, for example, [13–17], and the application of fractional-order derivatives in biological phenomena [18,19]. However, to our knowledge, literature dedicated to modeling honeybee population dynamics via fractional-order derivatives is quite scarce. For instance, to investigate the causes of colony collapse, the author of [20] proposed a fractional honeybee colony population model. We adopted this model to demonstrate the solution approach to the inverse parameter reconstruction problem.

The rest of this paper is structured as follows. In the next section, the necessary fractional calculus background is mentioned. In Section 3, the direct and inverse problems are formulated and interpreted. The numerical methods used to solve the direct problems are described in Section 4, while the adjoint equation optimization method, for solving the inverse problems, is presented in detail in Section 5, which is the main novelty of the study. The simulation results are discussed in Section 6 and the paper is concluded in Section 7.

This work is an extended version of the LSSC'21 conference paper [21]. There, the Caputo derivative model in the special case was studied when the identified parameters were $\boldsymbol{p} = \{m, n, \alpha, \sigma, \omega\}$ and they were raised to the power of one at the right hand-side of the system (3). Obviously, the current study extends the latter in two ways. Firstly, the coefficients at the right hand-side of the model system are raised to the poser of the fractional derivation, which is more meaningful, due to the preservation of the physical unit. Secondly, an investigation with the Caputo–Fabrizio fractional derivative is performed.

The main advantages of the application of the Caputo–Fabrizio derivative in the present context are two. To begin with, the smooth, non-singular kernel makes the numerical treatment easier. The mathematical expressions, derived from the Caputo derivative, are often cumbersome and tedious to derive. The Caputo–Fabrizio derivative is suitable for both temporal and spatial variables. The consequent formulae exhibit simplifications, which also make the analytical treatment lighter as well. What is more, the application of the Caputo derivative is more appropriate when the model is related to "plasticity, fatigue, damage and with electromagnetic hysteresis". Otherwise, it is useful to employ the Caputo–Fabrizio derivative [22].

2. Fractional Calculus Background

In this section some basic definitions and results from fractional calculus are introduced.

2.1. Caputo Derivative

For any function $v \in \mathcal{AC}[0,T]$, i.e., v is absolutely continuous on $[0,T]$, we define the left (forward) Riemann–Liouville integral for $p \in [0,1]$ [15]:

$$\left(J_{0+}^{p} v\right)(t) := \begin{cases} v(t), & p = 0, \\ \dfrac{1}{\Gamma(p)} \displaystyle\int_0^t \frac{v(s)}{(t-s)^{1-p}} \mathrm{d}s, & 0 < p \le 1, \end{cases} \quad t \in [0,T).$$

Then, the left (forward) Caputo derivative, as defined above, could be expressed in this way:

$${}^{\mathfrak{C}}\mathrm{D}_0^p v(t) = \left(J_{0+}^{1-p} \frac{\mathrm{d}v}{\mathrm{d}t}\right)(t) = \frac{1}{\Gamma(1-p)} \int_0^t \frac{1}{(t-s)^p} \frac{\mathrm{d}v}{\mathrm{d}t}(s) \mathrm{d}s.$$

The left (forward) Riemann–Liouville derivative is defined as

$$ {}^{\mathfrak{R}}\mathrm{D}_0^p v(t) = \frac{\mathrm{d}}{\mathrm{d}t}\left(J_{0^+}^{1-p} v\right)(t) = \frac{1}{\Gamma(1-p)}\frac{\mathrm{d}}{\mathrm{d}t}\int_0^t \frac{v(s)}{(t-s)^p}\mathrm{d}s. $$

The right (backward) integral is defined as

$$ \left(J_{T^-}^p v\right)(t) := \begin{cases} v(t), & p = 0, \\ \dfrac{1}{\Gamma(p)}\displaystyle\int_t^T \frac{v(s)}{(s-t)^{1-p}}\mathrm{d}s, & 0 < p \le 1, \end{cases} \quad t \in (0,T], $$

and, further, we define the right (backward) Caputo derivative as

$$ {}^{\mathfrak{C}}\mathrm{D}_T^p v(t) = -\left(J_{T^-}^{1-p}\frac{\mathrm{d}v}{\mathrm{d}t}\right)(t) = -\frac{1}{\Gamma(1-p)}\int_t^T \frac{1}{(s-t)^p}\frac{\mathrm{d}v}{\mathrm{d}t}(s)\mathrm{d}s. $$

$$ {}^{\mathfrak{R}}\mathrm{D}_T^p v(t) = \left(-\frac{\mathrm{d}}{\mathrm{d}t}\right)\left(J_{T^-}^{1-p} v\right)(t) = -\frac{1}{\Gamma(1-p)}\frac{\mathrm{d}}{\mathrm{d}t}\int_t^T \frac{1}{(s-t)^p}v(s)\mathrm{d}s. $$

There exists a relationship between the Caputo and Riemann–Liouville forward and backward derivatives

$$ {}^{\mathfrak{C}}\mathrm{D}_0^p f(t) = {}^{\mathfrak{R}}\mathrm{D}_0^p f(t) - \frac{f(0)}{\Gamma(1-p)}t^{-p},\ t \in (0,T], $$

$$ {}^{\mathfrak{C}}\mathrm{D}_T^p f(t) = {}^{\mathfrak{R}}\mathrm{D}_T^p f(t) - \frac{f(T)}{\Gamma(1-p)}(T-t)^{-p},\ t \in (0,T]. $$

For later use, we recall the following version of integration by parts, see e.g., [15].

Lemma 1. *Let $v_1(t), v_2(t) \in C^1[0,T]$. Then*

$$ \int_0^T \left({}^{\mathfrak{C}}\mathrm{D}_0^p v_1\right)v_2 \mathrm{d}t + v_1(0)\left(J_{T^-}^{1-p}v_2\right)(0) = \int_0^T v_1\left({}^{\mathfrak{C}}\mathrm{D}_T^p v_2\right)\mathrm{d}t + \left(J_{T^-}^{1-p}v_1\right)(T)v_2(T). \tag{1} $$

We use the *generalized mean value formula (GMF)* in the following form [15]. Suppose $f(t) \in C[a,b]$ and $\mathrm{D}_0^p f(t) \in C[a,b]$ for $0 < p \le 1$, then we have

$$ f(t) = f(0) + \frac{1}{\Gamma(p)}\mathrm{D}_0^p f(\xi)t^p \text{ with } 0 \le \xi \le t,\ \forall t \in [a,b]. $$

It is clear from this formula that if $\mathrm{D}_0^p f(t) \ge 0\ \forall t \in (a,b)$, then the function $f(t)$ is nondecreasing for each $t \in [a,b]$, and if $\mathrm{D}_0^p f(t) \le 0\ \forall t \in (a,b)$, then the function $f(t)$ is nonincreasing $\forall t \in [a,b]$.

2.2. Caputo–Fabrizio Derivative

In recent years, the results of many papers have demonstrated that fractional models describe natural phenomena in an accurate and systematic way, which is better than the classic integer-order counterparts ordinary time derivatives; see, for example, [23,24]. However, in some cases, a satisfactory duration may not be achieved in whole time duration due to the singularity in the traditional (namely, Caputo's) kernel; see, for example, [22]. This is one of the reasons the Caputo–Fabrizio derivative was used in [20].

Similarly to the Caputo case, if $v \in \mathcal{AC}[0,T]$, then for $p \in [0,1]$ we define the left (forward) Caputo–Fabrizio derivative in the Caputo and Riemann senses, respectively, as follows [22]:

$$ \begin{aligned} {}^{\mathfrak{CFC}}\mathrm{D}_0^p v(t) &= \frac{M(p)}{1-p}\int_0^t \exp\left(-\frac{p}{1-p}(t-s)\right)\frac{\mathrm{d}v}{\mathrm{d}t}(s)\mathrm{d}s, \\ {}^{\mathfrak{CFR}}\mathrm{D}_0^p v(t) &= \frac{M(p)}{1-p}\frac{\mathrm{d}}{\mathrm{d}t}\int_0^t \exp\left(-\frac{p}{1-p}(t-s)\right)v(s)\mathrm{d}s, \end{aligned} $$

where $M(p)$ is a normalization function such that $M(0) = M(1) = 1$.

Analogously, the right (backward) Caputo–Fabrizio derivative is defined as

$$
\begin{aligned}
{}^{\mathfrak{CFC}}\mathrm{D}_T^p v(t) &= -\frac{M(p)}{1-p}\int_t^T \exp\left(-\frac{p}{1-p}(s-t)\right)\frac{\mathrm{d}v}{\mathrm{d}t}(s)\mathrm{d}s, \\
{}^{\mathfrak{CFR}}\mathrm{D}_T^p v(t) &= -\frac{M(p)}{1-p}\frac{\mathrm{d}}{\mathrm{d}t}\int_t^T \exp\left(-\frac{p}{1-p}(s-t)\right)v(s)\mathrm{d}s.
\end{aligned}
$$

The relationship between the Caputo and Riemann senses of the Caputo–Fabrizio forward and backward derivatives is

$$
\begin{aligned}
{}^{\mathfrak{CFC}}\mathrm{D}_0^p f(t) &= {}^{\mathfrak{CFR}}\mathrm{D}_0^p f(t) - \frac{M(p)}{1-p}\exp\left(-\frac{p}{1-p}t\right),\ t \in (0,T], \\
{}^{\mathfrak{CFC}}\mathrm{D}_T^p v(t) &= {}^{\mathfrak{CFR}}\mathrm{D}_T^p v(t) - \frac{M(p)}{1-p}\exp\left(-\frac{p}{1-p}(T-t)\right),\ t \in (0,T].
\end{aligned}
$$

In order to derive the integration by parts for the Caputo–Fabrizio derivative, we introduce the Caputo–Fabrizio fractional integrals [25]:

$$
\begin{aligned}
\left({}^{\mathfrak{CF}}J_{0+}^p v\right)(t) &:= \frac{1-p}{M(p)}v(t) + \frac{p}{M(p)}\int_0^t v(s)\mathrm{d}s, \\
\left({}^{\mathfrak{CF}}J_{T-}^p v\right)(t) &:= \frac{1-p}{M(p)}v(t) + \frac{p}{M(p)}\int_t^T v(s)\mathrm{d}\,s.
\end{aligned}
$$

Now, we state the Caputo–Fabrizio integration by parts:

Lemma 2. *Let $v_1(t), v_2(t) \in C^1[0,T]$. Then*

$$
\begin{aligned}
&\int_0^T \left({}^{\mathfrak{CFC}}\mathrm{D}_0^p v_1\right)v_2\mathrm{d}t + \frac{M(p)}{1-p}v_1(0)\int_0^T \exp\left(-\frac{p}{1-p}t\right)v_2\mathrm{d}t = \\
&\qquad \int_0^T v_1\left({}^{\mathfrak{CFC}}\mathrm{D}_T^p v_2\right)\mathrm{d}t + \frac{M(p)}{1-p}v_2(T)\int_0^T \exp\left(-\frac{p}{1-p}(T-t)\right)v_1\mathrm{d}t. \quad (2)
\end{aligned}
$$

The *generalized mean value formula (GMF)* for the Caputo–Fabrizio fractional derivative is as follows [26]. Suppose $f(t) \in C[a,b]$ and ${}^{\mathfrak{CF}}\mathrm{D}_0^p f(t) \in C[a,b]$ for $0 < p \leq 1$, then we have

$$
f(t) = f(0) + \frac{1}{M(p)}\,{}^{\mathfrak{CFC}}\mathrm{D}_0^p f(\xi)\big((1-\alpha)+t\alpha\big) \text{ with } 0 \leq \xi \leq t,\ \forall t \in [a,b].
$$

For further detailed studies on the fractional calculus of the derivatives with the nonsingular kernel and its applications, the interested reader could refer to [22,25].

3. Models' Interpretations

In this section we introduce and discuss the two models with Caputo and Caputo–Fabrizio derivatives, respectively. Then we formulate the corresponding point-observation inverse problems and solve them by minimizing a least-square functional using the adjoint equation optimization approach.

3.1. Direct Problems

3.1.1. Model with Caputo Derivative

In [20] the following two-order fractional derivatives population model is proposed:

$$ {}^{\mathfrak{C}}\mathrm{D}_0^r H = L^r \frac{H+F}{\omega^r + H + F} - H\left(\alpha^r - \sigma^r \frac{F}{H+F}\right) - n^r H \equiv h(H,F;\boldsymbol{p}), \tag{3a} $$

$$ {}^{\mathfrak{C}}\mathrm{D}_0^q F = H\left(\alpha^r - \sigma^r \frac{F}{H+F}\right) - m^q F \equiv g(H,F;\boldsymbol{p}), \tag{3b} $$

$$ H(0) = H^0,\ F(0) = F^0, \quad t > 0, \tag{3c} $$

where $\mathrm{D}_0^p \mathfrak{f}$ $(p = r, q)$ denotes the fractional derivative of $\mathfrak{f}$ of order $0 < p \leq 1$. Here, H is the number of hive bees and the ones working outside the hive are the foragers F. The total number of bees in the colony is assumed to be $N = H + F$, since bees in compartments other than H and F do not contribute to the work in the hive. The workers are recruited to the forager class from the hive bee class and die with rate m. It is assumed that the maximal rate of eclosion is equivalent to the queen's laying rate L and it approaches the maximum as N increases. The constant parameter ω determines the rate at which $\mathcal{E}(H,F) = L^r(H+F)/(\omega^r + H + F)$ approaches L as N becomes large.

In the recruitment function $\mathcal{R}(H,F) = \alpha^r - \sigma^r F/(H+F)$, the parameter α represents the maximal rate at which hive bees become foragers when there are no foragers present in the colony, and σ is the rate of social inhibition. Following [20], the model (3a)–(3c) does not neglect the death rate n of the hive bees.

Theorem 1. *There exists a unique solution $(H,F)^\top \in C^1[0,T]$ to the initial-value problem* (3a)–(3c) *and it remains positive for $t \in [0,T]$ provided that the initial data is positive.*

Proof. The existence and uniqueness of the solution to the system (3a)–(3c) could be obtained on the base of the theory in [27], and some results in [28]. We need to show the positivity. On the contrary, let us assume that $H^0 > 0,\ F^0 > 0$ and let t^1 be the first time moment in which $H(t^1) = 0,\ F(t^1) > 0$. Then, from (3a), we have $\mathrm{D}_0^r H(t^1) = L^r \dfrac{F(t^1)}{\omega^r + F(t^1)} > 0$. However, from GMF the function $H(t)$ is non-decreasing for each $t \in [0, t^1]$ which contradicts the assumption. □

3.1.2. Model with Caputo–Fabrizio Derivative

Again in [20] the fractional population model with Caputo–Fabrizio derivatives follows:

$$ {}^{\mathfrak{CFC}}\mathrm{D}_0^r H = L^r \frac{H+F}{\omega^r + H + F} - H\left(\alpha^r - \sigma^r \frac{F}{H+F}\right) - n^r H \equiv h(H,F;\boldsymbol{p}), \tag{4a} $$

$$ {}^{\mathfrak{CFC}}\mathrm{D}_0^q F = H\left(\alpha^r - \sigma^r \frac{F}{H+F}\right) - m^q F \equiv g(H,F;\boldsymbol{p}), \tag{4b} $$

$$ H(0) = H^0,\ F(0) = F^0, \quad t > 0, \tag{4c} $$

The results for the existence and positivity of the solution, similar to Theorem 1, could be analogously proved. For results concerning uniqueness please refer to [20].

3.2. Inverse Problems

The functions $H(t), F(t)$ satisfy the *direct problem* (3a)–(3c) if the coefficients $p^1 = m$, $p^2 = n$, $p^3 = \alpha$, $p^4 = \sigma$, $p^5 = \omega$ are known. In practice, the parameters $m, n, \alpha, \sigma, \omega$ are not known, in general, and have to be identified. After their "fair" values are obtained, the model could be used for further robust analysis.

The main question is how to find the coefficients $\boldsymbol{p} \equiv \{m, n, \alpha, \sigma, \omega\}$ if we know the population size at certain times:

$$ H(t_k;\boldsymbol{p}) = X_k,\ k = 1,\ldots,K_H, \quad F(t_k;\boldsymbol{p}) = Y_k,\ k = 1,\ldots,K_F. \tag{5} $$

The estimation of the parameter $\boldsymbol{p}$ is referred to as an *inverse modeling problem*. This means adjusting the parameter values of a mathematical model in such a way as to reproduce measured data.

4. Numerical Solution to the Direct and Inverse Problems

The models (3a)–(3c) and (4), being nonlinear, do not suggest an analytical solution. In this section, we present the numerical schemes for solving the direct and inverse problems.

4.1. Model with Caputo Derivative

Firstly, we briefly recall the Adams–Bashford–Moulton method for forward fractional derivatives. We follow [29].

It is well known that a fractional initial value problem

$$ {}^{\mathfrak{C}}\mathrm{D}_0^p y(t) = f^p(t, y(t)), \qquad y(0) = y_0 $$

for $0 < p \leq 1$ is equivalent to the Volterra integral equation

$$ y(t) = y_0 + \frac{1}{\Gamma(p)} \int_0^t (t-s)^{p-1} f^p(s, y(s)) \mathrm{d}s \tag{6} $$

for $t \leq T$.

Introducing a uniform temporal mesh $\bar{\omega} = \{t_j = j\triangle t : j = 0, 1, \ldots, N\}$, where $\triangle t = T/N$ is the time step and $y_j \approx y(t_j)$, the approximate solution to (6) is:

$$ \begin{cases} y_{i+1}^P = y_0 + \dfrac{1}{\Gamma(p)} \displaystyle\sum_{j=0}^{i} b_{j,i+1} f^p(t_j, y_j), \\ y_{i+1} = y_0 + \dfrac{1}{\Gamma(p)} \left(\displaystyle\sum_{j=0}^{i} a_{j,i+1} f^p(t_j, y_j) + a_{i+1,i+1} f^p(t_{i+1}, y_{i+1}^P) \right) \end{cases} \quad \text{for } i = 0, 1, \ldots, N-1, \tag{7} $$

where

$$ a_{j,i+1} = \frac{\triangle t^p}{p(p+1)} \begin{cases} i^{p+1} - (i-p)(i+1)^p, & j = 0, \\ (i-j+2)^{p+1} - 2(i-j+1)^{p+1} + (i-j)^{p+1}, & 1 \leq j \leq i, \\ 1, & j = i+1 \end{cases} $$

and

$$ b_{j,i+1} = \frac{\triangle t^p}{p} \left((i-j+1)^p - (i-j)^p \right) \text{ for } j = 0, 1, \ldots, i. $$

In order to compute (3a)–(3c), we use (7) with $y := (H, F)^\top$ and $f^p := (h, g)^\top$.

As discussed in detail later, in order to solve the inverse problem, we need to solve the system of adjoint equations, which is backward. Therefore, we introduce the Adams–Bashford–Moulton formulae for backward fractional derivatives. They are derived analogously to the forward counterparts.

The fractional final value problem

$$ {}^{\mathfrak{C}}\mathrm{D}_T^p y(t) = f^p(t, y(t)), \qquad y(T) = y_T $$

for $0 < p \leq 1$ is equivalent to the Volterra integral equation

$$ y(t) = y_T + \frac{1}{\Gamma(p)} \int_t^T (s-t)^{p-1} f^p(s, y(s)) \mathrm{d}s \tag{8} $$

for $t \leq T$.

Using the mesh $\bar{\omega}$, the numerical solution to (8) follows:

$$ \begin{cases} y_{i-1}^P = y_T + \dfrac{1}{\Gamma(p)} \displaystyle\sum_{i}^{j=N} b_{j,i-1} f^p(t_j, y_j), \\ y_{i-1} = y_T + \dfrac{1}{\Gamma(p)} \left(\displaystyle\sum_{i}^{j=N} a_{j,i-1} f^p(t_j, y_j) + a_{i-1,i-1} f^p(t_{i-1}, y_{i_1}^P) \right) \end{cases} \quad \text{for } i = N, N-1, \ldots, 1, \tag{9} $$

where

$$a_{j,i-1} = \frac{\triangle t^p}{p(p+1)} \begin{cases} (N-i)^{p+1} - (N-i-p)(N-i+1)^p, & j = N, \\ (j-i+2)^{p+1} - 2(j-i+1)^{p+1} + (j-u)^{p+1}, & \leq j \leq N-1, \\ 1, & j = i-1 \end{cases}$$

and

$$b_{j,i-1} = \frac{\triangle t^p}{p}((j-i+1)^p - (j-i)^p) \text{ for } j = 0,1,\ldots,i.$$

Analogously, to solve (15), we use (9) and set $y := (\varphi_H, \varphi_F)^\top$.

4.2. Model with Caputo–Fabrizio Derivative

Similarly to the Caputo case, numerical approaches are developed for the Caputo–Fabrizio fractional derivative; see, for example, [14]. Here we employ a simple PECE (predict–evaluate–correct–evaluate) Adams-type method.

The fractional initial value problem

$$^{\mathfrak{CFC}}\mathrm{D}_0^p y(t) = f^p(t, y(t)), \qquad y(0) = y_0$$

for $0 < p \leq 1$ is equivalent to the integral equation

$$y(t) = y_0 + (1-p)f^p(t, y(t)) + p\int_0^t f^p(s, y(s))\mathrm{d}s \tag{10}$$

for $t \leq T$.

Using the same uniform temporal mesh $\bar{\omega}$, we write the approximate solution to (10):

$$\begin{cases} y_{i+1}^P = y_0 + (1-p)f^p(t_i, y_i) + p\triangle t \sum_{j=0}^{i} f^p(t_j, y_j), \\ y_{i+1} = y_0 + (1-p)f^p(t_{i+1}, y_{i+1}^P) + \frac{p\triangle t}{2}\left(f^p(t_0, y_0) + 2\sum_{j=1}^{i} f^p(t_j, y_j) + f^p(t_{i+1}, y_{i+1}^P)\right) \end{cases} \tag{11}$$

for $i = 0, 1, \ldots, N-1$.

Similarly, to compute (4), we apply (11) with $y := (H, F)^\top$ and $f^p := (h, g)^\top$.

The formulae for the backward system are as follows:

$$\begin{cases} y_{i-1}^P = y_T + (1-p)f^p(t_i, y_i) + p\triangle t \sum_{i}^{j=N} f^p(t_j, y_j), \\ y_{i-1} = y_T + (1-p)f^p(t_{i-1}, y_{i-1}^P) + \frac{p\triangle t}{2}\left(f^p(t_T, y_T) + 2\sum_{i}^{j=N-1} f^p(t_j, y_j) + f^p(t_{i-1}, y_{i-1}^P)\right) \end{cases} \tag{12}$$

for $i = N, N-1, \ldots, 1$.

To solve (15), we use (12) and set $y := (\varphi_H, \varphi_F)^\top$.

5. Adjoint Optimization Method

We solve the point observation problem (3a)–(3c) and (5) via minimization of the appropriate functional [28,30]. We minimize the least-square functional

$$J(\mathbf{p}) = J(m, n, \alpha, \sigma, \omega) = J_H(\mathbf{p}) + J_F(\mathbf{p}) = \sum_{k=1}^{K_H}(H(t_k; \mathbf{p}) - X_k)^2 + \sum_{k=1}^{K_F}(F(t_k; \mathbf{p}) - Y_k)^2. \tag{13}$$

5.1. Caputo Fractional Derivative Case

Theorem 2. *The gradient $J'_{\mathbf{p}} \equiv (J'_m, J'_n, J'_\alpha, J'_\sigma, J'_\omega)$ of the functional $J(\mathbf{p})$ is given by*

$$J'_m(\boldsymbol{p}) = qm^{q-1}\int_0^T \varphi_F F dt,\ J'_n(\boldsymbol{p}) = rn^{r-1}\int_0^T \varphi_H H dt,\ J'_\alpha(\boldsymbol{p}) = r\alpha^{r-1}\int_0^T (\varphi_H - \varphi_F) H dt,$$
$$J'_\sigma(\boldsymbol{p}) = r\sigma^{r-1}\int_0^T (\varphi_F - \varphi_H)\frac{HF}{H+F} dt,\ J'_\omega(\boldsymbol{p}) = r\omega^{r-1}L^r\int_0^T \varphi_H \frac{H+F}{(\omega+H+F)^2} dt, \tag{14}$$

where the functions $\{\varphi_H = \varphi_H(t),\ \varphi_F = \varphi_F(t)\}$ are the unique solution to the adjoint final-value problem

$$\begin{aligned}
&{}^{\mathfrak{C}}\mathrm{D}_T^r \varphi_H = a_{11}(H,F)\varphi_H + a_{12}(H,F)\varphi_F - 2\sum_{k=1}^{K_H}(H(t;p) - X(t))\delta(t-t_k),\\
&{}^{\mathfrak{C}}\mathrm{D}_T^q \varphi_F = a_{21}(H,F)\varphi_H + a_{22}(H,F)\varphi_F - 2\sum_{k=1}^{K_F}(F(t;p) - Y(t))\delta(t-t_k),\\
&\varphi_H(T) = 0,\ \varphi_F(T) = 0,
\end{aligned} \tag{15}$$

$$\begin{aligned}
a_{11}(H,F;\boldsymbol{p}) &= -\frac{\partial f}{\partial H} = L^r\frac{\omega^r}{(\omega^r+H+F)^2} + \sigma^r\frac{F}{H+F} - \sigma^r\frac{HF}{(H+F)^2} - (\alpha^r + n^r),\\
a_{21}(H,F;\boldsymbol{p}) &= -\frac{\partial f}{\partial F} = L^r\frac{\omega^r}{(\omega^r+H+F)^2} + \sigma^r\frac{H^2}{(H+F)^2},\\
a_{12}(H,F;\boldsymbol{p}) &= -\frac{\partial g}{\partial H} = \alpha^r - \sigma^r\frac{F}{H+F} + \sigma^r\frac{HF}{(H+F)^2},\\
a_{22}(H,F;\boldsymbol{p}) &= -\frac{\partial g}{\partial F} = -\sigma^r\frac{H^2}{(H+F)^2} - m^q,
\end{aligned}$$

and $X(t)$, $Y(t)$ are interpolants of the discrete functions, taking values X_k at $t = t_k$, $k = 1,\dots,K_H$ and Y_k at $t = t_k$, $k = 1,\dots,K_F$, respectively.

Proof. We denote $\delta\boldsymbol{p} = (\delta m, \delta n, \delta\alpha, \delta\sigma, \delta\omega)$, $\delta m = \varepsilon h_1$, $\delta n = \varepsilon h_2$, $\delta\alpha = \varepsilon h_3$, $\delta\sigma = \varepsilon h_4$, $\delta\omega = \varepsilon h_5$ and $\delta H(t;\boldsymbol{p}) = H(t;\boldsymbol{p}+\delta\boldsymbol{p}) - H(t;\boldsymbol{p})$, $\delta F(t;\boldsymbol{p}) = F(t;\boldsymbol{p}+\delta\boldsymbol{p}) - F(t;\boldsymbol{p})$. Then, we write the system (3a) and (3b) at $\boldsymbol{p} := \boldsymbol{p}+\delta\boldsymbol{p}$ for the pair $\{H(t;\boldsymbol{p}+\delta\boldsymbol{p}),\ F(t;\boldsymbol{p}+\delta\boldsymbol{p})\}$ with initial $\{H^0,\ F^0\}$. Next, we perform the differences between the corresponding equations to obtain a system for the pair $\{\delta H(t;\boldsymbol{p}),\ \delta F(t;\boldsymbol{p})\}$ with zero initial conditions. After a little algebraic manipulation, we obtain:

$$\begin{aligned}
{}^{\mathfrak{C}}\mathrm{D}_0^r \delta H &= a_{11}\delta H + a_{21}\delta F + o(\delta H) + o(\delta F) - r\alpha^{r-1}H\delta\alpha + r\sigma^{r-1}\frac{HF}{H+F}\delta\sigma\\
&\quad - r\omega^{r-1}L^r\frac{H+F}{(\omega^r+H+F)^2}\delta\omega - qn^{q-1}H\delta n + o(\delta\boldsymbol{p}),\quad \delta H(0) = 0,
\end{aligned} \tag{16a}$$

$$\begin{aligned}
{}^{\mathfrak{C}}\mathrm{D}_0^q \delta F &= a_{12}\delta H + a_{22}\delta F + o(\delta H) + o(\delta F)\\
&\quad - qn^{q-1}F\delta m + r\alpha^{r-1}H\delta\alpha - r\sigma^{r-1}\frac{HF}{H+F}\delta\sigma + o(\delta\boldsymbol{p}),\quad \delta F(0) = 0.
\end{aligned} \tag{16b}$$

For the increment of the functional $J(\boldsymbol{p})$ we find:

$$\begin{aligned}
J(\boldsymbol{p}+\delta p) - J(\boldsymbol{p}) &= \sum_{k=1}^{K_H}(\delta H(t_k;\boldsymbol{p}) + H(t_k;\boldsymbol{p}) - X_k)^2 - \sum_{k=1}^{K_H}(H(t_k;\boldsymbol{p}) - X_k)^2\\
&\quad + \sum_{k=1}^{K_F}(\delta F(t_k;\boldsymbol{p}) + F(t_k;\boldsymbol{p}) - Y_k)^2 - \sum_{k=1}^{K_F}(F(t_k;\boldsymbol{p}) - Y_k)^2 =\\
&\quad 2\sum_{k=1}^{K_H}\int_0^T \delta H(t;\boldsymbol{p})(H(t;\boldsymbol{p}) - X(t))\delta(t-t_k)\mathrm{d}t\\
&\quad + 2\sum_{k=1}^{K_F}\int_0^T \delta F(t;\boldsymbol{p})\big(F(t;\boldsymbol{p}) - Y(t)\big)\delta(t-t_k)\mathrm{d}t + o(\varepsilon).
\end{aligned} \tag{17}$$

Following the main idea of the adjoint equation method [28], we multiply Equation (16a) by a smooth function $\varphi_H(t)$, such that $\varphi_H(T) = 0$, and Equation (16b) by a function $\varphi_F(t)$, such that $\varphi_F(T) = 0$ (later these functions are completely reconstructed). We integrate both sides of the results from 0 to T and add them together:

$$\int_0^T (\varphi_H \, {}^{\mathfrak{C}}\mathrm{D}_0^r \delta H + \varphi_F \, {}^{\mathfrak{C}}\mathrm{D}_0^q \delta F)\mathrm{d}t = \int_0^T \varphi_H(a_{11}\delta H + a_{21}\delta F)\mathrm{d}t + \int_0^T \varphi_F(a_{12}\delta H + a_{22}\delta F)\mathrm{d}t$$
$$- r\alpha^{r-1}\delta\alpha \int_0^T \varphi_H H\mathrm{d}t + r\sigma^{r-1}\delta\sigma \int_0^T \varphi_H \frac{HF}{H+F}\mathrm{d}t - r\omega^{r-1}L^r\delta\omega \int_0^T \varphi_H \frac{H+F}{(\omega^r + H + F)^2}\mathrm{d}t$$
$$- rn^{r-1}\delta n \int_0^T \varphi_H H\mathrm{d}t - rm^{r-1}\delta m \int_0^T \varphi_F F\mathrm{d}t + r\alpha^{r-1}\delta\alpha \int_0^T \varphi_F H\mathrm{d}t$$
$$- r\sigma^{r-1}\delta\sigma \int_0^T \varphi_F \frac{HF}{H+F}\mathrm{d}t + o(\varepsilon). \quad (18)$$

Integrating, by parts, the left-hand side using formula (1) and using the facts that $\varphi_H(T) = 0$, $\delta H(0) = 0$ and $\varphi_F(T) = 0$, $\delta F(0) = 0$, we obtain

$$\int_0^T (\varphi_H \, {}^{\mathfrak{C}}\mathrm{D}_0^r \delta H + \varphi_F \, {}^{\mathfrak{C}}\mathrm{D}_0^q \delta F)\mathrm{d}t = \int_0^T \delta H \, {}^{\mathfrak{C}}\mathrm{D}_T^r \varphi_H \mathrm{d}t + \int_0^T \delta F \, {}^{\mathfrak{C}}\mathrm{D}_T^q \varphi_F \mathrm{d}t. \quad (19)$$

Then, placing the expressions for ${}^{\mathfrak{C}}\mathrm{D}_T^r\varphi_H$ and ${}^{\mathfrak{C}}\mathrm{D}_T^q\varphi_F$ from (15) in (19) and using (17) and (18), after some lengthy manipulations we find

$$J(\boldsymbol{p} + \delta\boldsymbol{p}) - J(\boldsymbol{p}) \equiv J(m + \varepsilon h_1, n + \varepsilon h_2, \alpha + \varepsilon h_3, \sigma + \varepsilon h_4, \omega + \varepsilon h_5) - J(m, n, \alpha, \sigma, \omega)$$
$$= qm^{q-1}\delta m \int_0^T \varphi_F F\mathrm{d}t + rn^{r-1}\delta n \int_0^T \varphi_H H\mathrm{d}t + r\alpha^{r-1}\delta\alpha \int_0^T (\varphi_H - \varphi_F) H\mathrm{d}t$$
$$+ r\sigma^{r-1}\delta\sigma \int_0^T (\varphi_F - \varphi_H) \frac{HF}{H+F}\mathrm{d}t + r\omega^{r-1}L^r\delta\omega \int_0^T \varphi_H \frac{H+F}{(\omega^r + H + F)^2}\mathrm{d}t. \quad (20)$$

Now, taking $\varepsilon_2 = \varepsilon_3 = \varepsilon_4 = \varepsilon_5 = 0$, dividing the both sides of (20) by εh_1 and passing to the limit $\varepsilon \to 0$, we obtain the formula for J'_m in (14). In the same manner one can check the validity of the other formulae in (14). □

5.2. Caputo–Fabrizio Fractional Derivative Case

To solve the point observation problem (4) and (5), we minimize the same cost functional $J(\boldsymbol{p})$ (13):

Theorem 3. *The gradient $J'_{\boldsymbol{p}} \equiv (J'_m, J'_n, J'_\alpha, J'_\sigma, J'_\omega)$ of the functional $J(\boldsymbol{p})$ is given by* (14), *where the functions $\{\varphi_H = \varphi_H(t),\ \varphi_F = \varphi_F(t)\}$ are the unique solution to the adjoint final-value problem*

$$^{\mathfrak{CFC}}\mathrm{D}_T^r\varphi_H = a_{11}(H,F)\varphi_H + a_{12}(H,F)\varphi_F - 2\sum_{k=1}^{K_H} (H(t;p) - X(t))\delta(t - t_k),$$
$$^{\mathfrak{CFC}}\mathrm{D}_T^q\varphi_F = a_{21}(H,F)\varphi_H + a_{22}(H,F)\varphi_F - 2\sum_{k=1}^{K_F} (F(t;p) - Y(t))\delta(t - t_k),$$
$$\varphi_H(T) = 0,\ \varphi_F(T) = 0,$$

and $X(t)$, $Y(t)$ are, again, interpolants of the discrete functions, taking values X_k at $t = t_k$, $k = 1, \dots, K_H$ and Y_k at $t = t_k$, $k = 1, \dots, K_F$, respectively.

The proof of Theorem 3 is analogous to that of Theorem 2.

6. Numerical Algorithm

Since the focus was to provide an adequate parameter identification study and simulation of the fractional-order model, we simply adopted the Volterra integral representation of the solution to obtain the numerical results.

In this section, we briefly comment on the numerical solution to the direct problem (3a)–(3c) and inverse problem (14) and (15). In general, such complex models do not posses a closed-form or an analytic solution at all, so one has to stick to a numerical approach. What is more, in our quasi-real framework, a solution to the direct problem is required in order to take measurements to test the algorithmic performance in solving the inverse problem.

Let us introduce the following piecewise–uniform mesh:

$$\overline{\omega}_\tau = \{t_0,\ t_i = t_{i-1} + \tau_i J_i,\ t_K = T\} \text{ for } i = 1, \ldots, K-1, \tag{21}$$

for $K \equiv K_N$ and $K \equiv K_F$, and the respective subinterval division $t_i^j = t_{i-1} + j\tau_i$, $j = 1, \ldots, J_i$, where $\forall i = 1, \ldots, K-1$, t_i are the time instances at which observations are taken; t_i^j, $j = 1, \ldots, J_i$ and τ_i are the time nodes and the time steps corresponding to $(t_{i-1}, t_i]$.

In the case of an integer–order model, there are many ways to solve it, and the issue has been extensively studied; see, for example, [31]. We followed the method described in [20], where the Volterra integral representation of (3a) and (3b) are discretized over the mesh (21) and approximated via the trapezoidal rule to obtain the respective numerical schemes. In an analogous manner, the backward system (15) is solved. In turn, the solution to the inverse problem (3a)–(3c) and (5) is sketched with the aid of Algorithm 1.

Algorithm 1 Adjoint Equation Optimization Method

Initialize $\boldsymbol{p}_0 \in \mathbb{S}_{\text{adm}}$ and $l = -1$.
repeat
  $l := l + 1$
  Solve the direct problem (3a)–(3c) at the current value $\boldsymbol{p}_l$. Then, define

$$H(t_k; \boldsymbol{p}_l) = X_k,\ k = 1, \ldots, K_H; \quad F(t_k; \boldsymbol{p}_l) = Y_k,\ k = 1, \ldots, K_F$$

  Solve the adjoint problem (15) via the method described in Section 5.1 (or Section 5.2)
  Compute $J'(\boldsymbol{p}_l)$ by means of the formulae (14)
  Define the optimization parameter $\boldsymbol{r} > 0$ and compute the new parameter value $\boldsymbol{p}_{l+1}$ by

$$\boldsymbol{p}_{l+1} = \boldsymbol{p}_l - \boldsymbol{r} J'(\boldsymbol{p}_l), \quad \boldsymbol{r} > 0,\ \boldsymbol{r} \in \mathbb{R}_5^+ \tag{22}$$

until $\|\triangle \boldsymbol{p}_l\| := \|\boldsymbol{p}_{l+1} - \boldsymbol{p}_l\| < \varepsilon_{\boldsymbol{p}}$
Set $\check{\boldsymbol{p}} := \boldsymbol{p}_{l+1}$

The numerical approximation of the sought parameter $\boldsymbol{p}$ is $\check{\boldsymbol{p}}$. In case there is no convergence, one should choose another $\boldsymbol{p}_0$ and start the iterations again. The user-prescribed tolerance $\varepsilon_{\boldsymbol{p}}$ is chosen according to the practical needs, and the value of the descent parameter $\boldsymbol{r}$ (22) is chosen empirically, as can be seen in the following aection.

7. Model Simulations

In this section, computational results are presented, which confirm the efficiency and robustness of the proposed approach. In our quasi-real test framework, we first solve the direct problem to demonstrate the model. Then, we use the result for measurements to solve the inverse problem.

7.1. Direct Problem

Let us solve the direct problem (3a)–(3c) with data from [20]. We set the number of eggs laid by the queen per day $L = 2000$ and the half-saturation constant ω = 27,000. What is more, the maximal recruitment rate is $\alpha = 0.25$ and the social inhibition coefficient is $\sigma = 0.75$. We assume relatively *low* forager mortality rate $m = 0.154$ and the hive mortality rate is $n = m/18$. We conduct experiments with two types of colonies, where the number of foragers is $F^0 = 0$ or $F^0 = 4500$, while, in both cases, $H^0 = 4500$. The considered time interval is the maximal foraging season from the end of the winter to the end of the summer, which equals $T = 250$ days. Finally, we use high values $r = q = 0.9$. The results are shown in Figure 1.

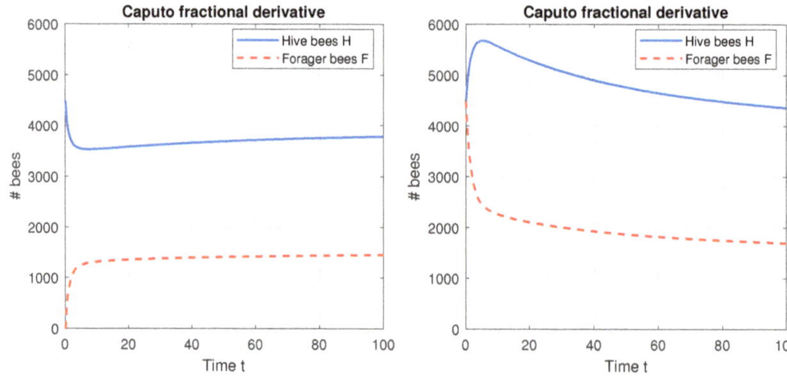

Figure 1. The colony population size for $H^0 = 4500$: $F^0 = 0$ (**left**), $F^0 = 4500$ (**right**), modeled by the Caputo derivative (3a)–(3c).

The colony survives well and is approaching a disease-free equilibrium state.

Now, we use the same setting, but we solve the problem (4). The results are plotted in Figure 2.

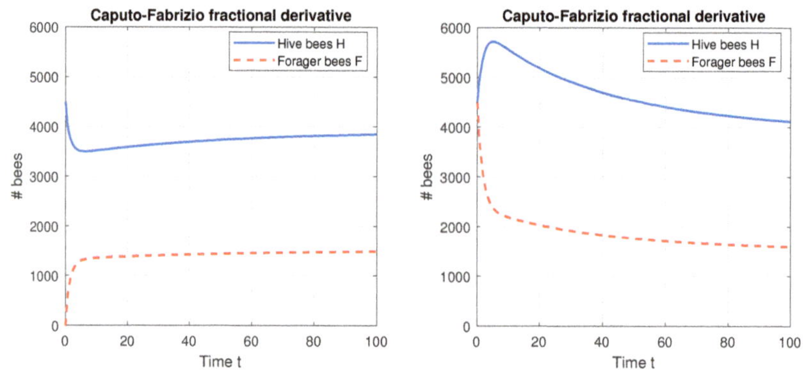

Figure 2. The colony population size for $H^0 = 4500$: $F^0 = 0$ (**left**), $F^0 = 4500$ (**right**), modeled by the Caputo–Fabrizio derivative (4).

They do not differ significantly from the results, obtained from the Caputo fractional derivative model.

To conclude the experiments, regarding the direct problem, we simulate the population dynamics with both models, when $r = q = 0.95$, as can be seen in Figure 3.

The difference between the two models is now more pronounced.

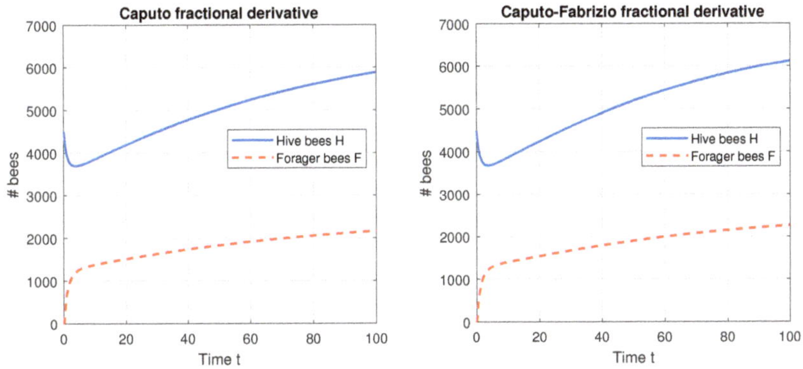

Figure 3. The colony population size for $H^0 = 4500$, $F^0 = 0$ and $r = q = 0.95$, modeled by the Caputo (3a)–(3c) (**left**) and Caputo–Fabrizio derivatives (4) (**right**).

7.2. Inverse Problem

Now, we solve the inverse problem. We follow the direct problem setting with $H^0 = 4500$ and $F^0 = 0$ and $r = q = 0.9$. We seek the unknown parameter $\boldsymbol{p}$, while provided with observations of type (5). Let us set $K_N = K_F = 11$, while the observation times are equidistantly distributed in the interval $[t_0, T]$. The true values of the unknown parameters are $\boldsymbol{p} = (m, n, \alpha, \sigma, \omega)^\top = (0.154, 0.0086, 0.25, 0.75, 27{,}000)^\top$. We test Algorithm 1 with initial approximation $\boldsymbol{p}_0 = (0.2, 0.01, 0.3, 0.7, 30{,}000)^\top$. The results are given in Table 1.

Table 1. Test with Caputo model (3a)–(3c).

Parameter	p_0^i	p^i	$\check{p}^i$	$\lvert p^i - \check{p}^i \rvert$	$\frac{\lvert p^i - \check{p}^i \rvert}{p^i}$	r^i
m	0.20	0.1540	0.1538	2.2148×10^{-4}	0.0014	3.40×10^{-13}
n	0.01	0.0086	0.0086	1.0541×10^{-5}	0.0012	3.25×10^{-15}
α	0.30	0.2500	0.2501	1.1786×10^{-4}	4.7145×10^{-4}	4.50×10^{-13}
σ	0.70	0.7500	0.7499	5.5183×10^{-5}	7.3578×10^{-5}	1.55×10^{-12}
ω	30,000	27,000	26,995	5.1638	1.9125×10^{-4}	2.55×10^{-3}

The values of $\boldsymbol{p}$ were accurately recovered. The relative errors were of magnitude 1×10^{-4}, which is acceptable. The gradient method required 52 iterations to converge. The differences (13) between the *observed* values $\{X_k, Y_k\}$ and the *implied* ones $\{H^{\text{obs}}(t_k; \check{\boldsymbol{p}}), F^{\text{obs}}(t_k; \check{\boldsymbol{p}})\}$ are as follows: $J_H(\check{\boldsymbol{p}}) = 16.7854$, $J_F(\check{\boldsymbol{p}}) = 42.5513$. The root mean squared errors were, respectively, $\text{RMSE}_H(\check{\boldsymbol{p}}) = 1.2353$ and $\text{RMSE}_F(\check{\boldsymbol{p}}) = 1.9668$, which again imply the accuracy of the results.

The convergence of the implied parameters $\boldsymbol{p}$ can be viewed of Figure 4. The last graph shows the implied population dynamics, i.e., simulation with the implied parameters. The difference is unnoticeable, as expected from the smallness of $J(\check{\boldsymbol{p}})$.

Now, we test Algorithm 1 on the model (4), with other settings staying the same. The results are presented in Table 2.

Table 2. Test with Caputo–Fabrizio model (4).

Parameter	p_0^i	p^i	$\check{p}^i$	$\lvert p^i - \check{p}^i \rvert$	$\frac{\lvert p^i - \check{p}^i \rvert}{p^i}$	r^i
m	0.20	0.1540	0.1536	3.5212×10^{-4}	0.0023	3.40×10^{-13}
n	0.01	0.0086	0.0086	1.4920×10^{-5}	0.0017	3.25×10^{-15}
α	0.30	0.2500	0.2502	2.4980×10^{-4}	9.9920×10^{-4}	4.60×10^{-13}
σ	0.70	0.7500	0.7503	3.0453×10^{-4}	4.0604×10^{-4}	1.60×10^{-12}
ω	30,000	27,000	27,023	22.9362	8.4949×10^{-4}	2.54×10^{-3}

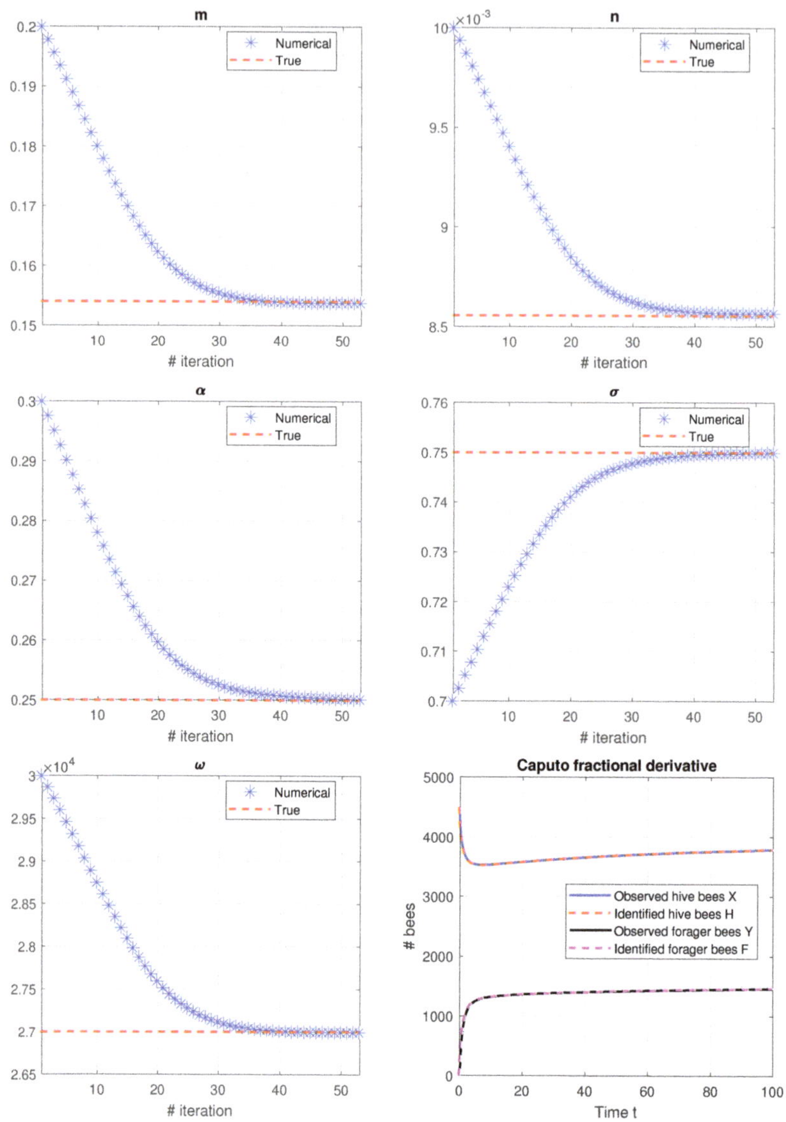

Figure 4. The convergence of $\boldsymbol{p} = (m, n, \alpha, \sigma, \omega)^\top$ and the implied population dynamics (**bottom right**).

In this case, 39 iterations were performed to reach convergence. The relative errors of the recovered parameters were a bit higher that those of the Caputo model, but the residuals $J_H(\check{\boldsymbol{p}}) = 16.1655$, $J_F(\check{\boldsymbol{p}}) = 32.9409$ were a bit smaller, as were the root mean squared errors $\text{RMSE}_H(\check{\boldsymbol{p}}) = 1.2123$ and $\text{RMSE}_F(\check{\boldsymbol{p}}) = 1.7305$, respectively. The two calibrations demonstrated similar results, which indicated that both the Caputo and the Caputo–Fabrizio derivatives are adequate for modeling the honeybee fractional population dynamics.

Now, we perform a computational experiment with different values of $p = 0.9$ and $q = 0.95$ [20]. The first to be tested was the Caputo model (3a)–(3c). The results are given in Table 3.

Table 3. Test with Caputo model (3a)–(3c) with different values of r and q.

Parameter	p_0^i	p^i	$\check{p}^i$	$\lvert p^i - \check{p}^i \rvert$	$\frac{\lvert p^i - \check{p}^i \rvert}{p^i}$	r^i
m	0.20	0.1540	0.1539	7.3542×10^{-5}	4.7754×10^{-4}	3.36×10^{-13}
n	0.01	0.0086	0.0086	6.0311×10^{-6}	7.0493×10^{-4}	3.34×10^{-15}
α	0.30	0.2500	0.2501	1.1972×10^{-4}	4.7887×10^{-4}	4.57×10^{-13}
σ	0.70	0.7500	0.7499	9.9080×10^{-5}	1.3211×10^{-4}	1.53×10^{-12}
ω	30,000	27,000	27,016	16.0889	5.9589×10^{-4}	2.63×10^{-3}

In total, 41 iterations were required for the algorithm to converge. The residuals were $J_H(\check{\mathbf{p}}) = 262.2052$, $J_F(\check{\mathbf{p}}) = 2.4509$, and the respective root mean squared errors were $\text{RMSE}_H(\check{\mathbf{p}}) = 4.8823$ and $\text{RMSE}_F(\check{\mathbf{p}}) = 0.4720$. The parameters were recovered in a precise manner.

Then, a test with the Caputo–Fabrizio model (4) is performed. The results are summarized in Table 4.

Table 4. Test with Caputo–Fabrizio model (4) with different values of r and q.

Parameter	p_0^i	p^i	$\check{p}^i$	$\lvert p^i - \check{p}^i \rvert$	$\frac{\lvert p^i - \check{p}^i \rvert}{p^i}$	r^i
m	0.20	0.1540	0.1541	7.8712×10^{-5}	5.1112×10^{-4}	3.30×10^{-13}
n	0.01	0.0086	0.0085	6.7634×10^{-6}	7.9053×10^{-4}	3.34×10^{-15}
α	0.30	0.2500	0.2501	1.0681×10^{-4}	4.2724×10^{-4}	4.61×10^{-13}
σ	0.70	0.7500	0.7504	4.1135×10^{-4}	5.4847×10^{-4}	1.56×10^{-12}
ω	30,000	27,000	26,690	10.0159	3.7096×10^{-4}	2.63×10^{-3}

Now, 34 iterations were needed for convergence, and the residuals, $J_H(\check{\mathbf{p}}) = 1.7525$, $J_F(\check{\mathbf{p}}) = 0.0625$, and the root mean squared errors, $\text{RMSE}_H(\check{\mathbf{p}}) = 0.3991$, $\text{RMSE}_F(\check{\mathbf{p}}) = 0.0754$, were very low. The parameters were accurately reconstructed as well. Simulations with the implied dynamics are plotted on Figure 5.

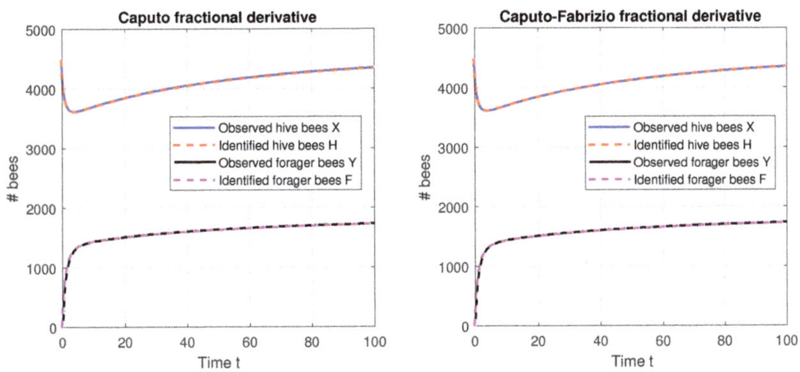

Figure 5. The implied population dynamics with $r = 0.9$ and $q = 0.95$, modeled by the Caputo (3a)–(3c) **(left)** and Caputo–Fabrizio derivatives (4) **(right)**.

At first glance, it might appear that there was no pronounced difference between the Caputo and Caputo–Fabrizio operators. Sometimes, this was, indeed, the case, as can be seen Figures 1 and 2 in [22], but, in other cases, there was a significant deviation, as can be seen in Figures 3 and 4, again in [22]. It was found that when the fractional order was closer to 1, the difference vanished. We visualized the Caputo–Fabrizio derivative against the Caputo one in the case of $r = q = 0.95$, compare Figure 6 (left) with Figure 3, and, in the case of $r = 0.9$, $q = 0.95$, compare Figure 6 (right), with Figure 5. In the first case, the difference was more pronounced, in contrast to the second case, where the difference was insignificant. These results do not act as a recommendation for or against the Caputo–Fabrizio derivative. They only show how the Caputo–Fabrizio derivative differs from the Caputo model in the particular cases. The Caputo–Fabrizio model is advantageous in view of prototyping and computational effort, since the Caputo–Fabrizio fractional integral is easier to implement and easier to perform numerical simulations with.

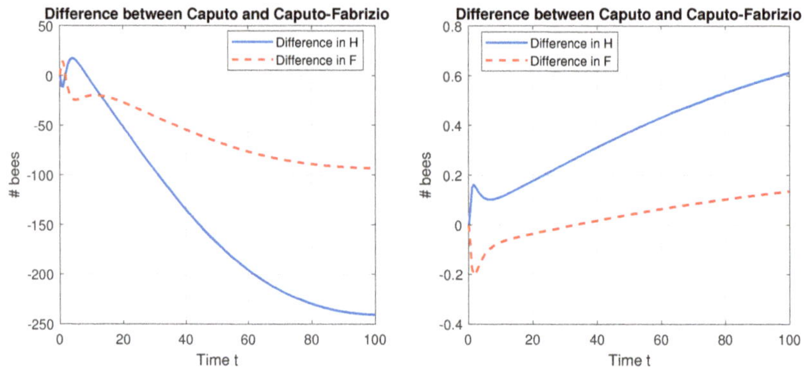

Figure 6. Differences between Caputo and Caputo–Fabrizio models with $r = q = 0.95$ (**left**) $r = 0.9$ and $q = 0.95$ (**right**).

In particular, when solving the direct problem with $r = q = 0.95$, the Caputo model required 0.53 s to finish, while the Caputo–Fabrizio needed 0.42 s, which yielded approximately 20% computational gain. When solving the inverse problem with $r = 0.9$ and $q = 0.95$, the algorithm for the Caputo model required 41 iterations to converge, while the Caputo–Fabrizio model required only 34 iterations, which again implies the computational efficiency of the latter.

For the sake of completeness, we conducted a test with an integer-order derivative model, meaning that $r = q = 1$ and the fractional derivatives in (3a)–(3c) and (4) are effectively substituted by a «regular» derivative with respect to time. The results are given in Table 5 and Figure 7. The residuals, $J_H(\check{\boldsymbol{p}}) = 21.1709$, $J_F(\check{\boldsymbol{p}}) = 133.9541$, and the root mean squared errors, $\text{RMSE}_H(\check{\boldsymbol{p}}) = 1.3873$, $\text{RMSE}_F(\check{\boldsymbol{p}}) = 3.4896$, were low, although higher than the simulations with fractional derivatives. This empirically confirmed the benefit of the fractional-order modeling.

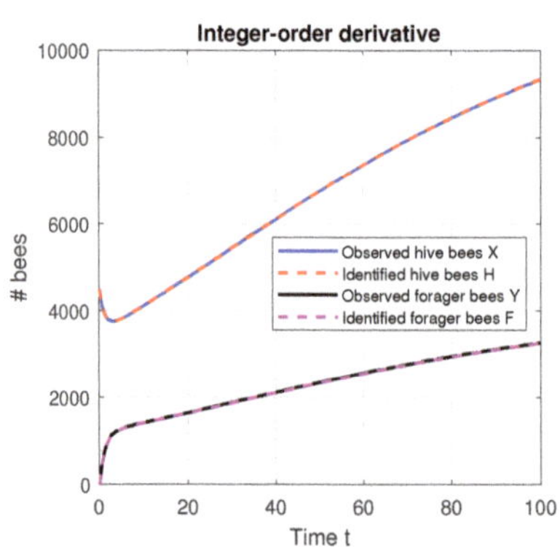

Figure 7. The implied population dynamics with the integer-order derivative model ($r = q = 1$).

Table 5. Test with the integer-order derivative model ($r = q = 1$).

Parameter	p_0^i	p^i	$\check{p}^i$	$\lvert p^i - \check{p}^i \rvert$	$\frac{\lvert p^i - \check{p}^i \rvert}{p^i}$	r^i
m	0.20	0.1540	0.1539	1.4229×10^{-4}	9.2398×10^{-4}	3.40×10^{-13}
n	0.01	0.0086	0.0086	1.4492×10^{-7}	1.6939×10^{-5}	3.15×10^{-15}
α	0.30	0.2500	0.2496	3.7857×10^{-4}	1.5143×10^{-3}	4.54×10^{-13}
σ	0.70	0.7500	0.7500	3.9556×10^{-6}	5.2741×10^{-6}	1.60×10^{-12}
ω	30,000	27,000	27,055	54.8891	2.0329×10^{-3}	2.66×10^{-3}

We concluded the experiments with a test of perturbed observations. In practice, each electronic device has a certain instrumental error, and sometimes this has a tremendous impact on the identifiability of the unknown parameters. To simulate this, we added Gaussian noise to the observations (5). It meant that, with 95% confidence, the bias in a single measurement did not go beyond 20%. We tested with such a high level of noise to validate the robustness of the algorithm. The results are shown on Table 6 and Figure 8.

Table 6. Test with Caputo model (3a)–(3c) and perturbed observations with 20% noise.

Parameter	p_0^i	p^i	$\check{p}^i$	$\lvert p^i - \check{p}^i \rvert$	$\frac{\lvert p^i - \check{p}^i \rvert}{p^i}$	r^i
m	0.20	0.1540	0.1543	2.5642×10^{-4}	0.0017	3.40×10^{-13}
n	0.01	0.0086	0.0086	1.5084×10^{-5}	0.0018	3.25×10^{-15}
α	0.30	0.2500	0.2497	3.0945×10^{-4}	0.0012	4.50×10^{-13}
σ	0.70	0.7500	0.7504	3.6251×10^{-4}	4.8335×10^{-4}	1.55×10^{-12}
ω	30,000	27,000	27,007	7.2513	2.6857×10^{-4}	2.55×10^{-3}

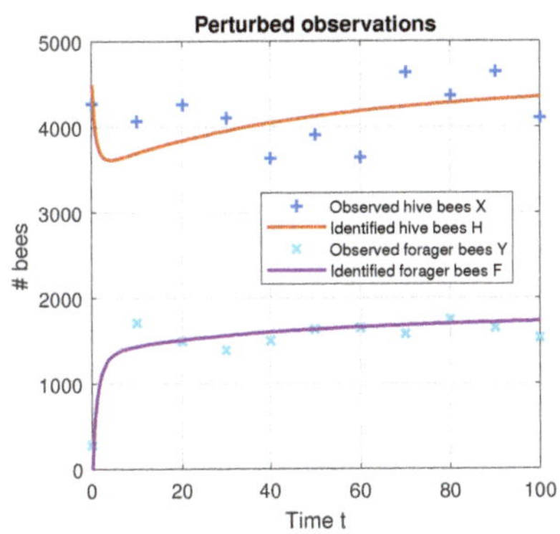

Figure 8. The implied population dynamics with model (3a)–(3c) and perturbed observations with 20% noise.

The number of iterations to convergence was 50 and, as expected, the residuals, $J_H(\check{\mathbf{p}}) = 11.9358$, $J_F(\check{\mathbf{p}}) = 97.0402$, were higher and so were the root mean squared errors $\mathrm{RMSE}_H(\check{\mathbf{p}}) = 1.0417$ and $\mathrm{RMSE}_F(\check{\mathbf{p}}) = 2.9702$. The relative parametric errors were of the order 1×10^{-3}, but they were not much larger than their counterparts from the exact observations cases. All of these facts imply that the approach is capable of working with real noisy data.

8. Conclusions

We employed a fractional-order model for honeybee population dynamics that balances simplicity and reality. The proposed adjoint state optimization approach allows one to find the unknown parameters in an accurate and robust way. This is achieved via solving a linear system of adjoint equations and minimizing a cost functional. The numerical simulations proved the sound foundations of the approach.

The implemented algorithm has several advantages. One is that it can work with scarce data, i.e., observations are not taken often and/or equidistantly. Another beneficial feature is the ability to cope with very noisy measurements. A limitation of the algorithm is that the optimization parameters $\boldsymbol{r}$ need to be adjusted. Some, though, may be given to develop a procedure for automatically tuning these parameters.

A possible continuation of the current work is to employ different fractional operators or more sophisticated models; as in, for example, [32,33]. Another interesting problem is obtaining reasonable values of the fractional orders. A way to achieve this is to use an approach similar to the bisection method [34]. Nevertheless, it is an open field to discover and might be a matter of further research. We believe the current and future algorithms give insight into managing honeybee colonies and help solve contemporary ecological and environmental issues.

Author Contributions: Conceptualization, L.V.; methodology, S.G. and L.V.; software, S.G.; validation, S.G.; formal analysis, L.V.; investigation, S.G. and L.V.; resources, S.G.; data curation, S.G.; writing—original draft preparation, S.G.; writing—review and editing, S.G. and L.V.; visualization, S.G.; supervision, L.V.; project administration, L.V.; funding acquisition, L.V. All authors have read and agreed to the published version of the manuscript.

Funding: This research was funded by the Bulgarian National Science Fund under Project KP-06-PN 46-7 "Design and research of fundamental technologies and methods for precision apiculture".

Data Availability Statement: Not applicable.

Acknowledgments: The authors are grateful to the anonymous referees for the useful suggestions and comments.

Conflicts of Interest: The authors declare no conflict of interest. The funders had no role in the design of the study; in the collection, analyses, or interpretation of data; in the writing of the manuscript; or in the decision to publish the results.

References

1. Atanasov, A.Z.; Georgiev, I.R. A multicriteria model for optimal location of honey bee colonies in regions without overpopulation. *AIP Conf. Proc.* **2021**, *2333*, 090008.
2. Booton, R.D.; Iwasa, Y.; Marshall, J.A.R.; Childs, D.Z. Stress-mediated Alle effects can cause the sudden collapse of honey bee colonies. *J. Theor. Biol.* **2017**, *420*, 213–219. [CrossRef] [PubMed]
3. Russel, S.; Barron, A.B.; Harris, D. Dynamics modelling of honeybee (Apis mellifera) colony growth and failure. *Ecol. Model.* **2013**, *265*, 138–169.
4. Harbo, J.R. Effect of brood rearing on honey consumption and the survival of worker honey bees. *J. Apic. Res.* **1993**, *32*, 11–17. [CrossRef]
5. Khoury, D.S.; Myerscough, M.R.; Barron, A.B. A quantitative model of honey bee colony population dynamics. *PLoS ONE* **2011**, *6*, e18491. [CrossRef]
6. Khoury, D.S.; Barron, A.B.; Meyerscough, M.R. Modelling food and population dynamics honey bee colonies. *PLoS ONE* **2013**, *8*, e0059084. [CrossRef]
7. Switanek, M.; Crailsheim, K.; Truhetz, H.; Brodschneider, R. Modelling seasonal effects of temperature and precipitation on honey bee winter mortality in a temperate climate. *Sci. Total Environ.* **2017**, *579*, 1581–1587. [CrossRef]
8. Le Conte, Y.; Ellis, M.; Ritter, W. Varroa mites and honey bee health: Can varroa explain part of the colony losses? *Apidologie* **2010**, *41*, 353–363. [CrossRef]
9. Hayes, J., Jr.; Underwood, R.M.; Pettis, J.; van Engelsdorp, D. A survey of honey bee colony losses in the US, fall 2007 to spring 2008. *PLoS ONE* **2008**, *3*, e4071.
10. Atanasov, A.Z.; Georgiev, S.G.; Vulkov, L.G. PParameters reconstruction in modeling of honeybee colonies infested with Varroa destructor. *AIP Conf. Proc.* **2022**, *2522*, 110005.
11. Chen, J.; DeGrandi-Hoffman, G.; Ratti, V.; Kang, Y. Review on mathematical modeling of honeybee population dynamics. *Math. Biosci. Eng.* **2021**, *18*, 9606–9650. [CrossRef]
12. Becher, M.A.; Osborne, J.L.; Thorbek, P.; Kennedy, P.J.; Grimm, V. Towards a systems approach for understanding honeybee decline: A stocktaking and synthesis of existing models. *J. Appl. Ecol.* **2013**, *50*, 868–880. [CrossRef] [PubMed]
13. Li, C.-P.; Tao, C.-X. On the fractional Adams method. *Comput. Math. Appl.* **2009**, *58*, 1573–1588. [CrossRef]

14. Akman, T.; Yıldız, B.; Baleanu, D. New discretization of Caputo–Fabrizio derivative. *Comput. Appl. Math.* **2018**, *37*, 3307–3333. [CrossRef]
15. Baleanu, D.; Diethelm, K.; Scalas, E.; Trujillo, J.J. Fractional Calculus. In *Models and Numerical Methods*; World Scientific: Singapore, 2017.
16. Li, C.-P.; Zeng, F.-H. The finite difference methods for fractional ordinary differential equations. *Numer. Funct. Anal. Optim.* **2013**, *34*, 149–179. [CrossRef]
17. Mahatekar, Y.; Scindia, P.S.; Kumar, P. A new numerical method to solve fractional differential equations in terms of Caputo-Fabrizio derivatives. *Phys. Scr.* **2023**, *98*, 024001. [CrossRef]
18. Ionescu, C.; Lopes, A.M.; Copot, D.; Machado, J.A.T.; Bates, J.H.T. The role of fractional calculus in modelling biological phenomena: A review. *Commun. Nonlinear Sci. Numer. Simul.* **2017**, *51*, 141–159. [CrossRef]
19. Magin, R.L. Fractional calculus in bioengineering, part 3. *Crit. Rev. Biomed. Eng.* **2004**, *32*, 195–377. [CrossRef]
20. Yıldız, T.A. A fractional dynamical model for honeybee colony population. *Int. J. Biomath.* **2018**, *11*, 1850063.
21. Georgiev, S.G.; Vulkov, L.G. Parameter identification approach for a fractional dynamics model of honeybee population. In *Lecture Notes in Computer Science*; Springer: Cham, Switzerland, 2022; Volume 13127, pp. 40–48.
22. Caputo, M.; Fabrizio, M. A new definition of fractional derivative without singular kernel. *Progr. Fract. Differ. Appl.* **2015**, *1*, 73–85.
23. Baleanu, D.; Jajarmi, A.; Mohammadi, H.; Rezapour, S. A new study on the mathematical modelling of human liver with Caputo–Fabrizio fractional derivative. *Chaos Solitons Fractals* **2020**, *134*, 109705. [CrossRef]
24. Kilbas, A.-A.; Srivastava, H.M.; Trujillo, J.J. *Theory and Applications of Fractional Differential Equations*; Elsevier B. V.: Amsterdam, The Netherlands, 2006.
25. Losada, J.; Nieto, J.J. Properties of a new fractional derivative without singular kernel. *Progr. Fract. Differ. Appl.* **2015**, *1*, 87–92.
26. Zine, H.; Lotfi, E.M.; Torres, D.F.M.; Yousfi, N. Taylor's formula for generalized weighted fractional derivatives with nonsingular kernels. *Axioms* **2022**, *11*, 231. [CrossRef]
27. Lin, W. Global existence theory and chaos control of fractional differential equations. *J. Math. Anal. Appl.* **2007**, *332*, 709–726. [CrossRef]
28. Marchuk, G.I.; Agoshkov, V.I.; Shutyaev, V.P. *Adjoint Equations and Perturbation Algorithms in Nonlinear Problems*; CRC Press: Boca Raton, FL, USA, 1996.
29. Diethelm, K.; Ford, N.J.; Freed, A.D. Detailed error analysis for a fractional Adams method. *Numer. Algor.* **2004**, *36*, 31–52. [CrossRef]
30. Kabanikhin, S.I. *Inverse and Ill-Posed Problems*; De Gruyter: Leipzig, Germany, 2012.
31. Atanasov, A.Z.; Georgiev, S.G. A numerical parameter estimation approach of the honeybee population. In *Modelling and Development of Intelligent Systems*; Springer: Cham, Switzerland, 2021; Volume 1341, pp. 349–362.
32. Atanasov, A.Z.; Georgiev, S.G.; Vulkov, L.G. Parameter identification of colony collapse disorder in honeybees as a contagion. In *Communications in Computer and Information Science*; Springer: Cham, Switzerland, 2021; Volume 1341, pp. 363–377.
33. Atanasov, A.Z.; Georgiev, S.G.; Vulkov, L.G. Reconstruction analysis of honeybee colony collapse disorder modeling. *Optim. Eng.* **2021**, *22*, 2481–2503. [CrossRef]
34. Georgiev, S.; Vulkov, L. Numerical coefficient reconstruction of time-depending integer- and fractional-order SIR models for economic analysis of COVID-19. *Mathematics* **2022**, *10*, 4247. [CrossRef]

fractal and fractional

MDPI

Article

Fractal Parameters as Independent Biomarkers in the Early Diagnosis of Pediatric Onset Inflammatory Bowel Disease

Vedrana Makević [1,†], Ivan D. Milovanovich [2,†], Nevena Popovac [2], Radmila Janković [3], Jelena Trajković [4,5], Andrija Vuković [1], Bojana Milosević [5], Jovan Jevtić [3], Silvio R. de Luka [1] and Andjelija Ž. Ilić [4,*]

[1] Faculty of Medicine, Department of Pathological Physiology, University of Belgrade, Dr Subotica 1, 11000 Belgrade, Serbia; vedrana.parlic@med.bg.ac.rs (V.M.); andrija.vukovic@med.bg.ac.rs (A.V.); silvio.de-luka@med.bg.ac.rs (S.R.d.L.)

[2] University Children's Hospital, University of Belgrade, Tiršova 10, 11000 Belgrade, Serbia; ivan.milovanovic@med.bg.ac.rs (I.D.M.); endoskopija@udk.bg.ac.rs (N.P.)

[3] Faculty of Medicine, Institute of Pathology, University of Belgrade, Dr Subotica 1, 11000 Belgrade, Serbia; radmila.jankovic@med.bg.ac.rs (R.J.)

[4] Institute of Physics Belgrade, University of Belgrade, Pregrevica 118, 11080 Belgrade, Serbia; jelena.trajkovic@ipb.ac.rs

[5] Faculty of Physics, University of Belgrade, 11000 Belgrade, Serbia; milosevicbojana96@gmail.com

* Correspondence: andjelijailic@ieee.org; Tel.: +381-113713164

† These authors contributed equally to this work.

Abstract: Inflammatory bowel disease (IBD), which encompasses two different phenotypes—Crohn's disease (CD) and ulcerative colitis (UC)—consists of chronic, relapsing disorders of the gastrointestinal tract. In 20–30% of cases, the disease begins in the pediatric age. There have been just a few studies that used fractals for IBD investigation, but none of them analyzed intestinal cell chromatin. The main aim of this study was to assess whether it is possible to differentiate between the two phenotypes in pediatric patients, or either of the phenotypes versus control, using the fractal dimension and lacunarity of intestinal cell chromatin. We analyzed nuclei from at least seven different intestinal segments from each group. In the majority of colon segments, both the fractal dimension (FD) and the lacunarity significantly differed between the UC group and CD group, and the UC group and control group. In addition, the ileocecal valve and rectum were the only segments in which CD could be differentiated from the controls based on the FD. The potential of the fractal analysis of intestinal cell nuclei to serve as an observer-independent histological tool for ulcerative colitis diagnosis was identified for the first time in this study. Our results pave the way for the development of computer-aided diagnosis systems that will assist the physicians in their clinical practice.

Keywords: fractal dimension; lacunarity; medical image analysis; nucleus chromatin architecture; inflammatory bowel disease

1. Introduction

Over the past two decades, medical image analysis has become an invaluable tool in the field of life sciences. Amongst other descriptors, fractal-based parameters have been used with success. As pointed out in [1], many natural and man-made objects can be characterized using the classical geometry and integer dimension; however, the random growth and/or branching of natural objects, at different scales, can be described in a sufficiently precise and concise way only by means of a non-integer fractal dimension. Some of the representative examples include a fern leaf, the branching in human lungs, a broccoli head, and the electric discharge in a storm [1]. In fractal objects, self-similarity at varying scales can be observed. Applications of fractal analysis to biomedical problems have been well established in ophthalmology, in exhibiting the fractal structure of vascular networks, and in the study of branching patterns of nerve dendrites, as well as in the studies of altered tissue and cell characteristics in cancers [1–6].

The dependences of the structural or functioning-related parameters of interest on the scale can be expressed by the power-law equations [1,7,8]. The fractal dimension (FD), which corresponds to the first-order mass moment of probability of finding a certain fractal measure amount at a certain scale [9,10], can be easily determined from the power-law dependence. In medical image analysis, the FD provides a statistical index that quantifies complexity and pattern reproducibility. As the biological specimens exhibit pronounced self-similarity at different scales, the FD is being increasingly used for diagnostic purposes in medicine [3]. Another parameter, which is often used alongside the FD, is the lacunarity (also sometimes referred to as "gappiness" or inhomogeneity). The lacunarity is calculated by taking into account the first-order and second-order mass moments of probability of finding a certain fractal measure amount at a certain scale [9]. It is a measure of heterogeneity and translational and rotational invariance that describes the space-filling property of fractals [9]. It is highly useful as an additional parameter to differentiate natural surfaces and textures with the same or similar fractal dimension [6,11].

In the field of medical science, the concept of fractals has been used for both image [1–6,12–14] and signal [15–18] analysis. The fractal feature-based image analysis employed so far in gastroenterology has shown promising results in cancer research [19–23] and has helped in the analysis of wireless capsule endoscopy [24] and colonoscopy images [25]. On the other hand, fractal-based signal analysis methods have been applied in gastroenterology in the study of digestion [26], colonic pressure [27], and intestinal sound analysis [28]. Although it produced very good results in the investigations of other intestinal pathologies, fractal-based methodology has rarely been used in inflammatory bowel disease (IBD) research [11,29,30].

The FD of nuclear chromatin [31,32] proved to be a sensitive parameter capable of the early detection of fine structural and textural changes in the cell nucleus. Nuclear chromatin FD changes have been found during the processes of cell differentiation, development, mitosis, apoptosis, aging, and cancer development [33,34]. Lacunarity has also been employed for chromatin structure evaluation in, among others, studies of apoptosis, postnatal development, and aging. In many of the studies, lacunarity has been inversely related to the FD, i.e., there has been a negative correlation between the FD and lacunarity, although, depending on the underlying processes, this association does not apply in general [33].

IBD, which encompasses two major phenotypes—Crohn's disease (CD) and ulcerative colitis (UC)—consists of chronic, relapsing disorders of the gastrointestinal tract [35,36]. Continuous mucosal inflammation that starts from the rectum and proceeds to more proximal colon segments, with variability in extent, is typical for UC [37]. On the other hand, discontinuous transmural granulomatous inflammation occurring at any part of the gastrointestinal tract characterizes CD [38]. The disease etiology is still not fully elucidated, but it has become clear that genetic factors, environment, diet, and changes in the microbiome are implicated in the pathogenesis. CD can affect any part of the gastrointestinal system, although it is most often evidenced in the terminal part of small intestine (terminal ileum) and the colon. On the other hand, UC is a disease restricted to the colon and rectum [35]. Both phenotypes sometimes display extraintestinal manifestations, which might stem from factors such as chronic inflammation or nutrient malabsorption [36]. In 20–30% of cases the disease begins in the pediatric age. We are currently witnessing an increase in incidence in the pediatric population [39]. Pediatric ulcerative colitis sometimes has an atypical endoscopic presentation like rectal sparing or patchy disease, which makes the differentiation between the two IBD phenotypes far more challenging [40]. The new European Crohn's and Colitis Organization (ECCO) guidelines [41] stress the importance of novel and possibly noninvasive biomarkers in diagnostics. The only recommended biomarker of intestinal inflammation so far is fecal calprotectin. Hence, there is a great demand for the invention of new efficient biomarkers for IBD, which could be combined with the standard medical procedures [42].

There have been just a few studies [11,29,30] which have employed fractals for IBD investigation. To the best of our knowledge, the fractals have not yet been applied in the analysis of the chromatin structure in the intestinal cells. However, there are indications that alterations in nuclear chromatin are very likely to occur in many functional gastrointestinal and motility disorders [43]. It has been demonstrated that the gene regulation by the microbiota is linked to DNA methylation and chromatin accessibility changes [44]. The underlying epigenetic mechanisms have recently been recognized as highly important in the pathogenesis of inflammatory bowel disease (IBD). Therefore, possible alterations of the fractal parameters describing the intestinal cell chromatin structure need to be investigated. The main aim of this study was to assess whether it is possible to differentiate between children with one of the two IBD phenotypes and children in a control group and to differentiate between the two phenotypes, based on the intestinal cell chromatin fractal dimension and lacunarity. Also, we checked the potential and the methods of application of fractal analysis as an observer-independent tool for IBD diagnosis.

2. Materials and Methods

2.1. Patients

The current study was conducted on children newly diagnosed with IBD (14 cases of CD and 10 cases of UC). The control group ($N = 16$) comprised children with irritable bowel syndrome (IBS) (without intestinal inflammation) or healthy controls. Seven tissue samples per patient were obtained by colonoscopy, corresponding to seven intestinal segments. Each sample contained one to four endoscopic biopsies. The samples belonged to the terminal ileum, cecum, ascending, transversal, descending, and sigmoid colon, and rectum, respectively. In cases when the ileocecal valve appeared affected, an additional 8th sample from the valve was obtained.

2.2. Intestinal Tissue Preparation and Staining

Intestinal tissue was fixed in 4% neutral buffered formaldehyde. The tissues were dehydrated in graded ethanol, according to the routine procedure, and then embedded in paraffin blocks and sectioned. The paraffin tissue blocks were cut into 4 µm thick sections and stained with hematoxylin and eosin.

2.3. Medical Image Preprocessing

The following image preprocessing procedure was employed for each intestinal segment. Four different micrographs containing at least one intestinal crypt each were acquired using the Olympus DP70 camera (Olympus BX50, Tokyo, Japan) and Analysis 5.0 software (SoftImaging System, Olympus, Tokyo, Japan). The total microscope magnification was 1000 times. All the micrographs were saved as TIFF files (dimensions 4080 × 3072 pixels, resolution 200 DPI, bit depth 24). Using the polygon tool of the ImageJ software (NIH, Bethesda, MD, USA), twenty crypt cell nuclei per segment were acquired for every patient and transferred to the white background images (500 × 500 pixels). Such newly acquired micrographs of nuclei were converted to monochromatic images using the Colour Deconvolution plugin of the ImageJ software [45,46], with an option denoted as H&E 2. The hematoxylin component (R: 0.49015734, G: 0.76897085, B: 0.41040173) is dominant for nuclei; it was recorded as an 8-bit grayscale image and used in further analyses.

2.4. Niblack Thresholding

Prior to fractal analysis, all the nuclei images underwent local Niblack thresholding and conversion to binary images. The local threshold value at each pixel was calculated by taking into account the neighborhood around that pixel and summing the neighborhood mean value of the grayscale intensity with the weighted standard deviation of the grayscale intensity. Both the window radius defining a neighborhood size and the weighting coefficient have to be adjusted empirically. The default value of the weighting coefficient is 0.2 for bright objects on a dark background and −0.2 for dark objects on a light background. In our case, the default coefficient provided very good results for all the images, and it was not changed. A window of a radius of $w = 6$ px, chosen empirically, was centered around each considered pixel. The local threshold at each pixel was then calculated according to the expression:

$$t_{Ni} = \mu(w) - 0.2 \cdot \sigma(w) \quad (1)$$

In (1), $\mu(w)$ and $\sigma(w)$ correspond to the mean and standard deviation of the grayscale intensities within a local neighborhood window of size w. Thus, a different threshold for every pixel is based on the grayscale properties of the neighboring pixels [47]; this was employed to better outline the spatial distribution of two types of chromatin—euchromatin (lighter) and heterochromatin (darker in appearance) [33]. Specifically, the altered spatial distribution of these regions seems to appear macroscopically mostly through altered nuclei texture.

2.5. Fractal Analysis

Fractal analysis was carried out on binary images using the FracLac plugin (A. Karperien, Charles Sturt University, Australia) for the ImageJ software [48]. The fractal dimension (D_b) was calculated using the box counting method as well as the cumulative mass method, with agreement of the results for the same sets of grids. We applied a scaled series 7/8, meaning that an enlargement of a consequent grid cell size was about 1/8. By using a scaled series, a sufficient number of relatively dense data points for fitting the regression lines was easily obtained. Here, a total of 18 grid cell sizes were used to obtain data points for fitting the regression curves to describe the scale–count power law dependence. Specifically, grid cells sized $\varepsilon \in \{5, 6, 7, 8, 9, 10, 12, 14, 16, 18, 20, 23, 27, 30, 35, 40, 46, 52\}$ px were used in both the box counting method and the cumulative mass method. Figure 1 shows an example binary image of a nucleus and also illustrates the typical nucleus size and the look of the chromatin texture, covered by grid cells of different sizes, ε. Typical grid cell arrangements are shown for four out of the eighteen utilized sizes, as denoted above each of the four plots. Twelve random grid origin positions per nucleus, per each grid cell size, were used.

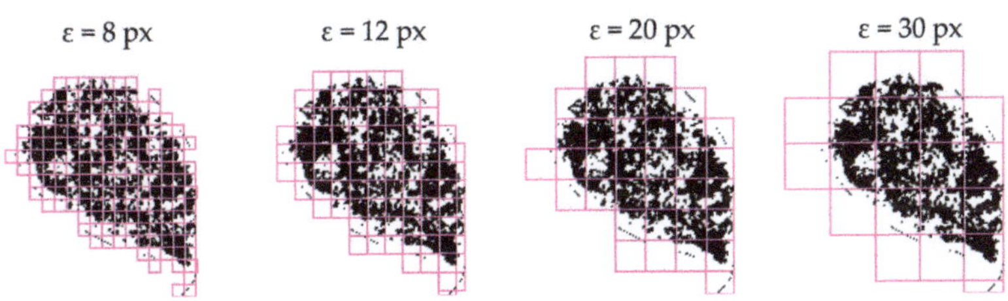

Figure 1. Grids of different grid cell sizes, ε, used to cover a binary two-dimensional (2D) object while obtaining data points for the scale–count dependence. The example nucleus shown corresponds to the 2nd patient in the CD group.

A change in the number of non-empty grid cells, $N(\varepsilon)$, with a change in the grid cell size, ε, was modeled by a best-fit regression line, whose slope served to estimate D_b.

$$D_b = -\lim_{\varepsilon \to 0} \frac{\ln N(\varepsilon)}{\ln \varepsilon} \quad (2)$$

The cumulative mass method makes an assessment of the probability of finding m pixels inside the cell of a size ε, $P(m,\varepsilon)$, by counting the pixels inside the grid cells and normalizing the obtained pixel count data for the total probability of one, $\sum_m P(m,\varepsilon) = 1$. The first-order mass moment, $M(\varepsilon)$, and the second-order mass moment, $M^2(\varepsilon)$, were obtained as:

$$M(\varepsilon) = \sum_m mP(m,\varepsilon), \; M^2(\varepsilon) = \sum_m m^2 P(m,\varepsilon) \quad (3)$$

The FD was then estimated from the (ε, $M(\varepsilon)$) data, as:

$$D_{\mathrm{m}} = \lim_{\varepsilon \to 0} \frac{\ln M(\varepsilon)}{\ln \varepsilon} \quad (4)$$

In both cases, the adequacy of the regression line fit was estimated based on the correlation coefficient, r^2, which was close to one in all cases, confirming almost linear data and high FD estimate accuracy. The lacunarity is calculated from the first-order and second-order mass moments as:

$$\lambda(\varepsilon) = \frac{\langle M^2(\varepsilon)\rangle - \langle M(\varepsilon)\rangle^2}{\langle M(\varepsilon)\rangle^2} \quad (5)$$

2.6. Statistical Analysis

The normality of distribution was tested with the Shapiro–Wilk test. Depending on the type of variables and the normality of the distributions, the results are presented as frequency (percent), mean (±SD), and median (range). Statistical hypotheses were tested using the ANOVA, Kruskal–Wallis, and Mann–Whitney tests and the chi square test. The statistical hypotheses were analyzed at the significance level of 0.05. Statistical data analysis was performed using IBM SPSS Statistics 22 (IBM Corporation, Armonk, NY, USA).

3. Results

3.1. Demographic and Clinical Characteristics

The demographic and clinical characteristics of the study participants, i.e., the pediatric patients used in this particular study, are shown in Table 1.

Table 1. Demographic and clinical characteristics of IBD groups and control patients.

Variable	Control	UC	CD	Overall *p*
Gender				
Male	60.0%	60.0%	78.6%	0.498
Female	40.0%	40.0%	21.4%	
Age	11.3 ± 5.1	14.4 ± 3.3	12.1 ± 4.8	0.271
PUCAI		32.5 ± 19.0		
PCDAI			17.5 ± 6.3	

Abbreviations: CD—Crohn's disease; UC—ulcerative colitis; PUCAI—Pediatric Ulcerative Colitis Activity Index; PCDAI—Pediatric Crohn's Disease Activity Index.

3.2. Histological Activity

The histological activities of UC and CD are represented with the corresponding regional histological activity score and are presented in Table 2 and Figure 2 (Nancy score for UC) and Table 3 and Figure 3 (GHAS score for CD).

Table 2. Regional Nancy score in six different colon segments.

Segment	Nancy 0, 1	Nancy 2	Nancy 3	Nancy 4
S2	1 (10.0%)	3 (30.0%)	5 (50.0%)	1 (10.0%)
S3	2 (20.0%)	4 (40.0%)	2 (20.0%)	2 (20.0%)
S4	2 (22.2%)	3 (33.3%)	4 (44.4%)	
S5	2 (20.0%)	3 (30.0%)	5 (50.0%)	
S6	1 (10.0%)	3 (30.0%)	5 (50.0%)	1 (10.0%)
S7	2 (20.0%)	2 (20.0%)	5 (50.0%)	1 (10.0%)

Segment notation: S2—cecum; S3—ascending colon; S4—transversal colon; S5—descending colon; S6—sigmoid colon; S7—rectum.

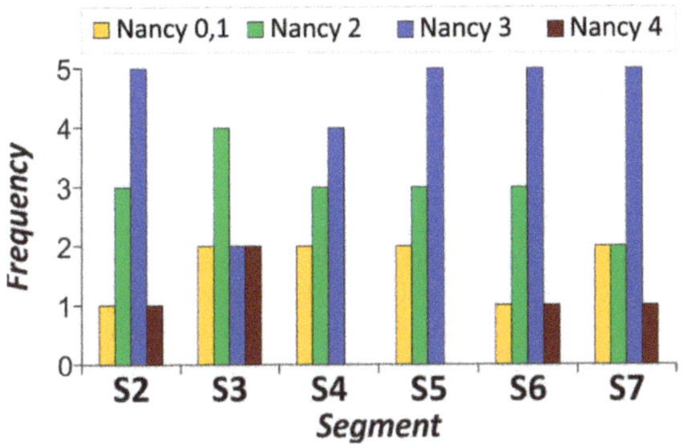

Figure 2. Regional Nancy score in six different colon segments.

Table 3. Regional GHAS score in seven different colon segments.

Segment	GHAS 1,2,3,4	GHAS 5,6,7	GHAS 8,9,10	GHAS 11–16
S1	3 (21.43%)	6 (42.86%)	4 (28.57%)	1 (7.14%)
S2	6 (42.86%)	5 (35.71%)	1 (7.14%)	2 (14.29%)
S3	6 (42.86%)	4 (28.57%)	2 (14.29%)	2 (14.29%)
S4	4 (28.57%)	4 (28.57%)	5 (35.71%)	1 (7.14%)
S5	7 (50.00%)	2 (14.29%)	2 (14.29%)	3 (21.43%)
S6	5 (35.71%)	4 (28.57%)	3 (21.43%)	2 (14.29%)
S7	7 (50.00%)	3 (21.43%)	4 (28.57%)	

Segment notation: S1—terminal ileum; S2—cecum; S3—ascending colon; S4—transversal colon; S5—descending colon; S6—sigmoid colon; S7—rectum.

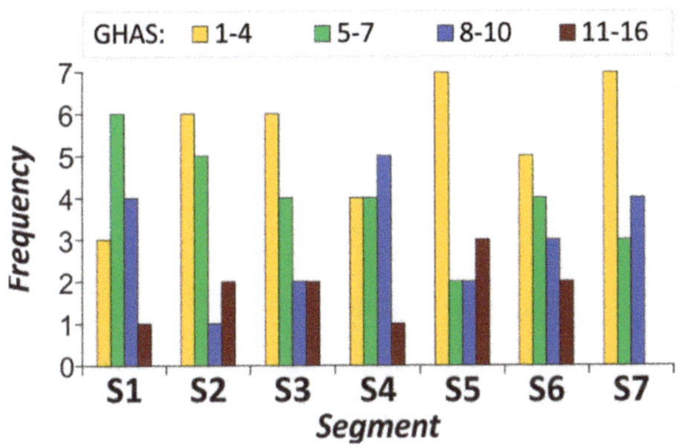

Figure 3. Regional GHAS score in seven different colon segments.

3.3. Fractal Dimension

We estimated the FD of the epithelial cell nuclei to assess potential differences in the chromatin organizational complexity between the two major IBD subtypes in the pediatric age. The same analysis was performed to assess differences in the intestinal cell chromatin complexity between either of the IBD phenotypes and the control subjects. A comparison was performed on seven different intestinal segments (terminal ileum, cecum, ascending, transversal, descending and sigmoid colon and rectum). The differences in the FDs of the investigated nuclei are shown in Figure 4 and Table 4. Figure 4 shows the mean ranks according to the nonparametric Kruskal–Wallis H test, where the mean rank is the arithmetic average of the positions in the sorted FD list for a total of 780 analyzed epithelial cell nuclei. The blue lines show the statistically significant mean rank differences. The children with UC had a significantly higher FD of the cell nuclei chromatin texture than the controls in all colonic segments except for the rectum ($p \leq 0.035$). Similar differences were revealed between the UC and CD children. Specifically, the UC patients had significantly higher FDs in comparison with the CD patients in every colon part except for the transversal colon ($p \leq 0.010$). On the other hand, the children with Crohn's disease had FDs that were statistically different from those of the controls only in the ileocecal valve and rectum ($p = 0.005$, $p = 0.014$; respectively), with lower median FD values in the CD patients. Interestingly, the terminal ileum of the CD patients, which is one of the most frequent localizations affected by the disease, had a statistically different nuclear FD only when compared with that of the UC patients.

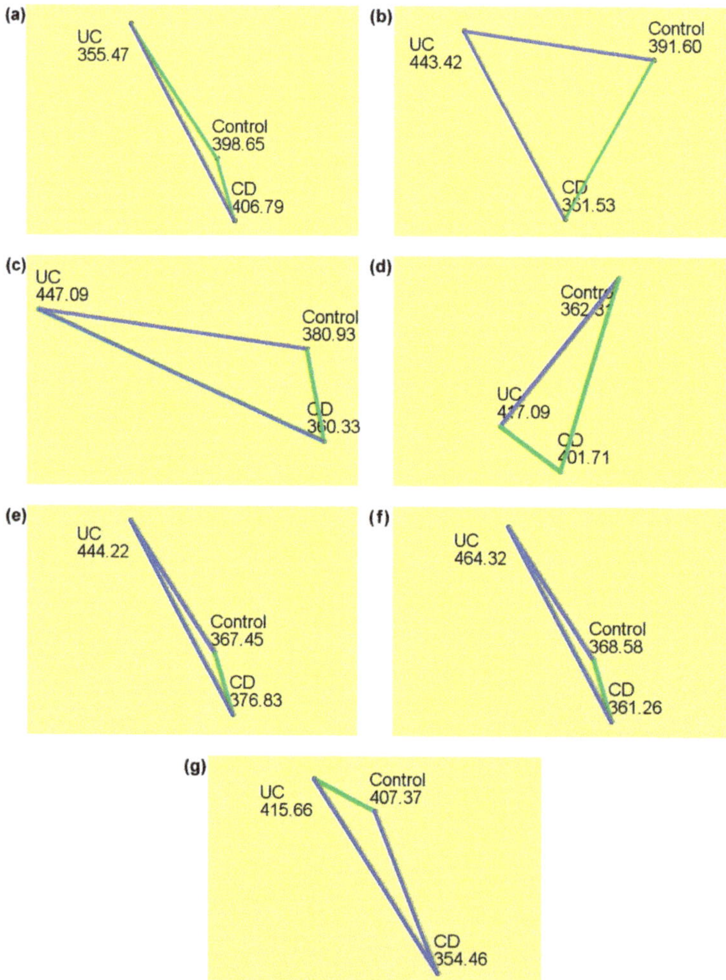

Figure 4. Fractal dimension mean rank comparison between CD, UC, and control group, for 7 different intestinal segments: (**a**) terminal ileum, (**b**) cecum, (**c**) ascending colon, (**d**) transversal colon, (**e**) descending colon, (**f**) sigmoid colon, (**g**) rectum.

Table 4. Fractal dimension comparison between CD, UC, and control group.

Intestinal Segment	Fractal Dimension (FD)			Statistical Signif. (p Values)
	Crohn's Disease (CD)	Ulcerative Colitis (UC)	Control Group	
S1	1.728(1.586–1.831)	1.722 (1.593–1.802)	1.728 (1.531–1.819)	**CD–UC (0.042)** CD–Control (1.000) UC–Control (0.107)
S2	1.732 (1.523–1.842)	1.755 (1.559–1.834)	1.741 (1.599–1.818)	**CD–UC (<0.0001)** CD–Control (0.097) **UC–Control (0.035)**
S3	1.732 (1.529–1.829)	1.752 (1.135–1.840)	1.736 (1.547–1.835)	**CD–UC (<0.0001)** CD–Control (0.814) **UC–Control (0.004)**
S4	1.736 (1.566–1.831)	1.738 (1.048–1.843)	1.728 (1.538–1.812)	CD–UC (1.000) CD–Control (0.106) **UC–Control (0.023)**
S5	1.734 (1.593–1.816)	1.747 (1.118–1.948)	1.734 (1.555–1.810)	**CD–UC (0.004)** CD–Control (1.000) **UC–Control (0.001)**
S6	1.722 (1.521–1.940)	1.749 (1.601–1.947)	1.727 (1.585–1.826)	**CD–UC (<0.0001)** CD–Control (1.000) **UC–Control (<0.0001)**
S7	1.719 (1.524–1.944)	1.733 (1.511–1.824)	1.730 (1.536–1.818)	**CD–UC (0.010)** **CD–Control (0.014)** UC–Control (1.000)
S8	1.731 (1.617–1.788)		1.749 (1.605–1.834)	**CD–Control (0.005)**

The results are presented as median (range). Segment notation: S1—terminal ileum; S2—cecum; S3—ascending colon; S4—transversal colon; S5—descending colon; S6—sigmoid colon; S7—rectum; S8—ileocecal valve.

3.4. Lacunarity

The size and spatial distribution of the gaps in the cell nuclei textures, their spatial diversity, and the level of the image deviation from the rotational and translational invariance was measured by determining the texture lacunarity. Lacunarity analysis revealed additional significant differences between the Crohn's disease and ulcerative colitis ($p \leq 0.001$), as well as between the ulcerative colitis and the control ($p \leq 0.002$) (Figure 5, Table 5). In Figure 5, the blue lines show the statistically significant mean rank differences for lacunarity. A statistically significant difference was present throughout the colon with the exception of the same segments as those in the FD comparison (the transversal part for the CD–UC and the rectum for the UC–control comparison). The difference in the terminal ileum nuclear lacunarity was not statistically significant among the compared groups. The colon enterocyte nuclear lacunarity was the lowest in the UC group.

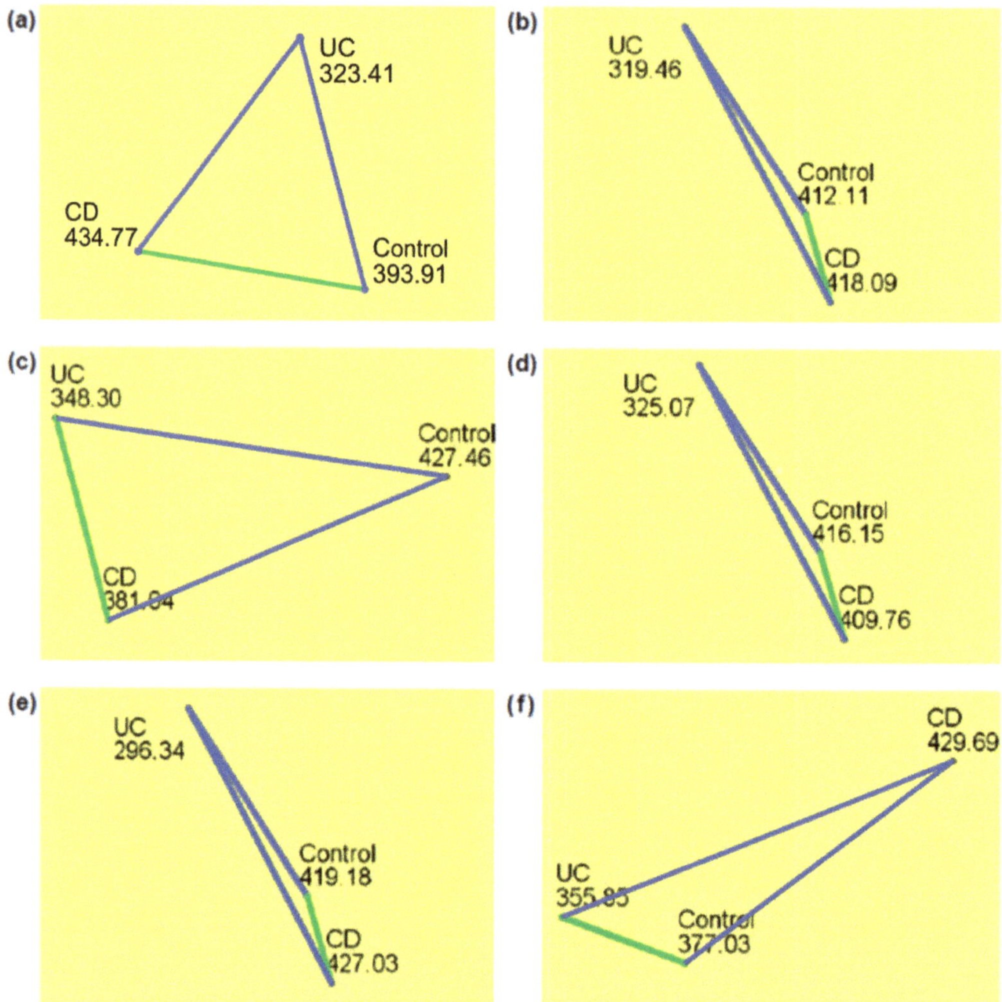

Figure 5. Lacunarity mean rank comparison between CD, UC, and control group for intestine segments: (**a**) cecum, (**b**) ascending colon, (**c**) transversal colon, (**d**) descending colon, (**e**) sigmoid colon, (**f**) rectum.

3.5. Intersegmental Comparison

Intersegmental comparisons of the fractal dimension and lacunarity of the cell nuclei texture are presented in Tables 6 and 7, respectively. One of the prominent results is a statistically lower rectal nuclear FD in comparison with the other segments (except for the sigmoid colon) in Crohn's disease patients. When the UC pediatric patients were considered, the nuclear FD proved highly useful in differentiating the colon (except for the rectum) and terminal ileum, the bowel part not affected by disease ($p < 0.002$). On the other hand, the FD across the control intestinal segments tended to be more uniform. As for the nuclear lacunarity, statistically significant differences were, with few exceptions, detected between the same segments as those in the case of the FD segment intercomparison.

Table 5. Lacunarity comparison between CD, UC, and control group.

Intestinal Segment	Lacunarity (Lac)			Statistical Signif. (p Values)
	Crohn's Disease (CD)	Ulcerative Colitis (UC)	Control Group	
S1	0.279 (0.172–0.430)	0.285 (0.209–0.455)	0.279 (0.197–0.517)	All groups (0.074)
S2	0.282 (0.163–0.470)	0.253 (0.167–0.422)	0.266 (0.178–0.407)	**CD–UC (<0.0001)** CD–Control (0.087) **UC–Control (0.002)**
S3	0.279 (0.174–0.460)	0.260 (0.175–0.404)	0.274 (0.192–0.481)	**CD–UC (<0.0001)** CD–Control (1.000) **UC–Control (<0.0001)**
S4	0.271 (0.184–0.442)	0.269 (0.181–0.554)	0.280 (0.198–0.482)	CD–UC (0.350) **CD–Control (0.039)** **UC–Control (<0.0001)**
S5	0.273 (0.273–0.430)	0.258 (0.037–0.365)	0.275 (0.191–0.475)	**CD–UC (<0.0001)** CD–Control (1.000) **UC–Control (<0.0001)**
S6	0.287 (0.042–0.510)	0.257 (0.038–0.378)	0.280 (0.190–0.467)	**CD–UC (<0.0001)** CD–Control (1.000) **UC–Control (<0.0001)**
S7	0.289 (0.040–0.480)	0.272 (0.183–0.450)	0.276 (0.182–0.504)	**CD–UC (0.001)** **CD–Control (0.015)** UC–Control (0.909)
S8	0.276 (0.221–0.396)		0.263 (0.199–0.418)	CD–Control (0.126)

The results are presented as median (range). Segment notation: S1—terminal ileum; S2—cecum; S3—ascending colon; S4—transversal colon; S5—descending colon; S6—sigmoid colon; S7—rectum; S8—ileocecal valve.

Table 6. Intersegmental comparison of nuclear fractal dimension.

Intestinal Segment	Fractal Dimension (FD)		
	Crohn's Disease (CD)	Ulcerative Colitis (UC)	Control Group
S1	1.728 (1.586–1.832)	1.723 (1.593–1.802)	1.728 (1.531–1.819)
S2	1.732 (1.524–1.843)	1.755 (1.559–1.834)	1.741 (1.600–1.819)
S3	1.732 (1.529–1.829)	1.752 (1.135–1.840)	1.736 (1.547–1.835)
S4	1.736 (1.567–1.831)	1.738 (1.048–1.843)	1.728 (1.538–1.812)
S5	1.734 (1.593–1.816)	1.747 (1.118–1.948)	1.734 (1.555–1.811)
S6	1.722 (1.521–1.940)	1.749 (1.601–1.948)	1.727 (1.585–1.826)
S7	1.719 (1.524–1.944)	1.733 (1.511–1.824)	1.729 (1.536–1.818)
Stat.sign. (p values)	**S7-S1, S7-S3, S7-S2, S7-S5, S7-S4** ($p < 0.025$)	**S1-S4, S1-S6, S1-S5, S1-S3, S1-S2** ($p < 0.002$) **S7-S6, S7-S5, S7-S3, S7-S2** ($p < 0.013$)	**S1-S2, S4-S2, S7-S2** ($p < 0.090$)

The results are presented as median (range). Segment notation: S1—terminal ileum; S2—cecum; S3—ascending colon; S4—transversal colon; S5—descending colon; S6—sigmoid colon; S7—rectum.

Table 7. Intersegmental comparison of cell nuclei texture lacunarity.

Intestinal Segment	Lacunarity (Lac)		
	Crohn's Disease (CD)	Ulcerative Colitis (UC)	Control Group
S1	0.279 (0.173–0.430)	0.285 (0.209–0.455)	0.279 (0.197–0.517)
S2	0.279 (0.163–0.470)	0.253 (0.167–0.422)	0.266 (0.178–0.407)
S3	0.279 (0.174–0.460)	0.259 (0.175–0.404)	0.274 (0.192–0.482)
S4	0.271 (0.184–0.442)	0.269 (0.181–0.555)	0.280 (0.198–0.482)
S5	0.273 (0.184–0.430)	0.258 (0.037–0.365)	0.275 (0.191–0.475)
S6	0.287 (.0420–0.510)	0.257 (0.038–0.378)	0.280 (0.190–0.467)
S7	0.289 (0.040–0.480)	0.272 (0.183–0.450)	0.276 (0.182–0.504)
Stat.sign. (p values)	**S2-S7, S3-S7, S4-S7, S5-S7** ($p < 0.022$)	**S2-S1, S3-S1, S4-S1, S6-S1** ($p < 0.0001$), **S2-S7, S3-S7, S6-S7** ($p < 0.011$) **S2-S4** ($p < 0.025$)	**S2-S1, S2-S4, S2-S6** ($p < 0.040$)

The results are presented as median (range). Segment notation: S1—terminal ileum; S2—cecum; S3—ascending colon; S4—transversal colon; S5—descending colon; S6—sigmoid colon; S7—rectum.

4. Discussion

Our results indicate that pediatric UC patients have a significantly increased nuclear structure and texture complexity, as measured with the FD, and decreased lacunarity compared to the children suffering from CD and the controls. This is a very important finding, given that the two IBD phenotypes are sometimes hard to distinguish. A significant difference was confirmed in most of the colon parts. In addition, the only intestinal segment with a significantly different nuclear fractal dimension and lacunarity between the CD patients and the controls was the rectum. However, the ileocecal valve of the CD children had a significantly decreased nuclear FD while the colon transversum had a statistically decreased lacunarity compared to the controls.

To the best of our knowledge, our study is the first which employed the calculations of the fractal dimension and lacunarity of intestinal cell nuclear chromatin in the IBD investigation. However, fractal analysis has previously been applied in the study of other intestinal pathologies. This methodology proved to be a promising aid in diagnosis [19,20] and therapy response [22,23] in intestinal carcinomas. Furthermore, a methodology based on fractal analysis was very accurate in abnormality detection in wireless capsule endoscopy (WCE) images [24]. Moreover, the differentiation between healthy and pathologic rectal mucosal vasculature can be accomplished with the fractal analysis of endoscopy images. The same analysis also proved to be useful for distinguishing between different rectal pathologies, e.g., colitis and vascular malformations [25]. Regarding IBD, fractals have been successful in ulcer identification from WCE images (caused by CD and UC, among other causes) [11] and bowel sounds detection in different intestinal pathologies, e.g., UC [30]. Finally, promising results were obtained in estimating the severity of intestinal fibrosis in a study conducted on histological slides stained with Masson's trichrome stain, which were derived from surgical specimens of CD patients. Specifically, an extracellular matrix (ECM) FD showed a significant correlation with a histological fibrosis score, and sections with different histological fibrosis scores had significantly different FDs. Thus, this investigation indicates that fibrosis progression in CD is more than a pure ECM accumulation and that it also includes structural ECM changes [29].

It should be mentioned, however, that our FD results, although they were consistent through the colon segments, still had some exceptions. Specifically, the nuclear chromatin FD of the transversal colon epithelial cells was similar in the CD and UC patients. In the CD patients, the median FD values were the highest in this segment. To better understand these intersegmental differences, we calculated regional scores that represented the histological disease activity for every segment. It appeared, in our group of patients with Crohn's disease, that in general its symptoms less often skipped the transversal segment than the other segments (fewer patients had GHAS < 4, indicating remission). Furthermore, in this segment more Crohn's disease patients had moderate active disease (GHAS 8–10) than in the others. So, it appears that CD was more active in this part of colon. This finding strongly suggests the possibility that differences in the pathophysiological disease activity might have some influence on the FD results. However, this does not make fractal analysis less attractive for future diagnostic applications since in routine pathohistological diagnostics all seven different intestinal segments are being evaluated. Looking at the results of all the segments comparatively, it was confirmed without any doubt that the UC fractal dimension differed in a statistically significant way from the controls, as well as from the CD patient group.

UC is known as a disease exclusive to the colon. Therefore, as expected, in these patients the nuclear chromatin FDs in the terminal ileum were significantly lower than those of the rest of the colon (the rectum was an exception). This finding proves once more that the FD could serve as a very good discriminator of the UC-affected tissue.

In our study, the nuclear FD in the rectum was higher in the UC patients than in the other groups; however, in this case the difference was not sufficiently pronounced to provide a statistically significant result. Furthermore, in the UC patients, the nuclear FD in this segment was statistically different from those of the other colon segments (apart from the transversal colon). In general, the rectum is affected in a large majority of UC patients, but in the pediatric population, rectal sparing is not unusual. Histological rectal sparing absolute (normal rectum) or relative (less severe inflammation than in other colon parts) rectal sparing is present in 30% of pediatric patients [49]. Among our patients, 20% had absolute rectal sparing (Nancy 0 or 1), which probably mitigated the results. Therefore, rectal biopsies, although the easiest to obtain, will not be sufficient for UC diagnostics based on the FD, at least not in the pediatric population.

The rectum was also an interesting segment for the CD patients. This was the only segment in which the nuclear FDs of these patients statistically differed from those of the controls. The Crohn FDs generally tended to be lower than in the other groups, indicating decreased complexity of textures for those nuclei. However, the FD in the rectum was the lowest of all. In the intersegmental comparison among the CD patients, the rectal FD was statistically lower than in any other segment except for the sigmoid colon ($p < 0.025$). This makes the rectal nuclear chromatin FD a feature with a potential to be exploited in CD diagnosis.

One possible explanation for the increased FD in most of the colon parts in the UC patients might be an increase in euchromatin ("open" chromatin) versus the heterochromatin ratio. "Open" DNA is less densely packed, resulting in less intense staining and lighter color. In a study exploring the effects of the chromatin physical structure on the transcription of genes [31], both the mathematical predictions and the experimental evidence pointed to a link between the increased heterogeneity of the chromatin structure (increased fractal dimension) and the increased variation of the gene expression for most biological processes. The chromatin heterogeneity is considered a ubiquitous hallmark of cancer aggressiveness in tumor research [2,3,31,33]. However, changes in protein binding and chromatin structure have also been shown to play a role in gastrointestinal diseases and disorders, including the pathogenesis of inflammatory bowel disease (IBD) [44]. It might be challenging to recognize the chromatin structural changes on standard HE-dyed tissue slides [2]; this is of primary interest given that only such slides are available for diagnostic purposes. On the other hand, open chromatin can be distinguished by applying fractal analysis as it gives higher nuclear FD values [2,50]. The results of our study suggest that UC patients have a predominantly increased euchromatin/heterochromatin ratio in enterocyte nuclei compared to the CD patients and controls. One of the epigenetic mechanisms causing chromatin to be in a more open state is histone acetylation. In this process, the enhanced unwrapping ("opening") of DNA allows transcription [51]. On the other hand, the opposite process, histone deacetylation, enables histone and DNA binding, limiting access to DNA again [52]. It has been demonstrated that certain enzymes responsible for histone deacetylation—Sirtuin (SIRT)1, SIRT6 and histone deacetylase (HDAC)9—are decreased in the inflamed colon tissue of UC patients compared to the same tissue of CD patients [53]. Decreased HDAC activity in UC patients might lead to enhanced histone acetylation and an increased amount of euchromatin, which in turn leads to a significantly higher FD compared to that of the CD patient group. Interestingly, HDAC inhibitors are seen as possible new drugs for UC considering their ability to decrease inflammation in colonic epithelial cells and dextran sulfate sodium-induced colitis [54].

According to the literature, the increase in chromatin lacunarity is often followed by the decrease in chromatin FD [33]. In this regard, our study is in line with the others. In colon tissue, nuclear lacunarity revealed the same statistically significant differences as the FD. However, lacunarity proved to be an even better colon CD discriminator than the FD since it was able to differentiate CD from the controls in more intestinal segments than the FD.

5. Conclusions

We conducted a detailed study of the fractal parameters corresponding to the altered textures of intestinal cell nuclei in pediatric patients as the prospective biomarkers for IBD. Although the changes in cell nuclei chromatin structure have been observed in cancers and have been observed to also coincide with the altered nuclei textures seen in histological samples [2,4,33], here, for the first time, a similar methodology was applied to IBD. The changes occurring in the protein binding and chromatin structure in gastrointestinal diseases motivated us to investigate the cell nuclei textures in IBD. We demonstrated that the intestinal nuclei of children suffering from UC compared with children with CD and a control group statistically increased the nuclear FD and decreased nuclear lacunarity. Furthermore, the current study provided evidence that in CD pediatric patients the rectum had a decreased nuclear FD and an increased lacunarity compared to the control group. Additionally, in the comparison between the segments, the rectum was different from almost all the other segments in terms of the nuclear FD and lacunarity. Therefore, the fractal analysis of intestinal cell nuclei was proven to have the potential to be an observer-independent histological tool for ulcerative colitis diagnosis. In addition, the rectum of CD pediatric patients also seems to be a very good candidate for the development of fractal-based diagnostics. Further studies are necessary to confirm our findings and to check on the consistency of the results in repeated trials. Furthermore, the inconsistency of the nuclear FD and lacunarity between the rectum and rest of the colon in children with CD is interesting, and it should be more thoroughly investigated. Our results pave the way for the development of computer-aided diagnosis systems that will assist in the clinical practice in gastroenterology.

Author Contributions: Conceptualization, A.Ž.I., S.R.d.L. and I.D.M.; methodology, A.Ž.I., S.R.d.L., I.D.M., R.J. and V.M.; software, A.Ž.I. and J.T.; validation, A.Ž.I. and I.D.M.; formal analysis, V.M., R.J., A.V., J.T. and B.M.; investigation, V.M., J.J., R.J. and A.V.; resources, I.D.M. and N.P.; data curation, V.M.; writing—original draft preparation, V.M. and I.D.M.; writing—review and editing, A.Ž.I. and S.R.d.L.; visualization, A.Ž.I. and V.M.; supervision, A.Ž.I. and S.R.d.L.; project administration, A.Ž.I. and S.R.d.L.; funding acquisition, S.R.d.L., I.D.M. and N.P. All authors have read and agreed to the published version of the manuscript.

Funding: This research was funded by the Faculty of Medicine, University of Belgrade, and the Institute of Physics Belgrade, University of Belgrade, through the grants by the Ministry of Science, Technological Development, and Innovations of the Republic of Serbia.

Institutional Review Board Statement: The study was conducted in accordance with the Declaration of Helsinki.

Informed Consent Statement: Informed consent was obtained from all subjects involved in the study.

Data Availability Statement: Fractal analysis and statistical data presented in this study are available on request from the corresponding author. Patient-related data cannot be shared due to ethical, legal, and privacy issues.

Acknowledgments: The authors acknowledge funding provided by the Faculty of Medicine, University of Belgrade, and the Institute of Physics Belgrade, University of Belgrade, through the grants by the Ministry of Science, Technological Development, and Innovations of the Republic of Serbia.

Conflicts of Interest: The authors declare no conflict of interest.

References

1. Husain, A.; Nanda, M.N.; Chowdary, M.S.; Sajid, M. Fractals: An eclectic survey, part II. *Fractal Fract.* **2022**, *6*, 379. [CrossRef]
2. de Mattos, A.C.; Florindo, J.B.; Adam, R.L.; Lorand-Metze, I.; Metze, K. The fractal dimension suggests two chromatin configurations in small cell neuroendocrine lung cancer and is an independent unfavorable prognostic factor for overall survival. *Microsc. Microanal.* **2022**, *28*, 522–526. [CrossRef]
3. Karri, S.; Aviel-Ronen, S.; Firer, M.A. Fractal and textural imaging identify new subgroups of patients with colorectal cancer based on biophysical properties of the cancer cells. *Pathol. Res. Pract.* **2022**, *238*, 154040. [CrossRef]
4. Dinčić, M.; Todorović, J.; Nešović-Ostojić, J.; Kovačević, S.; Dunđerović, D.; Lopičić, S.; Spasić, S.; Radojević-Škodrić, S.; Stanisavljević, D.; Ilić, A.Ž. The fractal and GLCM textural parameters of chromatin may be potential biomarkers of papillary thyroid carcinoma in Hashimoto's thyroiditis specimens. *Microsc. Microanal.* **2020**, *26*, 717–730. [CrossRef]
5. Dinčić, M.; Popović, T.B.; Kojadinović, M.; Trbovich, A.M.; Ilić, A.Ž. Morphological, fractal, and textural features for the blood cell classification: The case of acute myeloid leukemia. *Eur. Biophys. J.* **2021**, *50*, 1111–1127. [CrossRef] [PubMed]
6. Einstein, A.J.; Wu, H.-S.; Gil, J. Self-affinity and lacunarity of chromatin texture in benign and malignant breast epithelial cell nuclei. *Phys. Rev. Lett.* **1998**, *80*, 397–400. [CrossRef]
7. Ioelovich, M. Fractal dimensions of cell wall in growing cotton fibers. *Fractal Fract.* **2020**, *4*, 6. [CrossRef]
8. Arsac, L.M.; Weissland, T. Multifractality in the movement system when adapting to arm cranking in wheelchair athletes, able-bodied athletes, and untrained people. *Fractal Fract.* **2022**, *6*, 176. [CrossRef]
9. Smith, T.G., Jr.; Lange, G.D.; Marks, W.B. Fractal methods and results in cellular morphology—Dimensions, lacunarity and multifractals. *J. Neurosci. Methods* **1996**, *69*, 123–136. [CrossRef] [PubMed]
10. Tél, T. Fractals, multifractals, and thermodynamics: An introductory review. *Z. Naturforschung A* **1988**, *43*, 1154–1174. [CrossRef]
11. Charisis, V.S.; Hadjileontiadis, L.J.; Liatsos, C.N.; Mavrogiannis, C.C.; Sergiadis, G.D. Capsule endoscopy image analysis using texture information from various colour models. *Comput. Methods Programs Biomed.* **2012**, *107*, 61–74. [CrossRef]
12. Oprić, D.; Stankovich, A.D.; Nenadović, A.; Kovačević, S.; Obradović, D.D.; De Luka, S.; Nešović-Ostojić, J.; Milašin, J.; Ilić, A.Ž.; Trbovich, A.M. Fractal analysis tools for early assessment of liver inflammation induced by chronic consumption of linseed, palm and sunflower oils. *Biomed. Sign. Process. Control* **2020**, *61*, 101959. [CrossRef]
13. Stojić, D.; Radošević, D.; Rajković, N.; Marić, D.L.; Milošević, N.T. Classification by morphology of multipolar neurons of the human principal olivary nucleus. *Neurosci. Res.* **2021**, *170*, 66–75. [CrossRef]
14. Lyu, X.; Jajal, P.; Tahir, M.Z.; Zhang, S. Fractal dimension of retinal vasculature as an image quality metric for automated fundus image analysis systems. *Sci. Rep.* **2022**, *12*, 11868. [CrossRef]
15. Freeborn, T.J.; Fu, B. Fatigue-induced Cole electrical impedance model changes of biceps tissue bioimpedance. *Fractal Fract.* **2018**, *2*, 27. [CrossRef]
16. Gladun, K.V. Higuchi fractal dimension as a method for assessing response to sound stimuli in patients with diffuse axonal brain injury. *Sovrem. Tehnologii Med.* **2020**, *12*, 63. [CrossRef]
17. Naik, G.R.; Arjunan, S.; Kumar, D. Applications of ICA and fractal dimension in sEMG signal processing for subtle movement analysis: A review. *Australas. Phys. Eng. Sci. Med.* **2011**, *34*, 179–193. [CrossRef] [PubMed]
18. Stylianou, O.; Kaposzta, Z.; Czoch, A.; Stefanovski, L.; Yabluchanskiy, A.; Racz, F.S.; Ritter, P.; Eke, A.; Mukli, P. Scale-free functional brain networks exhibit increased connectivity, are more integrated and less segregated in patients with Parkinson's disease following dopaminergic treatment. *Fractal Fract.* **2022**, *6*, 737. [CrossRef]
19. Goh, V.; Sanghera, B.; Wellsted, D.M.; Sundin, J.; Halligan, S. Assessment of the spatial pattern of colorectal tumour perfusion estimated at perfusion CT using two-dimensional fractal analysis. *Eur. Radiol.* **2009**, *19*, 1358–1365. [CrossRef]
20. Streba, L.; Forţofoiu, M.C.; Popa, C.; Ciobanu, D.; Gruia, C.L.; Mogoantă, S.; Streba, C.T. A pilot study on the role of fractal analysis in the microscopic evaluation of colorectal cancers. *Rom. J. Morphol. Embryol.* **2015**, *56*, 191–196. [PubMed]
21. Watanabe, H.; Hayano, K.; Ohira, G.; Imanishi, S.; Hanaoka, T.; Hirata, A.; Kano, M.; Matsubara, H. Quantification of structural heterogeneity using fractal analysis of contrast-enhanced CT image to predict survival in gastric cancer patients. *Dig Dis Sci.* **2021**, *66*, 2069–2074. [CrossRef] [PubMed]
22. Dzik-Jurasz, A.; Walker-Samuel, S.; Leach, M.O.; Brown, G.; Padhani, A.; George, M.; Collins, D.J. Fractal parameters derived from analysis of DCE-MRI data correlates with response to therapy in rectal carcinoma. In Proceedings of the International Society for Magnetic Resonance in Medicine 11, ISMRM 12th Scientific Meeting, Kyoto, Japan, 15–21 May 2004; p. 2503.
23. Tochigi, T.; Kamran, S.C.; Parakh, A.; Noda, Y.; Ganeshan, B.; Blaszkowsky, L.S.; Ryan, D.P.; Allen, J.N.; Berger, D.L.; Wo, J.Y.; et al. Response prediction of neoadjuvant chemoradiation therapy in locally advanced rectal cancer using CT-based fractal dimension analysis. *Eur. Radiol.* **2022**, *32*, 2426–2436. [CrossRef]
24. Jain, S.; Seal, A.; Ojha, A.; Krejcar, O.; Bureš, J.; Tachecí, I.; Yazidi, A. Detection of abnormality in wireless capsule endoscopy images using fractal features. *Comput. Biol. Med.* **2020**, *127*, 104094. [CrossRef] [PubMed]

25. Gryglewski, A.; Henry, B.M.; Mrozek, M.; Żelawski, M.; Piech, K.; Tomaszewski, K.A. Sensitivity and specificity of fractal analysis to distinguish between healthy and pathologic rectal mucosa microvasculature seen during colonoscopy. *Surg. Laparosc. Endosc. Percutan. Tech.* **2016**, *26*, 358–363. [CrossRef] [PubMed]
26. Paramasivam, A.; Kamalanand, K.; Emmanuel, C.; Mahadevan, B.; Sundravadivelu, K.; Raman, J.; Jawahar, P.M. Influence of electrode surface area on the fractal dimensions of electrogastrograms and fractal analysis of normal and abnormal digestion process. In Proceedings of the 2018 International Conference on Recent Trends in Electrical, Control and Communication (RTECC 2018), Malaysia, Malaysia, 20–22 March 2018; pp. 245–250. [CrossRef]
27. Yan, R.; Guo, X. Nonlinear fractal dynamics of human colonic pressure activity based upon the box-counting method. *Comput. Methods Biomech. Biomed. Eng.* **2013**, *16*, 660–668. [CrossRef]
28. Dimoulas, C.; Kalliris, G.; Papanikolaou, G.; Kalampakas, A. Long-term signal detection, segmentation and summarization using wavelets and fractal dimension: A bioacoustics application in gastrointestinal-motility monitoring. *Comput. Biol. Med.* **2007**, *37*, 438–462. [CrossRef]
29. Weber, M.C.; Schmidt, K.; Buck, A.; Kasajima, A.; Becker, S.; Wilhelm, D.; Friess, H.; Neumann, P.A. P067 Fractal analysis of extracellular matrix as a new histological method for observer-independent quantification of intestinal fibrosis in Crohn's disease. *J. Crohn's Colitis* **2023**, *17* (Suppl. 1), i234. [CrossRef]
30. Hadjileontiadis, L.J.; Rekanos, I.T. Detection of explosive lung and bowel sounds by means of fractal dimension. *IEEE Signal Process. Lett.* **2003**, *10*, 311–314. [CrossRef]
31. Almassalha, L.; Tiwari, A.; Ruhoff, P.; Stypula-Cyrus, Y.; Cherkezyan, L.; Matsuda, H.; Dela Cruz, M.A.; Chandler, J.E.; White, C.; Maneval, C.; et al. The global relationship between chromatin physical topology, fractal structure, and gene expression. *Sci. Rep.* **2017**, *7*, 41061. [CrossRef]
32. Bancaud, A.; Lavelle, C.; Huet, S.; Ellenberg, J. A fractal model for nuclear organization: Current evidence and biological implications. *Nucl. Acids Res.* **2012**, *40*, 8783–8792. [CrossRef]
33. Metze, K.; Adam, R.; Florindo, J.B. The fractal dimension of chromatin—A potential molecular marker for carcinogenesis, tumor progression and prognosis. *Expert Rev. Mol. Diagn.* **2019**, *19*, 299–312. [CrossRef] [PubMed]
34. Vesković, M.; Labudović-Borović, M.; Zaletel, I.; Rakočević, J.; Mladenović, D.; Jorgačević, B.; Vučević, D.; Radosavljević, T. The effects of betaine on the nuclear fractal dimension, chromatin texture, and proliferative activity in hepatocytes in mouse model of nonalcoholic fatty liver disease. *Microsc. Microanal.* **2018**, *24*, 132–138. [CrossRef]
35. Ray, G.; Longworth, M.S. Epigenetics, DNA organization, and inflammatory bowel disease. *Inflamm. Bowel Dis.* **2019**, *25*, 235–247. [CrossRef]
36. Fedor, I.; Zold, E.; Barta, Z. Temporal relationship of extraintestinal manifestations in inflammatory bowel disease. *J. Clin. Med.* **2021**, *10*, 5984. [CrossRef] [PubMed]
37. Gajendran, M.; Loganathan, P.; Jimenez, G.; Catinella, A.P.; Ng, N.; Umapathy, C.; Ziade, N.; Hashash, J.G. A comprehensive review and update on ulcerative colitis. *Dis. Mon.* **2019**, *65*, 100851. [CrossRef] [PubMed]
38. Sathiyasekaran, M.; Shivbalan, S. Crohn's disease. *Indian J. Pediatr.* **2006**, *73*, 723–729. [CrossRef]
39. Fuller, M.K. Pediatric inflammatory bowel disease: Special considerations. *Surg. Clin. N. Am.* **2019**, *99*, 1177–1183. [CrossRef]
40. De Roche, T.C.; Xiao, S.Y.; Liu, X. Histological evaluation in ulcerative colitis. *Gastroenterol. Rep.* **2014**, *2*, 178–192. [CrossRef]
41. Torres, J.; Bonovas, S.; Doherty, G.; Kucharzik, T.; Gisbert, J.P.; Raine, T.; Adamina, M.; Armuzzi, A.; Bachmann, O.; Bager, P.; et al. ECCO Working Group. ECCO Guidelines on Therapeutics in Crohn's Disease: Medical Treatment. *J. Crohn's Colitis* **2020**, *14*, 4–22. [CrossRef]
42. Szymanska, E.; Wierzbicka, A.; Dadalski, M.; Kierkus, J. Fecal zonulin as a noninvasive biomarker of intestinal permeability in pediatric patients with inflammatory bowel diseases—Correlation with disease activity and fecal calprotectin. *J. Clin. Med.* **2021**, *10*, 3905. [CrossRef]
43. Ordog, T.; Syed, S.; Hayashi, Y.; Asuzu, D.T. Epigenetics and chromatin dynamics: A review and a paradigm for functional disorders. *Neurogastroenterol. Motil.* **2012**, *24*, 1054–1068. [CrossRef]
44. Ansari, I.; Raddatz, G.; Gutekunst, J.; Ridnik, M.; Cohen, D.; Abu-Remaileh, M.; Tuganbaev, T.; Shapiro, H.; Pikarsky, E.; Elinav, E.; et al. The microbiota programs DNA methylation to control intestinal homeostasis and inflammation. *Nat. Microbiol.* **2020**, *5*, 610–619. [CrossRef] [PubMed]
45. Ruifrok, A.C.; Johnston, D.A. Quantification of histochemical staining by color deconvolution. *Anal. Quant. Cytol. Histol.* **2001**, *23*, 291–299.
46. Landini, G.; Martinelli, G.; Piccinini, F. Colour deconvolution: Stain unmixing in histological imaging. *Bioinformatics* **2021**, *37*, 1485–1487. [CrossRef] [PubMed]
47. Singh, T.R.; Roy, S.; Singh, O.I.; Sinam, T.; Singh, K.M. A new local adaptive thresholding technique in binarization. *IJCSI Int. J. Comp. Sci.* **2011**, *8*, 271–277. [CrossRef]
48. Karperien, A.L.; Jelinek, H.F. Box-counting fractal analysis: A primer for the clinician. In *The Fractal Geometry of the Brain*; Di Ieva, A., Ed.; Springer: New York, NY, USA, 2016; pp. 91–108. [CrossRef]
49. Glickman, J.N.; Bousvaros, A.; Farraye, F.A.; Zholudev, A.; Friedman, S.; Wang, H.H.; Leichtner, A.M.; Odze, R.D. Pediatric patients with untreated ulcerative colitis may present initially with unusual morphologic findings. *Am. J. Surg. Pathol.* **2004**, *28*, 190–197. [CrossRef]

50. Bancaud, A.; Huet, S.; Daigle, N.; Mozziconacci, J.; Beaudouin, J.; Ellenberg, J. Molecular crowding affects diffusion and binding of nuclear proteins in heterochromatin and reveals the fractal organization of chromatin. *EMBO J.* **2009**, *28*, 3785–3798. [CrossRef] [PubMed]
51. Mobley, A.S. Chapter 4—Induced pluripotent stem cells. In *Neural Stem Cells and Adult Neurogenesi*; Mobley, A.S., Ed.; Academic Press: London, UK, 2019; ISBN 9780128110140. [CrossRef]
52. Chessum, N.; Jones, K.; Pasqua, E.; Tucker, M. Recent advances in cancer therapeutics. *Prog. Med. Chem.* **2015**, *54*, 1–63. [CrossRef]
53. De Bruyn, J.; Wichers, C.; Radstake, T.; Broen, J.; D'Haens, G. Histone deacetylases in inflammatory mucosa distinguish Crohn's disease from ulcerative colitis. *J. Crohn's Colitis* **2015**, *9* (Suppl. 1), S87–S88. [CrossRef]
54. Blanchard, F.; Chipoy, C. Histone deacetylase inhibitors: New drugs for the treatment of inflammatory diseases? *Drug. Discov. Today* **2005**, *10*, 197–204. [CrossRef] [PubMed]

fractal and fractional

MDPI

Article

Unsupervised Deep Learning Approach for Characterizing Fractality in Dried Drop Patterns of Differently Mixed Viscum album Preparations

Carlos Acuña [1], Maria Olga Kokornaczyk [2,3], Stephan Baumgartner [2,3,4] and Mario Castelán [1,*]

[1] Robotics and Advanced Manufacturing, Center for Research and Advanced Studies of the National Polytechnic Institute, Ramos Arizpe 25900, Mexico; carlos.acuna@cinvestav.mx

[2] Society for Cancer Research, 4144 Arlesheim, Switzerland; m.kokornaczyk@vfk.ch (M.O.K.); st.baumgartner@vfk.ch (S.B.)

[3] Institute of Integrative and Complementary Medicine, University of Bern, 3010 Bern, Switzerland

[4] Institute of Integrative Medicine, University of Witten-Herdecke, 58313 Herdecke, Germany

* Correspondence: mario.castelan@cinvestav.edu.mx

Abstract: This paper presents a novel unsupervised deep learning methodology for the analysis of self-assembled structures formed in evaporating droplets. The proposed approach focuses on clustering these structures based on their texture similarity to characterize three different mixing procedures (turbulent, laminar, and diffusion-based) applied to produce *Viscum album Quercus* 10^{-3} according to the European Pharmacopoeia guidelines for the production of homeopathic remedies. Texture clustering departs from obtaining a comprehensive texture representation of the full texture patch database using a convolutional neural network. This representation is then dimensionally reduced to facilitate clustering through advanced machine learning techniques. Following this methodology, 13 clusters were found and their degree of fractality determined by means of Local Connected Fractal Dimension histograms, which allowed for characterization of the different production modalities. As a consequence, each image was represented as a vector in $\mathbb{R}^{13}$, enabling classification of mixing procedures via support vectors. As a main result, our study highlights the clear differences between turbulent and laminar mixing procedures based on their fractal characteristics, while also revealing the nuanced nature of the diffusion process, which incorporates aspects from both mixing types. Furthermore, our unsupervised clustering approach offers a scalable and automated solution for analyzing the databases of evaporated droplets.

Keywords: unsupervised clustering; patterns from evaporated droplets; plant extract; mixing procedures

1. Introduction

Computerized microscopy image analysis is crucial in various fields, including materials science, pathology, drug discovery, and biomedical research [1]. However, this field faces challenges due to data complexity, as microscopic images contain intricate structures that require advanced analysis methods [2]. Traditional approaches, such as manual annotation [3], morphological operations [4], segmentation techniques [5], and feature extraction using descriptors [6], heavily rely on human intervention, leading to subjectivity and limited adaptability [7–9]. Nevertheless, recent advances in computer vision and deep learning have significantly impacted microscopic image analysis, providing more automated and accurate approaches for processing and interpretation [1,10]. In pharmaceutical research, microscopic image analysis is essential for examining pharmaceutical extracts and understanding their properties and quality [11]. The Droplet Evaporation Method (DEM) is a notable method used for this purpose, involving the deposition of a liquid sample onto a surface and studying patterns formed in the droplet residues dried under controlled conditions [12,13]. Recent work [14] revealed significant differences in DEM patterns of pharmaceutical preparations with varying mixing procedures, emphasizing the importance of precise mixing control to ensure product quality and stability [15]. In many studies, DEM images were analyzed exclusively through visual evaluation [16]. To improve this, researchers have introduced the use of fractal descriptors [17–20], GLCM properties [21], Gabor filters [22], and Fourier transform (FT) [23] for texture feature extraction. Notably, deep learning models, especially convolutional neural networks (CNNs), have shown remarkable capabilities in capturing and learning complex patterns and features from microscopic images, including textures [24].

In a previous study [25], we proposed a semi-supervised deep learning-based methodology for analyzing three different mixing procedures (turbulent, laminar, and diffusion-based) used to produce *Viscum album Quercus* 10^{-3} according to the European Pharmacopoeia guidelines for homeopathic remedies [26]. This approach was based on the clustering of full texture patches with a texture similarity criterion. The mixing procedure characterization was restricted to three clusters since each procedure was used as an input to the Dense Convolutional Neural Network (DenseNet) architecture. An approach to overcome this restriction is unsupervised deep learning clustering [27], one of which implements clustering algorithms on coded texture representations obtained as a result of the hierarchical processing of a CNN model [28]. To create these deep texture representations, a pre-trained CNN model, such as VGGNet, ResNet, or InceptionNet, is trained on a large-scale dataset (e.g., ImageNet). Although the CNN model is initially trained for a classification task, it can be reused for other purposes, such as texture representation [29].

In this paper, we propose a novel unsupervised deep learning methodology for clustering DEM patterns obtained from differently produced *Viscum album Quercus* 10^{-3} dilution variants [14]. With the aim of characterizing the mixing modalities used to produce pharmaceutical extracts, we propose a method based on Regions of Interest (ROI) analysis through four stages. The first stage consists of the automatic selection of patches that present a rich texture along the database. In the second stage, a Deep Texture Representation (DTR) of each patch is obtained through the processing of the convolutional neural network architecture VGG-19. During the third stage, the deep texture representations undergo dimensionality reduction through Principal Component Analysis (PCA) to cluster similar textures using hierarchical clustering. Finally, outliers are re-clustered by the Dense Convolutional Neural Network (DenseNet) in the fourth stage. This scheme allowed us to automatically identify and discriminate thirteen clusters of patches that share texture similarity in the DEM image database. Once the patches were clustered, we verified their fractal degree using Local Connected Fractal Dimension (LCFD) histograms. In addition, with this clustering methodology we were able to determine image patch composition for the purposes of classifying the three mixing procedures via support vector machines.

2. Materials and Methods

The utilization of plants in this study adheres to international institutional guidelines. The *Viscum album Quercus* extract used for DEM experimentation was obtained from ISCADOR AG in Arlesheim, Switzerland. *Viscum album* L. was collected from Quercus robur plants growing in their natural habitats in Switzerland, which belonged to ISCADOR AG; hence, no harvesting permission was required. The plants were identified by Mirio Grazi from the Society for Cancer Research in Arlesheim, Switzerland. A voucher specimen (C.H. Quaresma 18.329) was deposited at the Herbarium of the Faculdade de Formação de Professores, Universidade Estadual do Rio de Janeiro, Brazil. *Viscum album* preparations are used in medicine, including as supportive treatment for cancer [30–32].

The DEM image database analyzed here was generously provided by the Society for Cancer Research, Arlesheim, Switzerland under a data-sharing agreement. This valuable database, as detailed in reference [25], consists of 606 images in resolution of 960×720 pixels. These images were obtained using the droplet evaporation method applied to analyze three *Viscum album Quercus* 10^{-3} (VAQ) dilution variants produced using the following different mixing procedures:

1 Turbulent Flow (Variant T): The mixing process involves using a machine to apply vertical strokes. This set comprises a total of 206 images.
2 Laminar Flow (Variant L): The mixing process is carried out manually, inducing a sequence of vortex-like flows. This set comprises a total of 196 images.
3 Diffusion Control (Variant D): This set, consisting of 204 images, represents the control variant where the mixture remains as undisturbed as possible, relying on diffusion processes for dilution.

The Rolling Ball and Sliding Paraboloid technique was employed for background removal in all the images. This involved calculating a local background value for each pixel by averaging it over a large surrounding ball. Subsequently, this calculated value was subtracted from the original image, effectively eliminating significant spatial variations in background intensities [33]. This approach successfully reduced glare effects commonly observed in microscopic images due to their physical characteristics. It is worth noting that the database used for this process did not include images with saturated or blurred conditions, as these conditions could potentially reduce the model's ability to distinguish textures.

The proposed DEM image texture analysis method is shown in the flowchart of Figure 1. The next Sections of this paper are organized in accordance with the flowchart as follows: first, we explain our method for automatic full texture patch selection; the codified texture information obtained by CNN is described later; then, the clustering process is detailed in the last two stages; in the last sections, we provide characterization and classification results, as well as a discussion and concluding remarks.

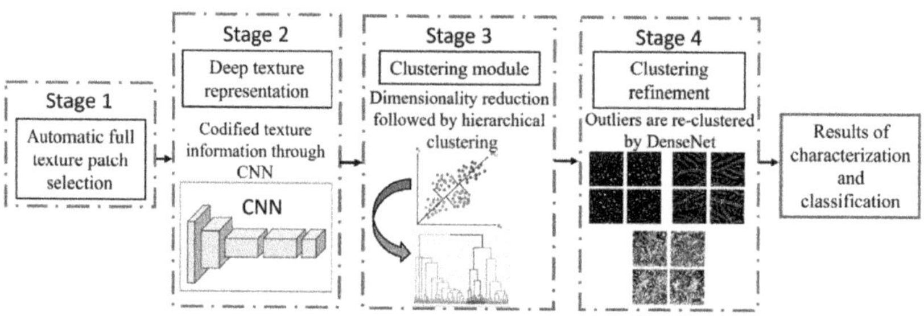

Figure 1. Flowchart of the proposed unsupervised learning approach for DEM image texture clustering. The texture analysis is based on four stages: (1) automatic selection of patches that observe rich texture along the database; (2) texture encoding through a VGG-19; (3) clustering of patches that share texture similarity; and (4) refinement of the clustering using DenseNet.

2.1. Automatic Full Texture Patch Selection

When encoding texture information through a CNN for a specific dataset, such as the VAQ database, it is important to consider regions of interest that exhibit full texture. This ensures that the network learns from all relevant image information and prevents biased learning, resulting in a more balanced and complete understanding of the data. To this end, we use the full texture patch selection method previously developed in [25], which consists of selecting patches of size 128×128 pixels that correspond to 108.4×108.4 μm to then undergo skewness analysis and PCA outlier removal to define patches observing full texture. Automatic selection of full texture patches (Stage 1) led to the formation of the patch database, containing 705 patches from each mixing procedure (D, diffusion control; T, turbulent flow; L, laminar flow), being used as inputs for the proposed unsupervised methodology in this paper. It is important to mention that our technique is not restricted to 128×128 size patches. Depending on hardware capabilities, larger sizes such as 256×256 and 512×512 could also be used.

2.2. Deep Texture Representation Using Convolutional Neural Network

The deep texture representation (DTR) used in this paper borrows ideas from [34], in which the texture encoding of the patch database was obtained through the sequential processing of the VGG-19 architecture, exhibiting advantages over other architectures. As VGG-19 was previously trained on large-scale Imagenet datasets for object recognition, it provides a wide variety of convolutional primitives for generalizing texture patterns. It is important to note that we did not train or fine-tune VGG-19 using the *Viscum album* dataset, as our aim was to obtain DTR from every image patch using the already-computed parameters and weights of VGG-19.

A linearly rectified convolution, with filters of size 3×3 and a maximum pooling in non-overlapping regions of 2×2, was used for the two fundamental computations of the used architecture. The deep texture representation was obtained by applying these computations in an alternating manner throughout five convolutions. Since the number of feature maps is doubled after the third pooling layer, the dimension of the DRT is 512×512. A schematic overview of the network process for obtaining the DRT is provided in Figure 2.

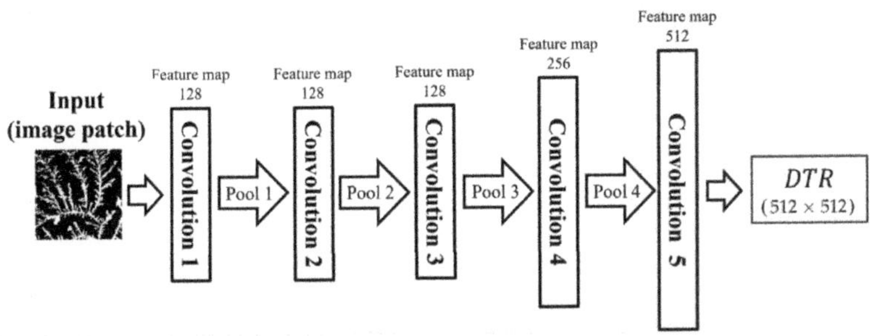

Figure 2. Deep texture representation process. The deep texture representation (DTR) is computed as the feature response of five convolutional layers of the VGG-19 architecture.

As the deep texture representation is obtained using the VGG-19 CNN architecture, the generated model provides a stationary description that fully specifies the texture of the input patches. This DTR matrix is the representation used for texture clustering purposes.

2.3. Dimensionality Reduction of the Deep Texture Representation

Since the dimension of the deep texture representation (512×512) is not tractable for clustering algorithms, dimensionality reduction is required. To this end, we performed a principal component analysis (PCA) of the DTR matrices database. Subsequently, we used DTR matrices to construct the training set data matrix, $\mathbf{T}_{k \times n} = [\mathbf{t}_{k,1} \mid \mathbf{t}_{k,2} \mid \cdots \mid \mathbf{t}_{k,n}]$, where $n = 2115$ (705 patches for each mixing procedure) is the number of patches and $k = 512 \times 512 = 262,144$ is the number of texture values encoded in each DTR matrix. The differences from the average $\bar{\mathbf{t}}$ are used to build the centered training data matrix $\bar{\mathbf{T}}_{k \times n} = [(\mathbf{t}_1 - \bar{\mathbf{t}}) \mid (\mathbf{t}_2 - \bar{\mathbf{t}}) \mid \cdots \mid (\mathbf{t}_n - \bar{\mathbf{t}})]$. The covariance matrix is calculated as $\mathbf{\Sigma}_{n \times n} = \bar{\mathbf{T}}^T \bar{\mathbf{T}}$. Given that $\mathbf{\Sigma}$ is symmetric, there always exists an orthogonal basis $\mathbf{U}_{n \times n}$ and a diagonal matrix $\mathbf{\Lambda}_{n \times n}$ that satisfies the relationship $\mathbf{\Sigma} = \mathbf{U} \mathbf{\Lambda} \mathbf{U}^T$, where $\mathbf{U}_{n \times n}$ is the eigenvector matrix and the eigenvalues of $\mathbf{\Sigma}$ are the diagonal elements of matrix $\mathbf{\Lambda}$.

Figure 3a shows that, with 35 components, the PCA model constructed from the DRT matrices achieves 95.96% variability. In contrast, Figure 3b shows that the PCA constructed directly from the pixel information of the patches (i.e., $k = 128 \times 128 = 16{,}384$) requires 1723 components to achieve 95.95% of the variability. This indicates that the variables in the DTR matrices are highly correlated and, therefore, can be effectively represented by a few principal components. We selected $l = 35$ principal components based on the variability achieved by the DTR model (see Figure 3a). The texture encoded information of the DTR matrices in the column space of U is given by $\mathbf{A}_{k \times l} = \mathbf{T}_{k \times n} \hat{\mathbf{U}}_{n \times l} \mathbf{\Lambda}_{l \times l}^{-1}$. The dimensionality reduction is defined by the orthogonal projection of the centered matrix $\bar{\mathbf{T}}$ in the column space of $\mathbf{A}$ by the expression $\hat{\mathbf{T}}_{l\times n} = \mathbf{A}_{k\times l}^{T}\bar{\mathbf{T}}_{k\times n}$. This expression allows movement from a dimension k = 262,144 (512 × 512) to a reduced-dimension space $l = 35$, which will facilitate, in the context of computational efficiency, the grouping of textures by means of hierarchical clustering.

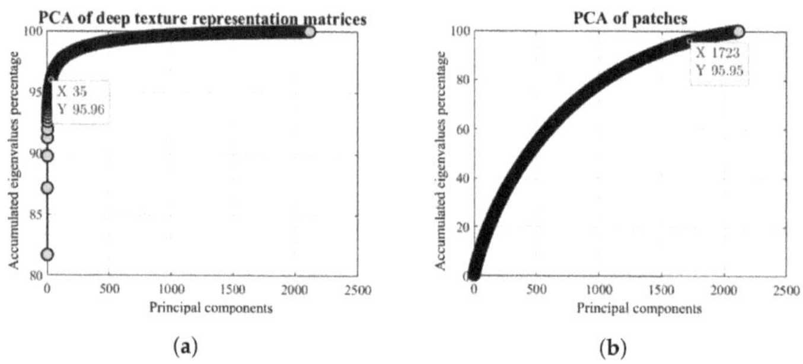

Figure 3. Percentage of variability reached by the models of two different pattern representations. (**a**) Accumulated eigenvalues percentage of DTR. (**b**) Accumulated eigenvalues percentage from pixel information.

Figure 4 shows the DTR matrices from representative patches of DEM images from differently mixed VAQ variants, as well as their respective reconstructions through the 35-dimensional PCA model.

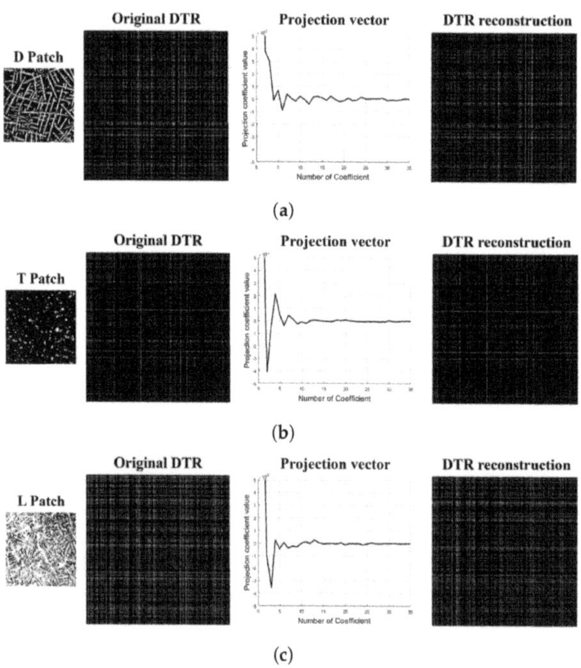

Figure 4. Representative patches of DEM images of differently mixed VAQ variants with their respective DTR matrices, projection vectors in $\mathbb{R}^{35}$, and PCA reconstructions. (**a**) DTR matrix and its reconstruction with 35 projection coefficient values from a representative D patch. (**b**) DTR matrix and its reconstruction with 35 projection coefficient values from a representative T patch. (**c**) DTR matrix and its reconstruction with 35 projection coefficient values from a representative L patch.

It is possible to notice that the coded information is denser in patch L (see Figure 4c) compared to patch T (see Figure 4b), which is in agreement with the visual information of each patch.

2.4. DTR Clusterization in the Reduced-Dimension Space

In order to cluster projections of DTR matrices on the reduced space, we used the hierarchical clustering algorithm [35] since it provides reproducible results and is not limited to the spheroidal shape of the data [36]. However, because the algorithm is sensitive to outliers [37], PCA outlier removal was performed before clustering.

By analyzing the first 35 principal components, 369 outliers were extracted considering a standard deviation of 2, and the remaining 1746 patches (textures) were clustered. In other words, we used the matrix $\hat{\mathbf{T}}_{l\times n-m}$ as input to the hierarchical clustering, where m corresponds to the 369 outliers and $l = 35$ is the encoded texture information represented in the reduced-dimension space.

The number of clusters was determined through the elbow method [38] which iterates over the number of clusters and obtains the intra-cluster variance of each iteration. The optimal number of clusters for our database was 13, i.e., beyond that point (see Figure 5a), increasing the number of clusters did not lead to a significant reduction in the distortion score. Clustering results are presented in Figure 5b as a distribution of patches along the 13 clusters. The orange portion of the bars indicates the number of patches that are considered outliers based on the analysis of their principal components. In total, 925 outliers were extracted, 369 before hierarchical clustering and 556 after; the latter can be attributed to the inherent limitations of the hierarchical clustering algorithm, primarily due to its reliance on the Euclidean distance metric and its proximity-based clustering approach. In certain cases, if an outlier is in close proximity to a cluster, it may be merged with that cluster, even if it does not exhibit significant similarity with the majority of data points [39].

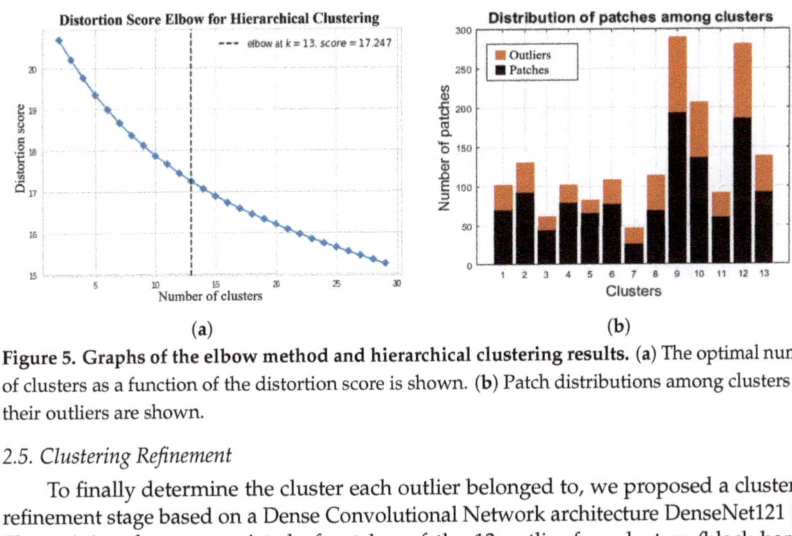

(a) (b)

Figure 5. Graphs of the elbow method and hierarchical clustering results. (**a**) The optimal number of clusters as a function of the distortion score is shown. (**b**) Patch distributions among clusters and their outliers are shown.

2.5. Clustering Refinement

To finally determine the cluster each outlier belonged to, we proposed a clustering refinement stage based on a Dense Convolutional Network architecture DenseNet121 [40]. The training dataset consisted of patches of the 13 outlier-free clusters (black bars in Figure 5b). With the aim of reducing learning bias, we trained DenseNet121 with the same number of samples per cluster by increasing the training database through 5 rotations: 30°, 60°, 90°, 120°, and 150°. Since cluster 7 was the one with the lowest number of patches, it limited data augmentation for the rest of clusters, which were randomly selected until the same number of patches as (augmented) cluster 7 was achieved.

Testing data consisted of the outliers, which were reorganized into the 13 clusters using the DenseNet121 architecture. The results presented in Figure 6 show that, after clustering refinement, there was a significant reduction in the number of final outliers, having only 31, representing 1.46% of the total patch database, revealing increased cluster cohesiveness after clustering refinement.

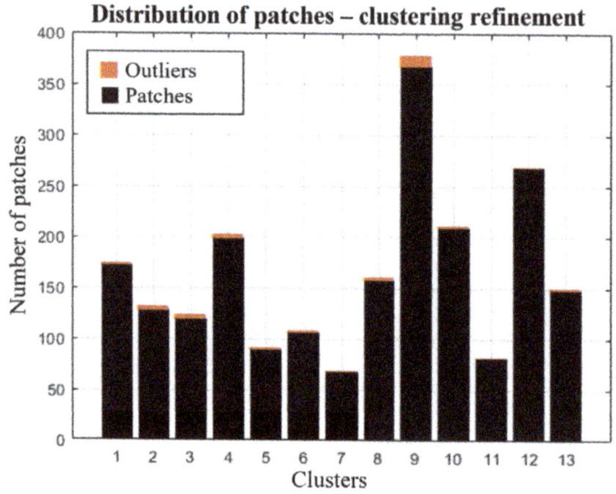

Figure 6. Patch distribution among the 13 classes. Noticeable reduction in outliers after clustering refinement.

To assess the fractality of each cluster, we calculated the weighted area under the curve (WAUC) of the average LCFD histogram for each cluster, as illustrated in Figure 7. In other words, WAUC was obtained as a result of the inner product of the frequency and the Local Connected Fractal Dimension for each of the 13 average LCFD histograms. This enabled us to arrange the clusters in ascending order based on their fractality degree.

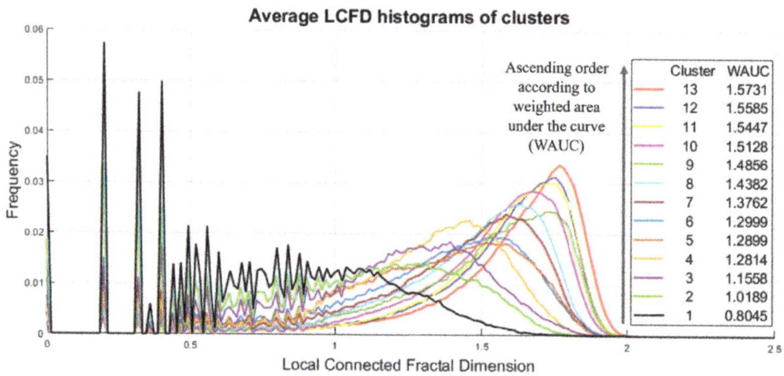

Figure 7. Average LCFD histograms of clusters. The average LCFD histograms are shown in ascending order, i.e., cluster 13 exhibits the highest fractality degree and cluster 1 exhibits the lowest fractality degree.

In Figure 8 we present patch samples of each cluster, in ascending order according to their degree of fractality. It is noteworthy that each cluster can be visually differentiated. In the samples of cluster 1, there is a great dispersion of the particles; in clusters 6 and 7, the particles are joining to generate structures that determine a greater fractality; and in the last clusters, complex patterns with intricate details are observed.

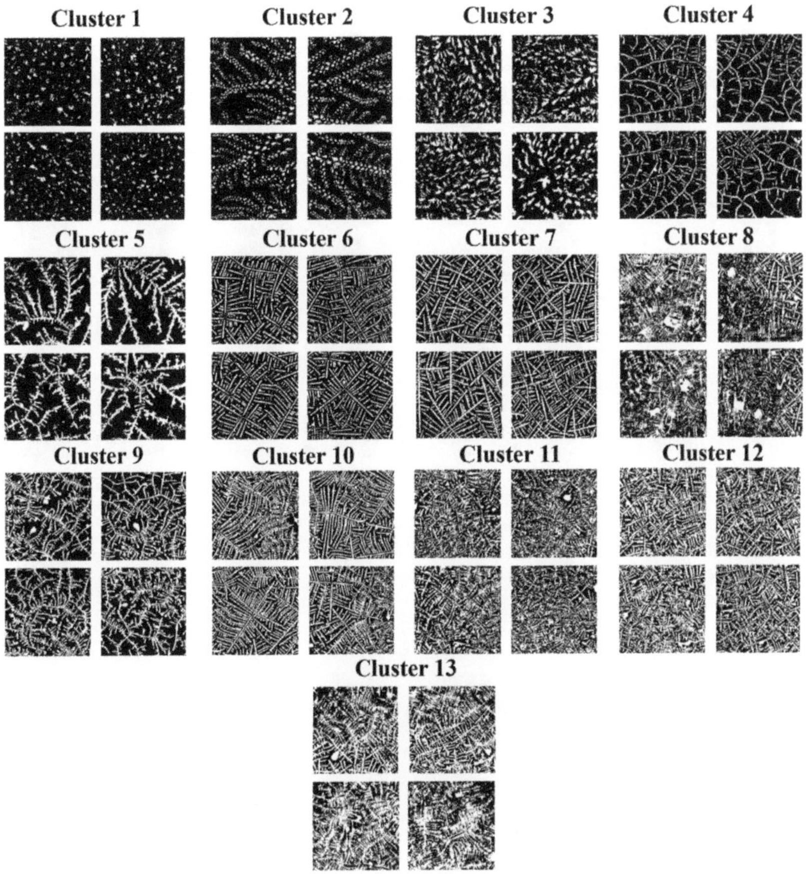

Figure 8. Samples of the thirteen clusters defined through the proposed unsupervised framework. The samples of the clusters are ordered according to their fractal degree, i.e., cluster 1 being the least fractal and cluster 13 the most fractal. The size of the patches is 128 × 128 pixels which corresponds to 108.4 × 108.4 μm.

3. Results at the Image Level

Figure 9 exhibits the distribution of patches with respect to the DEM image of each mixing procedure. The x-axis corresponds to the image number, while the y-axis corresponds to the number of clusters, ordered from least to most fractal. The cells, represented in grayscale, refer to the number of patches in each cluster, where white pixels indicate the highest number of patches and black pixels the absence of patches. Note how the distribution of patches in the turbulent mixing procedure shows a bias toward the bottom part (Figure 9b), revealing that this procedure tends to simplify fractal composition, reducing the complexity and intricacy that are often associated with fractal patterns. This may be attributed to the turbulent nature of the mixing process, which may lead to a more chaotic and disordered distribution of elements within the image. On the other hand, Figure 9c shows that the patches of the laminar mixing procedure accumulate towards the top, revealing that inducing a vortex-like flow results in a higher degree of fractality. Finally, the distribution of patches in the diffusion mixing procedure (Figure 9a), presents a uniform behavior, that is, the images of this mixing procedure tend to exhibit patches along the whole fractal spectrum.

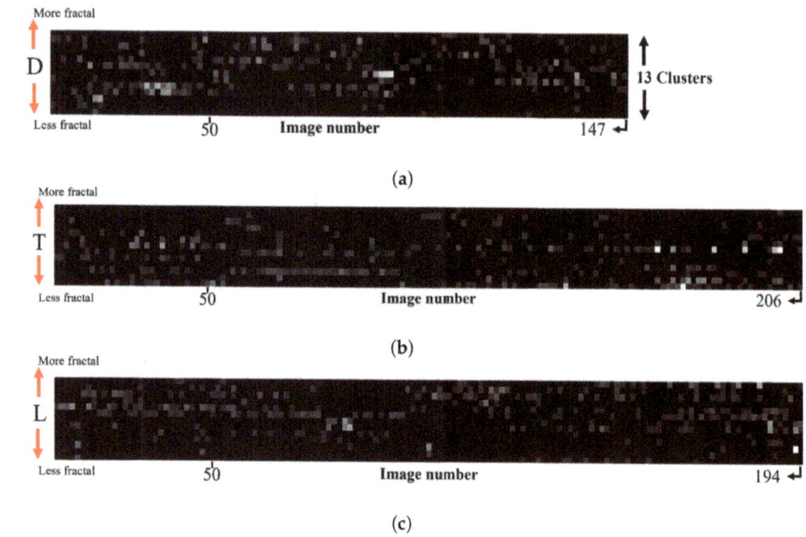

Figure 9. Patch distribution at image level. (**a**) Distribution of patches in the images of D mixing procedure. (**b**) Distribution of patches in the images of T mixing procedure. (**c**) Distribution of patches in the images of L mixing procedure.

As a result of clustering refinement, each image can be represented as a vector in $\mathbb{R}^{13}$, which characterizes the patch composition of the image. These vectors were used for classification purposes by means of a support vector machine (SVM). To this end, 60% of the vectors were considered for training and the remaining 40% for testing. Results are shown as a confusion matrix in Figure 10, where it is revealed that the best classification was obtained in turbulent flow with 72% accuracy, followed by 60% for laminar flow, and the lowest accuracy corresponded to the diffusion mixing procedure with 33%. These results are congruent with the patch distribution shown in Figure 9 since the distributions of mixing procedures T and L exhibit a particular footprint that allows for separability. However, mixing procedure D presents a uniform distribution, resulting in 43% confusion regarding turbulent flow and 24% regarding laminar flow. These results suggest that mixing procedure D holds the base fractal footprint of the pharmaceutical extract, with a greater similarity to procedure T than to procedure L.

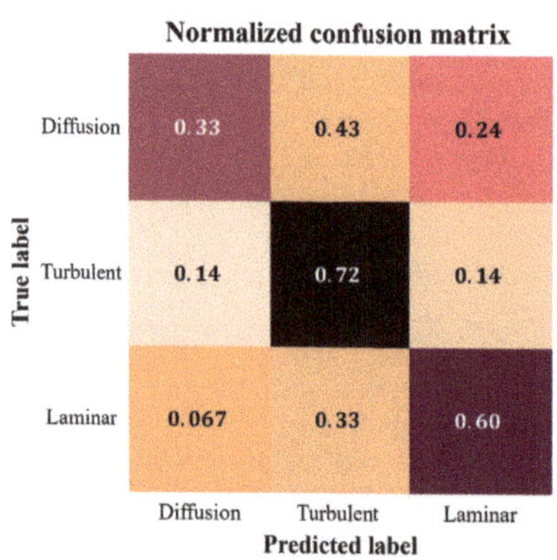

Figure 10. Confusion matrix. Results of the classification task between mixing procedures using a support vector machine are shown.

4. Discussion

The analysis of DEM patterns obtained from differently mixed variants of *Viscum album Quercus* 10^{-3} (turbulent, laminar, and diffusion-based mixing) present several challenges due to the complexity and variability of the micrographs. As the DEM patterns of the three VAQ variants originate from the same plant extract, a diverse range of textures is observed, making their differentiation a challenging task. Traditional techniques applied directly such as Gabor filters, Gray Level Co-occurrence Matrix (GLCM), and fractal-based measures do not succeed in determining the imprint of each mixing procedure. In a previous study [25], we introduced an analysis using a semi-supervised deep learning framework, leveraging a Dense Convolutional Network architecture to characterize the mixing procedures. Through this approach, we successfully identified three distinct groups of textures. However, one area of improvement worth considering is the restriction of categorizing the patterns only using three texture groups. This constraint restricts missing subtle variations or additional patterns that could be relevant to understand and differentiate plant extract's behavior under different mixing conditions.

Motivated by this, the present study explores an unsupervised learning solution. By employing the proposed methodology, we successfully identified and defined thirteen distinct texture groups found within the VAQ database. These texture groups were organized based on their fractality degree, determined by calculating the weighted area under the curve of the average Local Connected Fractal Dimension histograms. The results obtained through this approach provided a much more detailed characterization of the patterns, enabling us to gain valuable insights into the fractal distribution across the DEM images of VAQ variants obtained by different mixing procedures. This deeper understanding of the fractal composition sheds light on the underlying structures and variations present in the microscopic textures of dried droplets. Moreover, we leveraged the $\mathbb{R}^{13}$ vectors, which describe the fractal composition of each image, to perform classification using a support vector machine (SVM). By adopting an unsupervised learning strategy, we overcame the limitations of relying on predefined labels and allowed the data to reveal the inherent structures naturally. This data-driven approach not only provided a more comprehensive characterization, but also facilitated the discovery of previously unnoticed patterns and relationships within the VAQ database.

5. Conclusions

Through this paper we have shown that it is possible to characterize the DEM images of the VAQ dataset as vectors of 13 values, thus assessing classification attributes, per image, at the level of mixing procedures. We found that turbulent and laminar mixing modalities are more separable between them than they are with diffusion, i.e., diffusion exhibits features that are characteristic of both laminar and turbulence motions. These findings provide more detailed evidence that there may be an original DEM imprint in the diffusion state, which either becomes stronger (more fractal) with laminar motion or debilitates its fractality (is destructed—becomes less fractal) with turbulent motion. Our study suggests that the proposed unsupervised methodology for texture clustering provides a systematic and efficient approach to identify distinct DEM texture patterns within a set of pharmaceutical extract micrographs. This approach improves how succussions can be understood and interpreted in the context of solution preparations, which is relevant for homeopathy basic research as well as the manufacturing and distribution of pharmaceutical preparations.

Finally, we must note that clustering through deep learning techniques has gained much attention in the community. An example of a major clustering work is [41], which applies generative adversarial networks to generate deep representations. Compared to ours, such representations would demand a higher computational cost and more specialized hardware. Additionally, our work is the first to consider a refinement module such as the one based on DenseNet proposed in this paper. For a recent review in clustering methods see [42].

Author Contributions: M.O.K. and S.B. designed the experimental set-up of the study. Data were extracted by M.O.K. The proposed methodology to analyze the patterns of evaporated droplets of *Viscum album* extracts was developed by C.A. and M.C. The manuscript was written mainly by C.A. with contributions from the rest of the co-authors. All authors have read and agreed to the published version of the manuscript.

Funding: The unsupervised deep learning approach developed in this paper was funded by the National Council of Humanities, Science and Technology (CONAHCYT) under project CF-2023-G-454.

Data Availability Statement: Correspondence and requests for programming codes and database should be addressed to the corresponding author.

Acknowledgments: C.A. thanks CONAHCYT for studentship 765760.

Conflicts of Interest: The authors declare no conflict of interest.

Abbreviations

The following abbreviations are used in this manuscript:

VAQ	*Viscum album Quercus*
CNN	Convolutional Neural Network
DTR	Deep Texture Representation
DEM	Droplet Evaporation Method
PCA	Principal Component Analysis
DenseNet	Dense Convolutional Neural Network
WAUC	Weighted Area Under the Curve
LCFD	Local Connected Fractal Dimension
SVM	Support Vector Machine
GLCM	Gray Level Co-occurrence Matrix

References

1. Xing , F.; Xie, Y.; Su, H.; Liu, F.; Yang, L. Deep Learning in Microscopy Image Analysis: A Survey. *IEEE Trans. Neural Netw. Learn. Syst.* **2018**, *29*, 4550–4568. [CrossRef] [PubMed]
2. Razzak, M.I.; Naz, S.; Zaib, A. Deep Learning for Medical Image Processing: Overview, Challenges and Future. *arXiv* **2017**, arXiv:1704.06825
3. Englbrecht, F.; Ruider, I.E.; Bausch, A.R. Automatic image annotation for fluorescent cell nuclei segmentation. *PLoS ONE* **2021**, *16*, e0250093. [CrossRef]
4. Weeks, A.R. Morphological operations on color images. *J. Electron. Imaging* **2001**, *10*, 548. [CrossRef]
5. Sharma, N.; Ray, A.; Shukla, K.; Sharma, S.; Pradhan, S.; Srivastva, A.; Aggarwal, L. Automated medical image segmentation techniques. *J. Med. Phys.* **2010**, *35*, 3. [CrossRef]
6. Salau, A.O.; Jain, S. Feature Extraction: A Survey of the Types, Techniques, Applications. In Proceedings of the 2019 International Conference on Signal Processing and Communication (ICSC), Noida, India, 7–9 March 2019. [CrossRef]
7. Almeida-Prieto, S.; Blanco-Méndez, J.; Otero-Espinar, F.J. Microscopic image analysis techniques for the morphological characterization of pharmaceutical particles: Influence of process variables. *J. Pharm. Sci.* **2006**, *95*, 348–357. [CrossRef]
8. Raje, C.; Rangole, J. Detection of Leukemia in microscopic images using image processing. In Proceedings of the 2014 International Conference on Communication and Signal Processing, Melmaruvathur, India, 3–5 April 2014. [CrossRef]
9. Cruz, D.; Jennifer, C.; Valiente; Castor, L.C.; Mendoza, C.M.T.; Jay, B.A.; Jane, L.S.C.; Brian, P.T.B. Determination of blood components (WBCs, RBCs, and Platelets) count in microscopic images using image processing and analysis. In Proceedings of the 2017 IEEE 9th International Conference on Humanoid, Nanotechnology, Information Technology, Communication and Control, Environment and Management (HNICEM), Manila, Philippines, 1–3 December 2017. [CrossRef]
10. Liu, Z.; Jin, L.; Chen, J.; Fang, Q.; Ablameyko, S.; Yin, Z.; Xu, Y. A survey on applications of deep learning in microscopy image analysis. *Comput. Biol. Med.* **2021**, *134*, 104523. [CrossRef]
11. Galata, D.L.; Mészáros, L.A.; Kállai-Szabó, N.; Szabó, E.; Pataki, H.; Marosi, G.; Nagy, Z.K. Applications of machine vision in pharmaceutical technology: A review. *Eur. J. Pharm. Sci.* **2021**, *159*, 105717. [CrossRef]
12. Kokornaczyk, M.O.; Trebbi, G.; Dinelli, G.; Marotti, I.; Bregola, V.; Nani, D.; Borghini, F.; Betti, L. Droplet evaporation method as a new potential approach for highlighting the effectiveness of ultra high dilutions. *Complement. Ther. Med.* **2014**, *22*, 333–340. [CrossRef]
13. Kokornaczyk, M.O.; Würtenberger, S.; Baumgartner, S. Impact of succussion on pharmaceutical preparations analyzed by means of patterns from evaporated droplets. *Sci. Rep.* **2020**, *10*, 570. [CrossRef] [PubMed]

14. Kokornaczyk, M.O.; Kunz, C.; Baumgartner, S. Impact of vertical succussion strokes vs. vortex potentization on droplet evaporation patterns obtained from Iscador Quercus 3x potency. *Int. J. High Dilution Res.* **2021**, *18*, 3. [CrossRef]
15. Abdul-Fattah, A.M.; Kalonia, D.S.; Pikal, M.J. The Challenge of Drying Method Selection for Protein Pharmaceuticals: Product Quality Implications. *J. Pharm. Sci.* **2007**, *96*, 1886–1916. [CrossRef]
16. Scherr, C.; Bodrova, N.B.; Baumgartner, S.; Kokornaczyk, M. Phase-Transition-Induced Pattern Formation Applied to Basic Research on Homeopathy: A Systematic Review. *Homeopathy* **2018**, *107*, 181–188. [CrossRef]
17. Crivoi, A.; Duan, F. Evaporation-induced formation of fractal-like structures from nanofluids. *Phys. Chem. Chem. Phys.* **2012**, *14*, 1449–1454. [CrossRef] [PubMed]
18. Hossain, A.; Akhtar, M.N.; Navascués, M.A. Fractal Dimension of Fractal Functions on the Real Projective Plane. *Fractal Fract.* **2023**, *7*, 510. [CrossRef]
19. Pantic, I.; Valjarevic, S.; Cumic, J.; Paunkovic, I.; Terzic, T.; Corridon, P.R. Gray Level Co-Occurrence Matrix, Fractal and Wavelet Analyses of Discrete Changes in Cell Nuclear Structure following Osmotic Stress: Focus on Machine Learning Methods. *Fractal Fract.* **2023**, *7*, 272. [CrossRef]
20. Urgilez-Clavijo, A.; Rivas-Tabares, D.A.; Martín-Sotoca, J.J.; Alfonso, A.M.T. Local Fractal Connections to Characterize the Spatial Processes of Deforestation in the Ecuadorian Amazon. *Entropy* **2021**, *23*, 748. [CrossRef]
21. Carreón, Y.J.P.; Díaz-Hernández, O.; Santos, G.J.E.; Cipriano-Urbano, I.; Solorio-Ordaz, F.J.; González-Gutiérrez, J.; Zenit, R. Texture Analysis of Dried Droplets for the Quality Control of Medicines. *Sensors* **2021**, *21*, 4048. [CrossRef]
22. Zuñiga, A.G.; Florindo, J.B.; Bruno, O.M. Gabor wavelets combined with volumetric fractal dimension applied to texture analysis. *Pattern Recognit. Lett.* **2014**, *36*, 135–143. [CrossRef]
23. Scoutaris, N.; Ross, S.; Douroumis, D. Current Trends on Medical and Pharmaceutical Applications of Inkjet Printing Technology. *Pharm. Res.* **2016**, *33*, 1799–1816. [CrossRef] [PubMed]
24. Sachar, S.; Kumar, A. Deep ensemble learning for automatic medicinal leaf identification. *Int. J. Inf. Technol.* **2022**, *14*, 3089–3097. [CrossRef] [PubMed]
25. Acuña, C.; y Terán, A.M.; Kokornaczyk, M.O.; Baumgartner, S.; Castelán, M. Deep learning applied to analyze patterns from evaporated droplets of *Viscum album* extracts. *Sci. Rep.* **2022**, *12*, 15332. [CrossRef]
26. Monograph, T. European Pharmacopoeia. In *European Directorate for the Quality of Medicine & Health Care of the Council of 376 Europe (EDQM)*, 9th ed.; Communications and Events Division: Strasbourg, France, 2017; Volume 9, pp. 3104–3105.
27. Malhi, U.S.; Zhou, J.; Yan, C.; Rasool, A.; Siddeeq, S.; Du, M. Unsupervised Deep Embedded Clustering for High-Dimensional Visual Features of Fashion Images. *Appl. Sci.* **2023**, *13*, 2828. [CrossRef]
28. Fard, M.M.; Thonet, T.; Gaussier, E. Deep k-Means: Jointly clustering with k-Means and learning representations. *Pattern Recognit. Lett.* **2020**, *138*, 185–192. [CrossRef]
29. Ren, Y.; Pu, J.; Yang, Z.; Xu, J.; Li, G.; Pu, X.; Yu, P.S.; He, L. Deep Clustering: A Comprehensive Survey. *arXiv* **2022**, arXiv:2210.04142.
30. Stauder, G.M.; Matthes, H.; Friedel, W.E.; Bock, P.R. Use of fermented mistletoe (*Viscum album* L.) extract from oak tree (Quercus) as supportive treatment for patients with pancreatic cancer. *J. Clin. Oncol.* **2009**, *27*, e15656. [CrossRef]
31. Tröger, W.; Galun, D.; Reif, M.; Schumann, A.; Stanković, N.; Milićević, M. Quality of Life of Patients with Advanced Pancreatic Cancer During Treatment with Mistletoe. *Dtsch. Ärzteblatt Int.* **2014**, *111*, 493. [CrossRef]
32. Thronicke, A.; Schad, F.; Debus, M.; Grabowski, J.; Soldner, G. *Viscum album* L. Ther. Oncol. Update Curr. Evidence.*Complement. Med. Res.* **2022**, *29*, 362–368. [CrossRef]
33. Kelley, J.B.; Paschal, B.M. Fluorescence-based quantification of nucleocytoplasmic transport. *Methods* **2019**, *157*, 106–114. [CrossRef]
34. Gatys, L.A.; Ecker, A.S.; Bethge, M. Texture Synthesis Using Convolutional Neural Networks. *arXiv* **2015**, arXiv:1505.07376.
35. Nielsen, F. Hierarchical Clustering. In *Introduction to HPC with MPI for Data Science*; Springer International Publishing: Basel, Switzerland, 2016; pp. 195–211. [CrossRef]
36. Huang, Q.; Gao, R.; Akhavan, H. An ensemble hierarchical clustering algorithm based on merits at cluster and partition levels. *Pattern Recognit.* **2023**, *136*, 109255. [CrossRef]
37. Murtagh, F.; Contreras, P. Algorithms for hierarchical clustering: An overview. *WIREs Data Min. Knowl. Discov.* **2011**, *2*, 86–97. [CrossRef]
38. Zambelli, A.E. A data-driven approach to estimating the number of clusters in hierarchical clustering. *F1000Research* **2016**, *5*, 2809. [CrossRef] [PubMed]
39. Zhao, Y.; Karypis, G.; Fayyad, U. Hierarchical Clustering Algorithms for Document Datasets. *Data Min. Knowl. Discov.* **2005**, *10*, 141–168. [CrossRef]
40. Huang, G.; Liu, Z.; van der Maaten, L.; Weinberger, K.Q. Densely Connected Convolutional Networks. *arXiv* **2016**, arXiv:1608.06993.
41. de Mello, D.; Assunção, R.; Murai, F. Top-Down Deep Clustering with Multi-generator GANs. In Proceedings of the AAAI Conference on Artificial Intelligence, Virtual, 22 February–1 March 2022; AAAI Press: Palo Alto, CA, USA, 2021. [CrossRef]
42. Zhou, S.; Xu, H.; Zheng, Z.; Chen, J.; Li, Z.; Bu, J.; Wu, J.; Wang, X.; Zhu, W.; Ester, M. A Comprehensive Survey on Deep Clustering: Taxonomy, Challenges, and Future Directions. *arXiv* **2022**, arXiv:2206.07579.

fractal and fractional

MDPI

Article

Analysis of the Corneal Geometry of the Human Eye with an Artificial Neural Network

Waseem [1], Asad Ullah [2,3,*], Fuad A. Awwad [4] and Emad A. A. Ismail [4]

1 School of Mechanical Engineering, Jiangsu University, 301, Xuefu Road, Jingkou District, Zhenjiang 212013, China; waseem@ujs.edu.cn
2 School of Finance and Economics, Jiangsu University, 301, Xuefu Road, Jingkou District, Zhenjiang 212013, China
3 Department of Mathematical Sciences, University of Lakki Marwat, Lakki Marwat 28420, Khyber Pakhtunkhwa, Pakistan
4 Department of Quantitative Analysis, College of Business Administration, King Saud University, P.O. Box 71115, Riyadh 11587, Saudi Arabia; fawwad@ksu.edu.sa (F.A.A.); emadali@ksu.edu.sa (E.A.A.)
* Correspondence: asad@ujs.edu.cn

Abstract: In this paper, a hybrid cuckoo search technique is combined with a single-layer neural network (BHCS-ANN) to approximate the solution to a differential equation describing the curvature shape of the cornea of the human eye. The proposed problem is transformed into an optimization problem such that the L_2-error remains minimal. A single hidden layer is chosen to reduce the sink of the local minimum values. The weights in the neural network are trained with a hybrid cuckoo search algorithm to refine them so that we obtain a better approximate solution for the given problem. To show the efficacy of our method, we considered six different corneal models. For validation, the solution with Adam's method is taken as a reference solution. The results are presented in the form of figures and tables. The obtained results are compared with the fractional order Darwinian particle swarm optimization (FO-DPSO). We determined that results obtained with BHCS-ANN outperformed the ones acquired with other numerical routines. Our findings suggest that BHCS-ANN is a better methodology for solving real-world problems.

Keywords: nonlinear biosystem; corneal geometry; neural network; artificial intelligence; cuckoo search; medical image; human eye

1. Introduction

Eyesight is an indispensable sense for every organism that does not only connect with their surrounding but also keeps them safe and regulate mental sharpness. In the eye, the cornea is the outer transparent layer tissue which help us to see clearly and serves as a barrier against various infections. Corneal disorders lead to severe eyesight problems including keratitis, myopia, corneal dystrophy, dry eye, astigmatism, etc. To understand the underlying topography of corneal mechanisms, mathematical models can provide value insight for ophthalmologists. The basic mechanism of the eye is well known to everyone. The main functions and working procedures of the eye are explained at the high-school level. We all know that the cornea works like a window for the eye. When a light beam is focused on an eye, it directly passes through the cornea, which has a diameter of 0.5 inches. The geometry of the human eye is described in Figure 1. The mathematical form of the n-dimensional equation for the mean curvature is given as follows:

$$\begin{aligned} &\operatorname{div}\left(\frac{\nabla\psi(t)}{\sqrt{1+|\nabla\psi(t)|^2}}\right) = c\psi - \frac{d}{\sqrt{1+|\nabla\psi(t)|^2}} \quad \text{in } \Omega \\ &\psi(t) = 0 \text{ on } \partial\Omega. \end{aligned} \tag{1}$$

Here, $c, d > 0$, and $\Omega \subset R^n$, $n \geq 2$ is the bounded Lipschitz domain. Recently, Corsato et al. [1] studied Equation (1) for describing regularity, existence, and uniqueness. They described the mean anisotropic curvature considering the Dirichlet conditions. The one-dimensional analysis of Equation (1) was carried out by Okrasiński and Płociniczak [2]. They used the linearization technique on the divergence control operator by considering $[0,1]$ as a bounded domain. Their relationship to the cornea is described as follows:

$$\begin{array}{l} \left(\frac{\psi'(t)}{\sqrt{1+\psi'^2(t)}}\right)' - c\psi(t) + \frac{d}{\sqrt{1+\psi'^2(t)}} = 0, \quad t \in [0,1] \\ \psi'(0) = \psi(1) = 0 \end{array} . \tag{2}$$

A more detailed analysis related to Equation (2) can be found in Coelho et al. [3]. In the early 1990s, Komai and Ushiki [4] analyzed the three-dimensional collagen fibrils in the human eye. Later on, this work was extended by Peh et al. [5] and Almubrad and Akhtar [6]. They discussed the various impacts and briefly described the expansion of the cornea and its effects on tree shrews.

The exact solution to nonlinear problems is always a point of interest for researchers; however, due to nonlinearity and complexity including high dimensionality, closed-form solutions are very rare to find. One of the best attempts to explain the closed-form solution is made by Okrasiński and Płociniczak [2]. In addition to their unique analysis, they showed that their results are quite impressive, up to 1% absolute error. In this work, they approximated nonlinearity through a hyperbolic cosine function. The work of Płociniczak et al. [7] opened the door to the application of semianalytical methods. He [8] introduced a new idea to these methods by adding Taylor's series. This suggestion has made great improvements in the solution as well as in the reduction of the absolute error. Methods like Adomian decomposition [9], spline interpolation [10], variational iteration [11], Green's function approach [12], and differential transformation [9] are normally considered very effective for boundary value problems (BVPs). Płociniczak et al. [13] further explained the formulation of the corneal curvature with the help of pseudo-time derivatives. The transformed partial differential equations (PDEs) are further solved numerically, and the results are compared with the available literature. Griffiths et al. [14] analyzed the radial basis function by considering the mesh-free approach. A brief survey can be found in the references [15–17]. Researchers frequently use Green's function-based approaches to solve BVPs. For instance, Zur [18–20] provided a series of works employing Green's and quasi-Green's functions to investigate the vibration of thin circular plates, thin circular plates with variable thickness, and elastically supported functionally graded annular plates. The exact Green's function for each given rectangular potential was determined by Andrade [21]. The Ahyoune et al. [22] method of solving quasi-static partial element equivalent circuits made use of a weighted combination of 2D and 3D analytical Green's functions. The BVPs arise in heat transfer, strong nonlinear oscillation, electroanalytical chemistry, and Bratu problems, and are solved using linked Green's function with a fixed-point iteration approach [16,23].

In recent years, artificial-intelligence-based methods have been introduced in the literature for solving various complex problems [24]. The applications of artificial neural networks (ANNs) can be seen in circuit and electromagnetic theory [25,26], the fuel ignition model [27], motor induction models [28], the Thomas–Fermi model [29], doubly singular nonlinear systems [28], nanotechnology [30], nanofluidics [31], nonlinear prey–predator models [32], nonlinear equations [33], Troesch's problem [34], optimal control [35], signal processing [36], and the modeling and control of particle accelerators [37]. Pinsky and Datye [38] used the finite element method for the analysis of the incised cornea of the human eye. Pandolfi and Manganiello [39] analyzed the corneal shape model (CSM) by using a numerical procedure. Płociniczak et al. [7] studied the nonlinear CSM and presented a detailed description of the CSM-based boundary value problem (BVP). Ahmad et al. [40] studied the nonlinear CSM by using the neuroevolution-based approach. Płociniczak and Okrasiński [41] presented a detailed overview of the CSM model and explained the physical impact of each parameter encountered in the study. Recently, Erturk et al. [42]

used the concept of fractional derivatives to analyze the noninteger behavior of the CSM. Sáez-Gutiérrez et al. [43] investigated the surface geometry of the cornea by using the evolutionary algorithm. The use of machine learning is increasing day by day and has covered a substantial area of research [44]. Aziz et al. [45] used the cuckoo search (CS) algorithm for the analysis of the fish image. A more recent survey on CS can be found in the references [46–48].

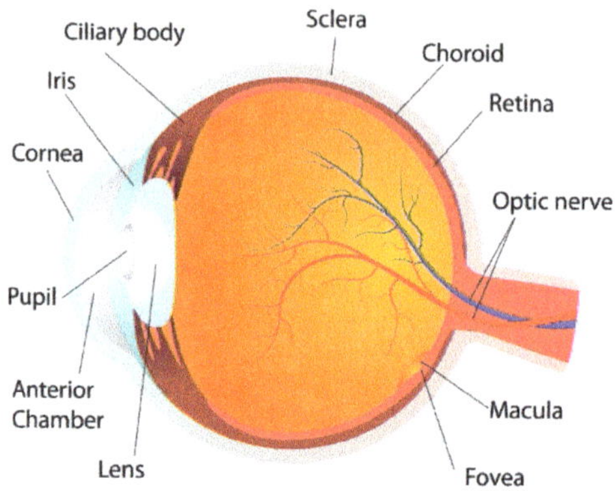

Figure 1. Geometryof human corneal model.

This evidence inspired the authors of this paper to design new computing standards for solving the CSM based on the power of artificial intelligence (AI) using neural network (NN) modeling, and hybrid cuckoo search (BHCS) as a global search algorithm.

2. Our Contribution

In view of the above literature, we propose a new methodology known as BHCS-ANN, which has the following features.

- To the best of our knowledge, this is the first study to tackle the curvature model of the eye by using the hybrid cuckoo search with the neural network.
- The proposed BHCS-ANN is applied to six different corneal geometries to show the accuracy of the method.
- The proposed BHCS-ANN is more accurate as compared to other state-of-the-art.
- Based on statistical analysis performed, BHCS-ANN outperformed other techniques.

Section 3 of this article explains the model proposed and the corresponding methodology that we chose for solution purposes. The results are described through statistical parameters presented in Section 5. The results achieved are displayed through graphs and tables in Section 6. Finally, the conclusion is provided in Section 7.

3. Mathematical Model

The description of a physical problem always asks for a mathematical relation that best describes certain parameters describing the problem. These problems are normally complex in nature, describing the nonlinear phenomenon, as shown in Figure 1. Researchers are well interested in the solution of these problems. The literature presented above shows that various semianalytical and numerical techniques are adopted for the solution of such types of problems. The proposed problem in this study is given by Equation (1). In our research, we separated our methodology into two distinct parts. First, we transformed the CSM differential equation into an optimization problem together with its boundary conditions. In the second phase, BHCS is used to minimize the mean squared error that assists ANN in determining the unknown weights in the network. This whole procedure is explained in Figures 2 and 3, which depict the abstract and the architecture of ANN for CSM.

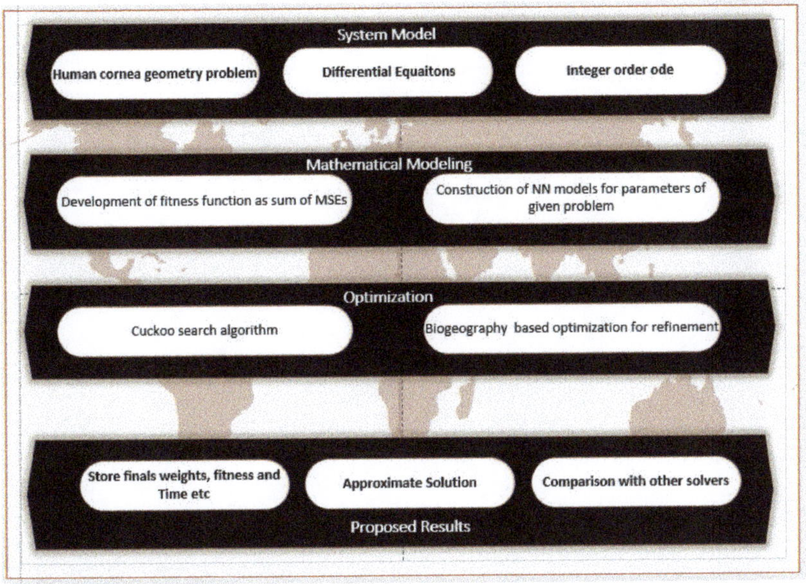

Figure 2. Graphical abstract.

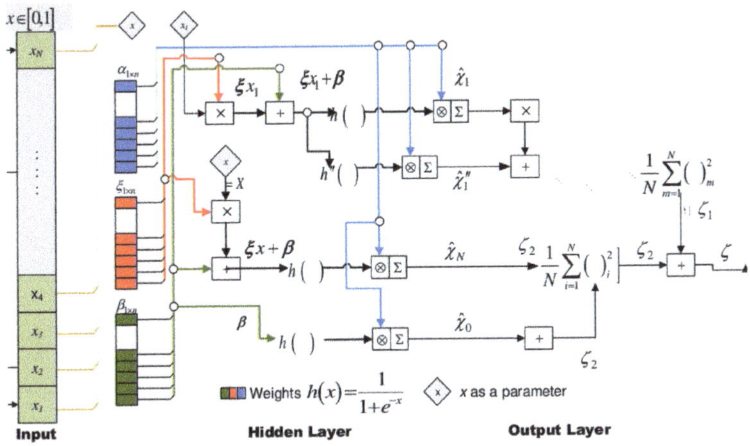

Figure 3. The neural network modeling.

Neural Network Modeling for Differential Equations

ANN is widely used for approximating the solution of differential equations [49]. The use of ANN is extended to fractional and some other nonlinear problems, as shown in the references [50,51]. We take continuous mapping by addressing the derivatives in the form of a series.

$$\hat{\psi}(t) = \sum_{i=1}^{M} \tilde{\alpha}_i \sigma(\phi_i t + \beta_i), \tag{3}$$

$$\hat{\psi}^{(m)}(t) = \sum_{i=1}^{M} \tilde{\alpha}_i \sigma^{(m)}(\phi_i t + \beta_i), \tag{4}$$

where $\hat{\psi}(t)$ is the approximate solution and ϕ, β, and $\tilde{\alpha}$ are weights. Similarly, M is the number of neurons and m is the order of the derivative. The radial basis function given by $\sigma(t) = \frac{1}{1+e^{-t}}$ is introduced into Equations (3) and (4), and we have

$$\hat{\psi}(t) = \sum_{i=1}^{M} \tilde{\alpha}_i \left(\frac{1}{1+e^{-(\phi_i t+\beta_i)}}\right), \tag{5}$$

$$\hat{\psi}^{(m)}(t) = \sum_{i=1}^{M} \tilde{\alpha}_i \frac{d^m}{dt^m} \left(\frac{1}{1+e^{-(\phi_i t+\beta_i)}}\right), \tag{6}$$

for $m = 2$, we have

$$\hat{\psi}''(t) = \sum_{j=1}^{M} \tilde{\alpha}_j \phi_j^2 \left[\frac{2e^{-2(\phi_j t+\beta_j)}}{\left(1+e^{-(\phi_j t+\beta_j)}\right)^3} - \frac{e^{-(\phi_j t+\beta_j)}}{\left(1+e^{-(\phi_j t+\beta_j)}\right)^2} \right]. \tag{7}$$

We need to reduce the L_2 error; therefore, using the above equations for constructing the optimization function as given below,

$$\epsilon = \epsilon_1 + \epsilon_2, \tag{8}$$

where the L_2 for the equations and the boundary conditions are given by ϵ_1 and ϵ_2, and are defined as under

$$\begin{aligned} &\epsilon_1 = \tfrac{1}{N} \textstyle\sum_{k=1}^{M} \left(\sqrt{1+\psi'^2(t)}\hat{\psi}_k''(t) - c\sqrt{1+\psi'^2(t)}\hat{\psi}(t) + d \right)^2, \\ &M = \tfrac{1}{h}, \quad \hat{\psi}_k = \hat{\psi}(t_k), \quad t_k = kh, \end{aligned} \tag{9}$$

$$\epsilon_2 = \frac{1}{2}\left((\hat{\psi}_0')^2 + (\hat{\psi}_M)^2 \right). \tag{10}$$

4. Proposed Algorithm

4.1. Proposed BHCS Algorithm

In this work, we use the biogeography-based heterogeneous cuckoo search (BHCS) technique that utilizes the Lévy flights' approach in search by adopting the cuckoo search (CS) algorithm. The biogeography-based approach utilizes the migration operator, which is particularly adopted in the local area, to produce new solutions.

The heterogeneous cuckoo search algorithm uses the Lévy flights approach. This technique was introduced by Ding et al. [52] and further extended by Cheung et al. [53] and is explained under

$$t_i^{\text{new}} = \left\{ \begin{array}{ll} t_i^{\text{old}} + \tilde{\alpha} \cdot (t_i - t_g) \oplus \text{Lévy}(\beta) & \frac{2}{3} < sr \le 1 \\ \bar{t} + L \cdot (\bar{t} - t_i^{\text{old}}) & \frac{1}{3} < sr \le \frac{2}{3} \\ t_i^{\text{old}} + \varepsilon \cdot (t_g - t_i^{\text{old}}) & \text{else,} \end{array} \right\} \tag{11}$$

Here, the $\varepsilon = \delta e^{\eta}, L = \delta \ln(1/\eta), t_g$ represents the best solution in the present version; $\bar{t} = \frac{1}{MP}\sum_{i=1}^{MP} t_i$ symbolizes the mean of all options. As random numbers in the range $[0,1]$, η, and sr, $\tilde{\alpha}$ is a constant. Equation (11) shows that three distinct updating equations with equal probabilities are used in heterogeneous BHCS. The Lévy flight serves as the foundation for the first update equation in the original CS. The second and third updating equations, on the other hand, are based on the quantum mechanism. Using inhomogeneous updating limitations can generate multiple possibilities for expanding the flying and search toward the actual global region in an optimistic manner.

4.2. Biogeography-Based Revelation Operator

The second phase of BHCS shows an impact of changing the search operator for the development of unique solutions.

A biogeography-based migration operator enables the host bird to recognize alien eggs with a high degree of certainty, abandon old nests, and produce new nests. Following that, the population is ranked from best to worst, and emigration rates are ascribed to each response. Here, emigration rates μ are defined as

$$\mu_i = E\frac{S_i}{MP}. \tag{12}$$

In the above equation, the maximum emigration rate is $E = 1$ and the number of species in the solution is $S_i = MPI$. The first algorithm describes the biogeography-based operator for discovering the ith solution. Solutions with higher fitness might share more characteristics with other solutions in the biogeography-based discovery operator, which is beneficial for exploitation enhancement.

5. Statistical Evaluation

This section will introduce some statistical concepts and formulas for explaining the performance and other graphical explanations. Some of the well-known concepts are the mean absolute deviation (*MAD*), global mean absolute deviation (*GMAD*), *GFIT*, *TIC*, *ENSE*, and *GENSE*. In this study, the *TIC*, *ENSE*, and *MAD* performance matrices are considered for each CSM scenario. In addition, we conducted a statistical analysis of our findings by employing minimum, mean, and standard deviation. To demonstrate the robustness of our methodology, 100 separate runs are conducted to estimate the performance of *GFIT* , *GMAD* , *GTIC* , and *GENSE* .

$$\text{MAD} = \frac{1}{l}\sum_{m=1}^{l}|\psi(t_m) - \widehat{\psi}(t_m)| \tag{13}$$

$$\text{TIC} = \frac{\sqrt{\frac{1}{l}\sum_{m=1}^{l}\left(\psi(t_m) - \widehat{\psi}(t_m)\right)^2}}{\sqrt{\frac{1}{l}\sum_{m=1}^{l}(\widehat{\psi}(t_m))^2} + \sqrt{\frac{1}{l}\sum_{m=1}^{l}(\widehat{\psi}(t_m))^2}} \tag{14}$$

$$\text{NSE} = \left\{1 - \frac{\sum_{m=1}^{l}\left(\psi(t_m) - \widehat{\psi}(t_m)\right)^2}{\sum_{m=1}^{l}\left(\psi(t_m) - \bar{\psi}(t_m)\right)^2}, \right. \tag{15}$$

$$\bar{\psi}(t_m) = \frac{1}{l}\sum_{m=1}^{l}\psi(t_m)$$

$$\text{E}_{\text{NSE}} = 1 - \text{NSE} \tag{16}$$

$$GMAD = \frac{1}{R}\sum_{r=1}^{R}\left(\frac{1}{m}\sum_{i=1}^{m}(|\psi(t_i) - \hat{\psi}(t_i)|)\right) \tag{17}$$

$$GFIT = \frac{1}{R}\sum_{r=1}^{R}e_r \tag{18}$$

$$GENSE = \frac{1}{R}\sum_{r=1}^{R}\left(\sqrt{\frac{1}{m}\sum_{i=1}^{m}(\psi(t_i) - \hat{\psi}(t_i))^2}\right) \tag{19}$$

TIC, MAD, and ENSE values approach zero for the best approximation solution that is close to the exact answer.

6. Results and Discussions

The section is devoted to the analysis of the results obtained for varying parameters c and d in Equation (2). We present this analysis by considering six different cases:

Case 1: Taking $c = d = 0.1$, we have, from Equation (2),

$$\begin{aligned} \psi''(t) - 0.1\psi(t) + \frac{0.1}{\sqrt{1+\psi'^2(t)}} &= 0, \\ \psi'(0) = \psi(1) = 0, \ \ t &\in [0,1]. \end{aligned} \tag{20}$$

The corresponding objective function takes the form

$$\begin{aligned} \zeta = \tfrac{1}{M}\textstyle\sum_{k=1}^{M}\big(\sqrt{1+\psi'^2(t_k)}\hat{\psi}''(t_k) - 0.1\sqrt{1+\psi'^2(t_k)}\psi(\hat{t}_k) + 0.1\big)^2 \\ +\tfrac{1}{2}\Big(\big(\hat{\psi}'_0\big)^2 + \big(\hat{\psi}_M\big)^2\Big). \end{aligned} \tag{21}$$

Similarly, the remaining cases are given below:

Case 2: $d = 0.1, c = 0.2$.

Case 3: $d = 0.1, c = 0.3$.

Case 4: $d = 0.2, c = 0.1$.

Case 5: $d = 0.3, c = 0.1$.

Case 6: $d = 0.4, c = 0.1$.

The results for each case considered above are presented in Figure 4 for the state variable ψ. The solution in each case is compared with the exact. The approximate solution and the exact solution comparison show that the proposed methodology has a high level of accuracy. In case 1, the solution curve drops down from 0.05 to 0 on the unit time interval. A quite similar trend can be observed in cases 2 and 3. The remaining cases 4, 5, and 6 are starting from different points of the state variables 0.099, 0.14, and 0.189, respectively. The trend of the approximate and the exact solution remains the same. From the analysis shown in case 5, we see that the radius of the cornea, and intramuscular pressure of the eye ($c = 0.1$, and $d = 0.3$) have the global minimal value 0.14 at $t = 0$ of the corneal curvature. The numerical results for all these cases are presented in the form of Tables 1 and 2. In the tables, the minimum values of the objective functions are compared with the standard deviation and the mean values for each scenario. The standard deviation shows a deviation of 10^{-9}, 10^{-10}, and 10^{-10} for cases 1, 2, and 3, respectively. The remaining cases 4, 5, and 6 have the same standard deviations up 10^{-7}. The minimum values of the state variable vary from 10^{-9} to 10^{-15}, which is a very small quantity. This reduction is possible only due to the applied BHCS that minimizes the L_2-error.

In Figure 5, the weight plots of the neural network are presented. In case 1, there are 9 neurons and 3 weight functions that range up to 4 in the third weight. In case 2, the number of neurons is 10, with the same number of weight functions that range up to 2. In cases 3 and 4 there are 7 neurons and three weight functions that are up to 4 and 2, respectively. Also, cases 5 and 6 have the same scenario but their ranges are different. These weights are chosen directly by the neural network for searching the best possible outcome for the objective function.

The absolute error in each case has been provided in Figure 6. The absolute errors in all six cases are very small and even vary up to 10^{-10}; for example, see case 4. In all six cases, the absolute error is computed at the grid points. The error in each case shows the accuracy of our implemented technique and its convergence.

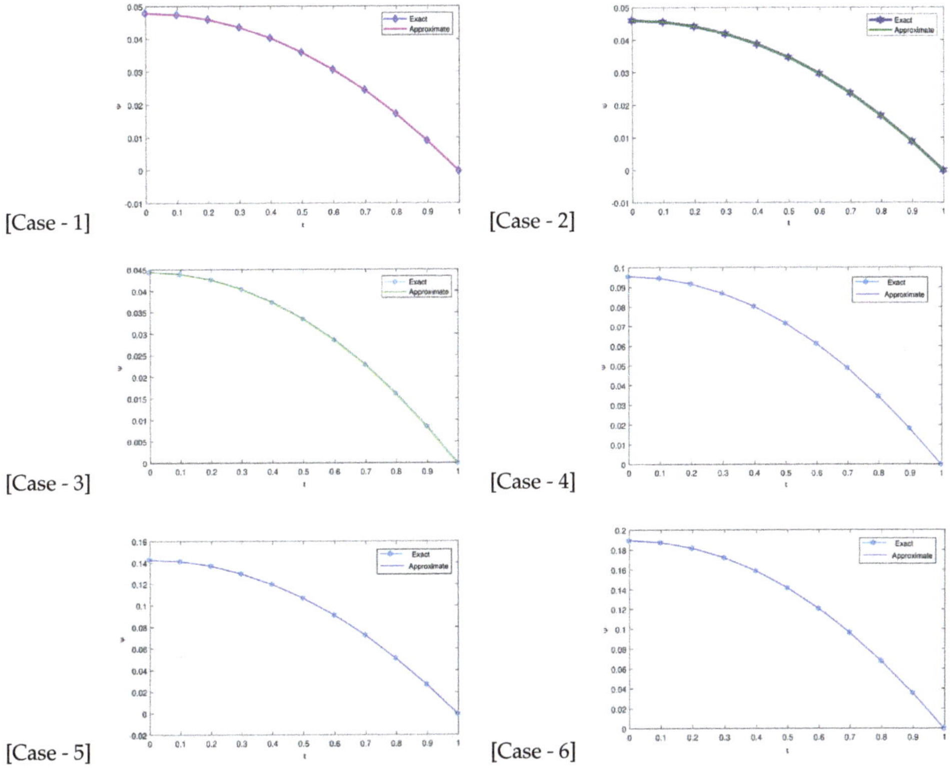

Figure 4. Solution plots for various cases.

The fitness function, MAD, TIC, and ENSE are all displayed in Figure 7 for all the cases. The fitness function minimum values in all the cases approach 10^{-11}, while the worst of all the cases approach 10^{-4}. The mean of all the values for the fitness function is also displayed through bar graphs. The mean is also observed to approach 10^{-6}. The statistical analysis of the present results is also presented through bar graphs. The minimal results for the MAD remain below 10^{-6}, while the mean values almost approach these points. In MAD, the worst cases are not too far from the mean and remain very near it. The bars of TIC and ENSE approach 10^{-6} and 10^{-7} in some cases, respectively. In the case of 4, these variations are very large, where the minimal values for ENSE approach 10^{-9}. All this analysis shows that the fitness function, MAD, TIC, and ENSE are stable at various iterations and the range in each case shows the total performance of the computational process.

The fitness function is plotted with a bar graph by using the normal distribution, as shown in Figure 8 for each case. The number of independent runs is plotted on the $y-$axis, while the fitness is shown on the $x-$axis. In case 1, the values remain greater than zero and below 0.25×10^{-5}. A maximum of the values remain inside the middle of the bill shape. A quite similar trend can be seen in the case of 5. In case 2, the fitness function has variations up to 10^{-6}, and the data remain inside the uniform distribution. In cases 3 and 4 again, the date remains inside the uniform bill and the variation extends up to 10^{-4} and 10^{-5}, respectively. In the last case 6, all the values are contained in the uniform bill, while the fitness function varies up to 10^{-4}.

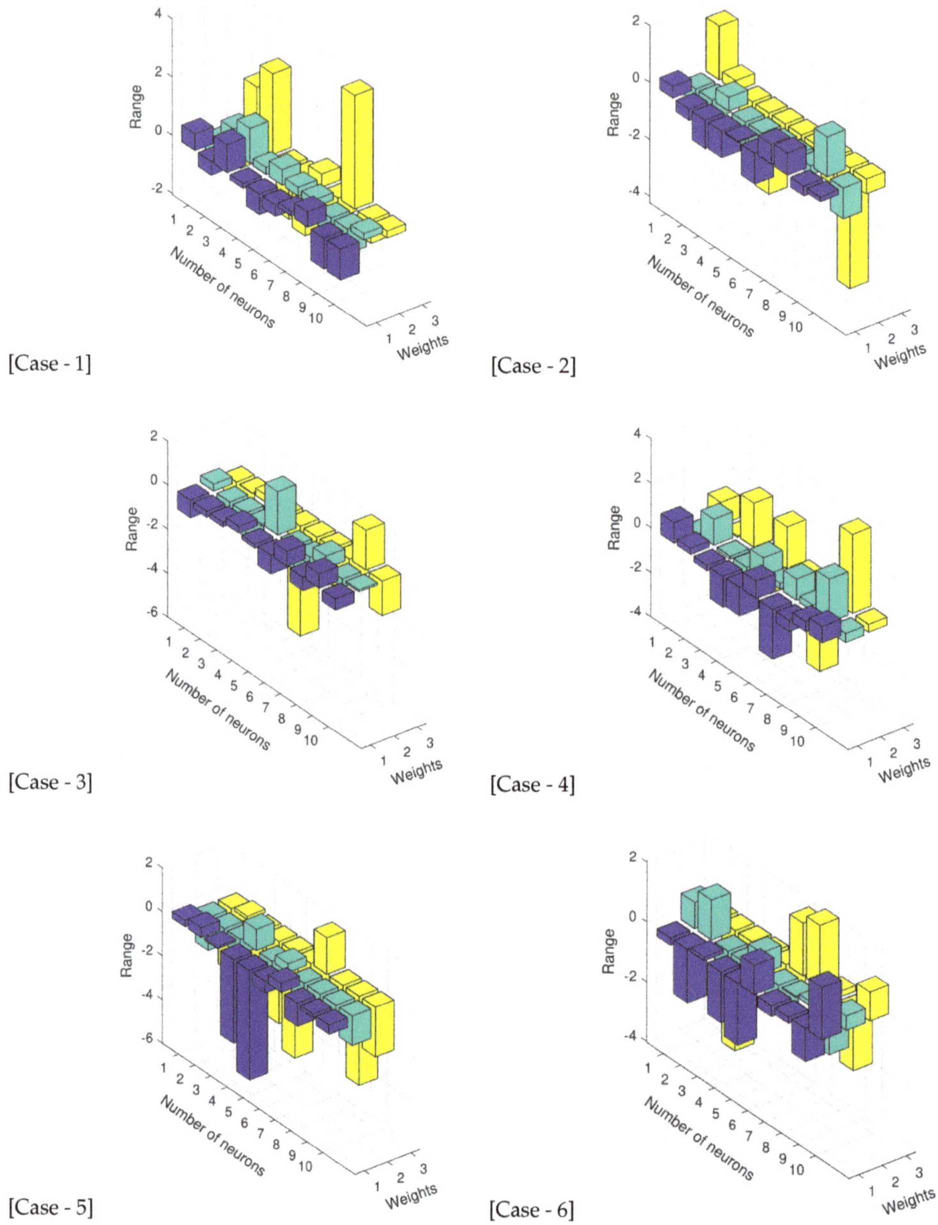

Figure 5. Weights plot for various cases.

The normal plots for MAD, TIC, and ENSE are presented in Figures 9–11. All six cases are comprehensively discussed against the number of runs. The results for MAD vary up to 10^{-5} for cases 1, 2, 4, and 5, respectively. The results for MAD remain inside the uniform distribution for all the cases and approach the midpoint. The results for cases 3 and 6 remain inside the range 10^{-4}. The TIC and ENSE plots are shown in Figures 10 and 11. The results for TIC remain inside the unit bill and approach 10^{-5} in cases 2, 4, and 5 respectively. Similarly, the results for cases 1 and 6 are bounded in 10^{-4}, while for the remaining case 3, it lies in 10^{-3}. The normal plots describing the bill shape distribution of the data for the ENSE show a variation up to 10^{-5} for cases 1, 2, 4, and 6. In case 3, this variation is 10^{-3}, while in case 5 it is 10^{-6}.

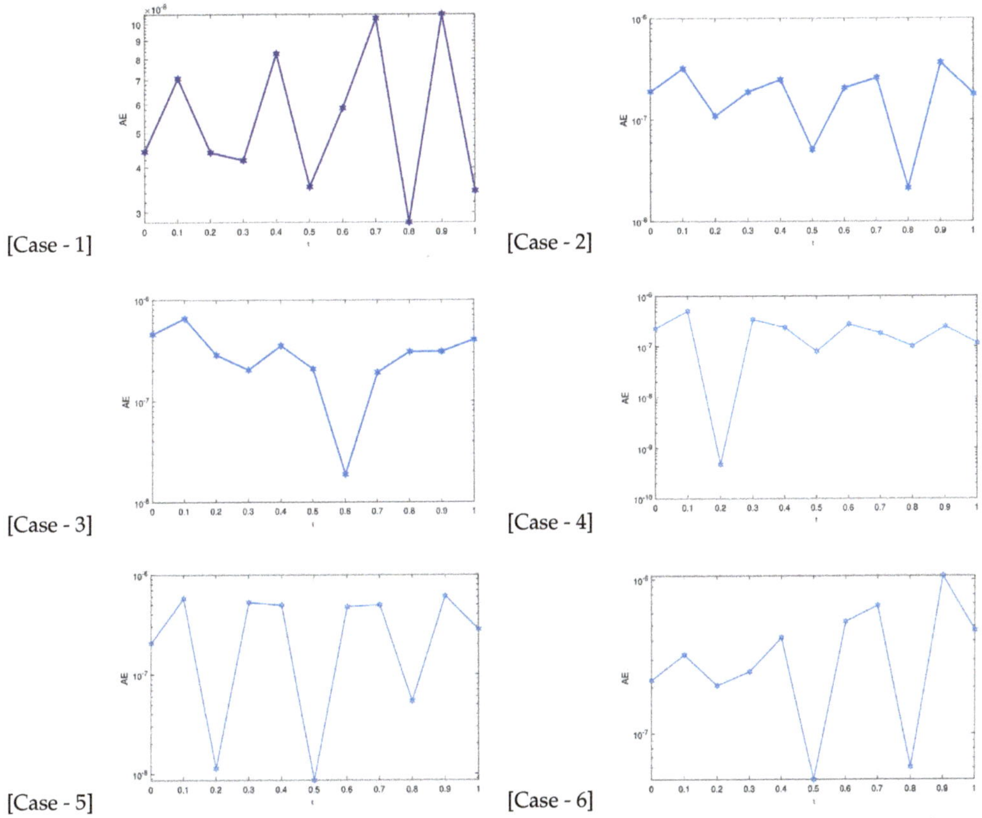

Figure 6. Absolute error obtained for various case studies.

Table 1. The statistical findings for every instance of the corneal shape model.

	Case 1			Case 2			Case 3		
t	Min	Mean	STD	Min	Mean	STD	Min	Mean	STD
0.0	4.04×10^{-12}	1.79×10^{-9}	1.08×10^{-8}	3.88×10^{-13}	1.29×10^{-9}	1.22×10^{-9}	2.09×10^{-14}	5.21×10^{-10}	1.11×10^{-9}
0.1	1.03×10^{-11}	6.19×10^{-10}	1.59×10^{-9}	1.09×10^{-12}	5.10×10^{-10}	1.19×10^{-9}	5.51×10^{-14}	6.79×10^{-10}	5.58×10^{-9}
0.2	1.18×10^{-13}	1.19×10^{-9}	6.11×10^{-9}	1.28×10^{-13}	5.89×10^{-10}	1.09×10^{-9}	2.09×10^{-14}	5.79×10^{-10}	1.81×10^{-9}
0.3	2.08×10^{-12}	1.78×10^{-9}	1.67×10^{-8}	3.91×10^{-13}	6.11×10^{-11}	1.32×10^{-10}	1.10×10^{-14}	2.49×10^{-10}	1.67×10^{-9}
0.4	7.19×10^{-13}	2.78×10^{-9}	2.51×10^{-8}	6.67×10^{-13}	2.79×10^{-10}	6.31×10^{-10}	7.49×10^{-14}	2.31×10^{-10}	4.38×10^{-10}
0.5	1.44×10^{-13}	3.14×10^{-9}	2.36×10^{-8}	2.91×10^{-14}	5.73×10^{-10}	1.11×10^{-9}	1.41×10^{-14}	5.92×10^{-10}	2.52×10^{-9}
0.6	4.93×10^{-13}	1.84×10^{-9}	1.38×10^{-8}	4.71×10^{-13}	2.48×10^{-10}	3.85×10^{-10}	3.81×10^{-14}	2.82×10^{-10}	1.08×10^{-9}
0.7	4.19×10^{-14}	3.68×10^{-10}	2.73×10^{-9}	7.29×10^{-13}	7.17×10^{-11}	1.37×10^{-10}	1.21×10^{-13}	1.61×10^{-10}	8.11×10^{-10}
0.8	3.17×10^{-14}	1.21×10^{-9}	3.10×10^{-9}	5.00×10^{-15}	6.72×10^{-10}	1.19×10^{-9}	8.68×10^{-15}	7.10×10^{-10}	3.38×10^{-9}
0.9	5.76×10^{-15}	5.29×10^{-9}	4.73×10^{-8}	1.52×10^{-12}	5.67×10^{-10}	8.68×10^{-10}	1.30×10^{-13}	4.87×10^{-10}	1.78×10^{-9}
1	2.10×10^{-15}	1.87×10^{-8}	1.77×10^{-7}	3.48×10^{-13}	7.11×10^{-10}	1.42×10^{-9}	1.26×10^{-14}	1.13×10^{-9}	4.52×10^{-9}

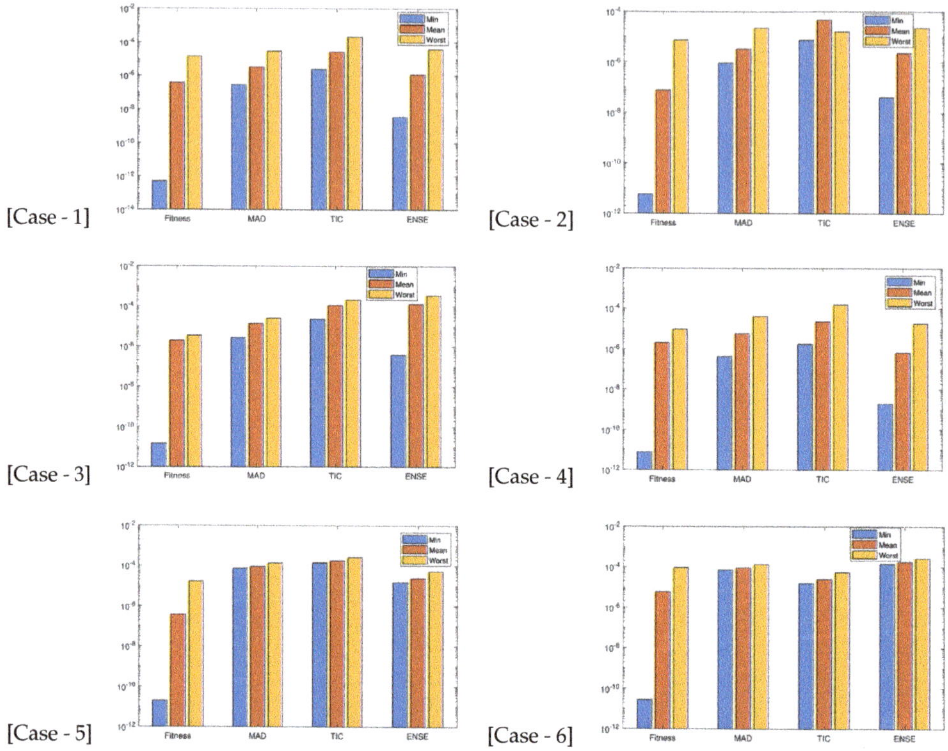

Figure 7. Various cases for best, worst, and mean.

Table 2. The statistical findings for every instance of the corneal shape model.

	Case 4			Case 5			Case 6		
t	**Min**	**Mean**	**STD**	**Min**	**Mean**	**STD**	**Min**	**Mean**	**STD**
0.0	4.38×10^{-10}	2.31×10^{-7}	5.42×10^{-7}	1.18×10^{-10}	2.76×10^{-7}	2.51×10^{-6}	7.58×10^{-10}	1.10×10^{-7}	4.87×10^{-7}
0.1	1.11×10^{-9}	2.43×10^{-7}	4.17×10^{-7}	7.68×10^{-11}	6.28×10^{-10}	7.52×10^{-7}	8.78×10^{-10}	1.41×10^{-7}	3.69×10^{-7}
0.2	8.43×10^{-11}	1.59×10^{-7}	3.37×10^{-7}	9.67×10^{-11}	3.68×10^{-7}	3.47×10^{-7}	6.58×10^{-10}	1.09×10^{-7}	2.58×10^{-7}
0.3	1.99×10^{-9}	1.12×10^{-7}	2.25×10^{-7}	7.71×10^{-13}	1.08×10^{-7}	3.35×10^{-7}	1.34×10^{-12}	1.11×10^{-7}	2.67×10^{-7}
0.4	2.36×10^{-9}	1.64×10^{-7}	2.75×10^{-7}	7.18×10^{-11}	9.23×10^{-8}	5.77×10^{-7}	3.53×10^{-10}	1.00×10^{-7}	2.37×10^{-7}
0.5	4.59×10^{-10}	1.52×10^{-7}	2.53×10^{-7}	1.72×10^{-10}	2.81×10^{-7}	7.58×10^{-7}	5.12×10^{-10}	1.00×10^{-7}	2.41×10^{-7}
0.6	4.69×10^{-10}	9.18×10^{-8}	1.72×10^{-7}	1.62×10^{-10}	1.98×10^{-7}	7.18×10^{-7}	1.32×10^{-7}	7.34×10^{-8}	1.81×10^{-7}
0.7	3.34×10^{-9}	1.38×10^{-7}	2.88×10^{-7}	1.09×10^{-10}	3.84×10^{-7}	6.41×10^{-7}	3.19×10^{-11}	1.41×10^{-7}	2.10×10^{-7}
0.8	4.12×10^{-9}	3.04×10^{-7}	4.13×10^{-7}	7.11×10^{-11}	3.00×10^{-7}	5.69×10^{-7}	2.87×10^{-10}	2.32×10^{-7}	5.06×10^{-7}
0.9	6.45×10^{-10}	1.59×10^{-7}	2.09×10^{-7}	1.41×10^{-12}	4.91×10^{-7}	2.39×10^{-7}	1.62×10^{-10}	7.31×10^{-8}	1.69×10^{-7}
1	4.57×10^{-9}	4.79×10^{-7}	7.69×10^{-7}	7.09×10^{-10}	4.38×10^{-7}	2.08×10^{-6}	1.43×10^{-10}	4.81×10^{-7}	1.11×10^{-6}

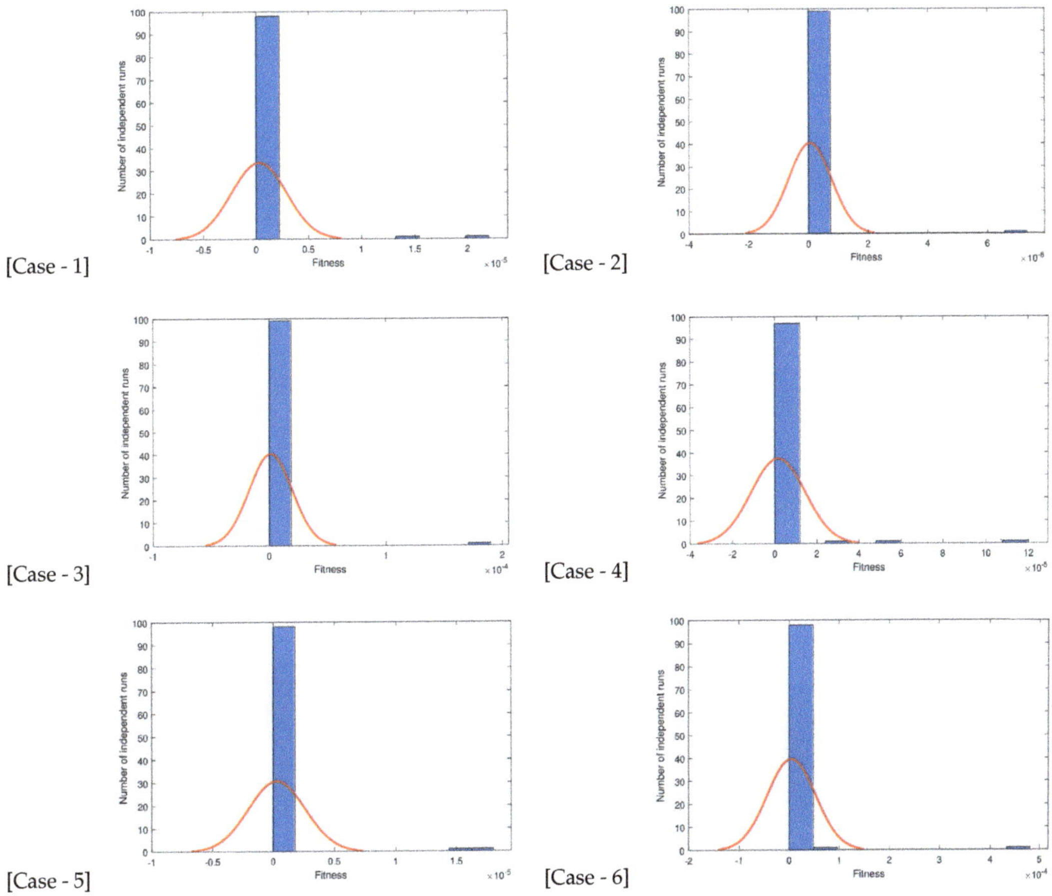

Figure 8. Normal plot of fitness function for different cases.

The fitness function minimum, mean, and standard deviation values for each are presented in Table 1. All these variations are shown for a step size of 0.1. In case 1, the minimum value for the fitness function is 2.10×10^{-15}, while the standard deviation remains up to 1.59×10^{-9}. In case 2, the minimum value is 5.00×10^{-15}, while the standard deviation touches 1.32×10^{-10}. Similarly, in cases 3–6, the minimum values of the fitness functions are 8.68×10^{-15}, 8.43×10^{-11}, 7.71×10^{-13}, and 1.34×10^{-12}, respectively. The standard deviations for all these cases touch 10^{-10} and 10^{-7}.

The global performances of TIC, MAD, FIT, and ENSE are shown in Table 3. The minimum value of GTIC exists in the case of 6, which is 2.38×10^{-5}, These values for GMAD, GFIT, and GENSE are 3.19×10^{-6}, 2.38×10^{-5}, 7.69×10^{-8}, and 6.71×10^{-7}. All these show the mean of the minimum values. The corresponding standard deviation for each case is plotted to check the stability.

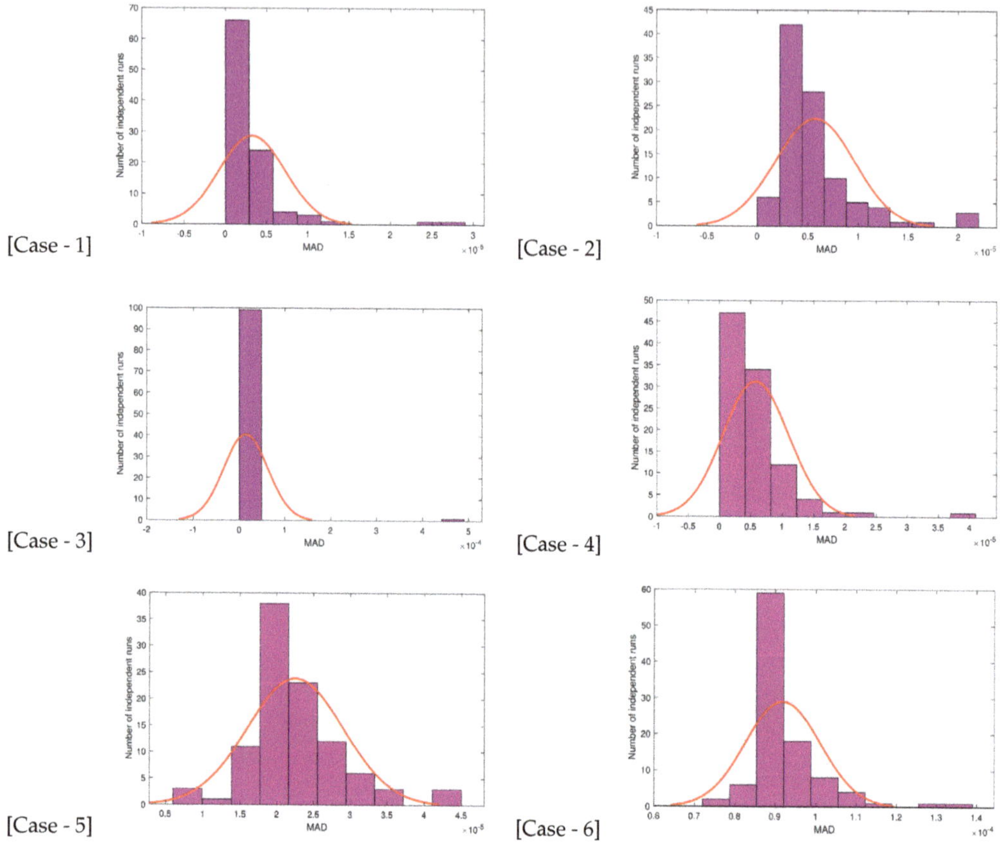

Figure 9. Normal plots of MAD for different cases.

Table 3. Corneal shape model's global performance indices and their respective results.

Case	GTIC		GMAD		GFIT		GENSE	
	Mean	**STD**	**Mean**	**STD**	**Mean**	**STD**	**Mean**	**STD**
1	2.63×10^{-5}	2.00×10^{-5}	3.19×10^{-6}	2.92×10^{-5}	3.68×10^{-7}	1.45×10^{-5}	1.17×10^{-6}	3.71×10^{-5}
2	4.59×10^{-5}	1.58×10^{-5}	3.19×10^{-6}	2.21×10^{-5}	7.69×10^{-8}	7.19×10^{-6}	2.30×10^{-6}	2.31×10^{-5}
3	1.20×10^{-4}	2.09×10^{-4}	1.39×10^{-5}	2.58×10^{-5}	1.88×10^{-6}	3.37×10^{-6}	1.31×10^{-4}	3.48×10^{-4}
4	2.24×10^{-5}	1.48×10^{-4}	5.68×10^{-6}	4.11×10^{-5}	2.02×10^{-6}	9.41×10^{-6}	6.71×10^{-7}	1.84×10^{-5}
5	1.81×10^{-4}	2.59×10^{-4}	9.16×10^{-5}	1.29×10^{-4}	3.62×10^{-7}	1.73×10^{-5}	2.39×10^{-5}	5.38×10^{-5}
6	2.38×10^{-5}	5.39×10^{-5}	9.18×10^{-5}	1.29×10^{-4}	5.68×10^{-6}	9.60×10^{-5}	1.81×10^{-4}	2.59×10^{-4}

The execution time and the number of executed functions are presented in Table 4. For validity, the standard deviation is also presented. A total of 200,010 functions for each case were computed with a minimal mean time of 17.7791 for case 1. The generation means remains 2000 in all the cases.

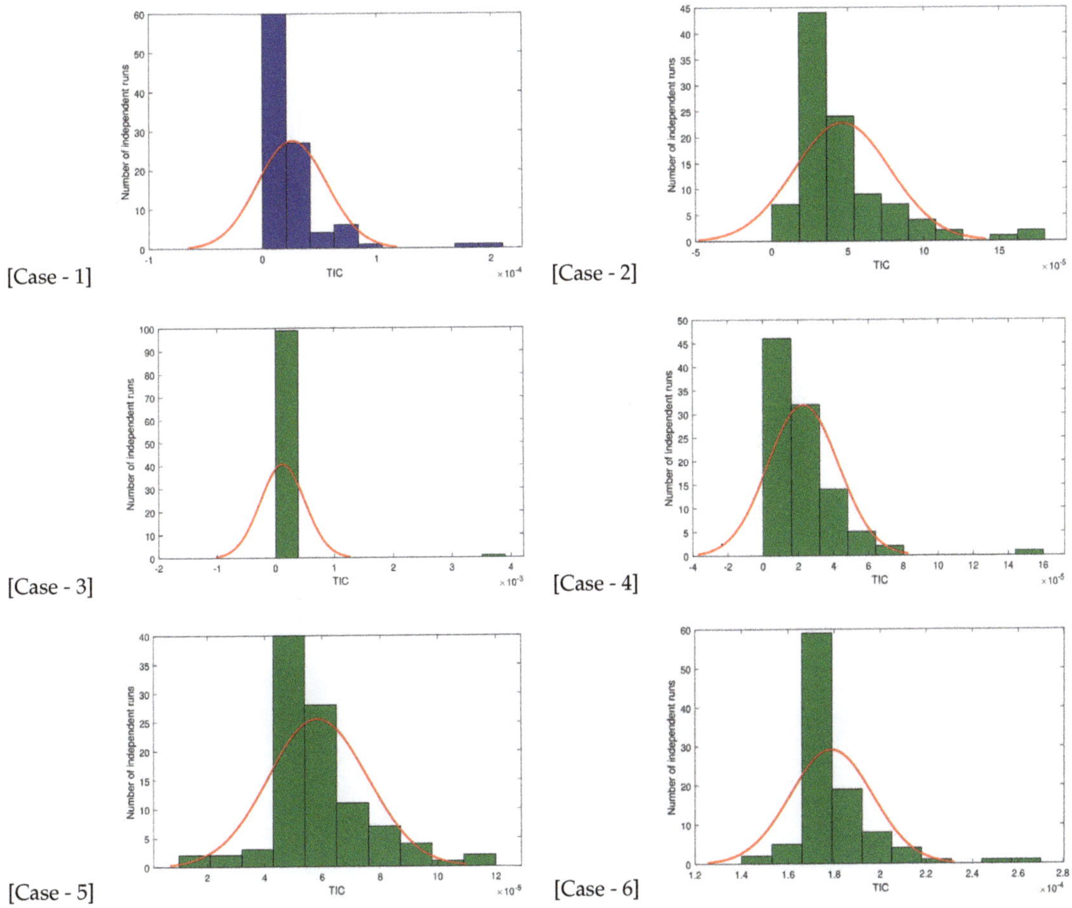

Figure 10. Normal plots of TIC for different cases .

Table 4. Complexity analysis for each corneal shape model case.

Case	Execution Time		Generation		Function Counts	
	Mean	STD	Mean	STD	Mean	STD
1	17.7791	3.0599	2000	0	200,010	0
2	27.5776	2.9333	2000	0	200,010	0
3	27.1637	2.448	2000	0	200,010	0
4	27.421	3.0261	2000	0	200,010	0
5	26.8823	3.2615	2000	0	200,010	0
6	27.0509	3.888	2000	0	200,010	0

The proposed BHCS-ANN has better performance as compared to the available results of FO-DPSO presented by Waseem et al. [54]. In their work, they compared their results with the PSO-ASA. In this study, the BHCS-ASA results are compared with FO-DPSO in Tables 5 and 6. In each case, our results are better than the available literature that proves the performance of our implemented method.

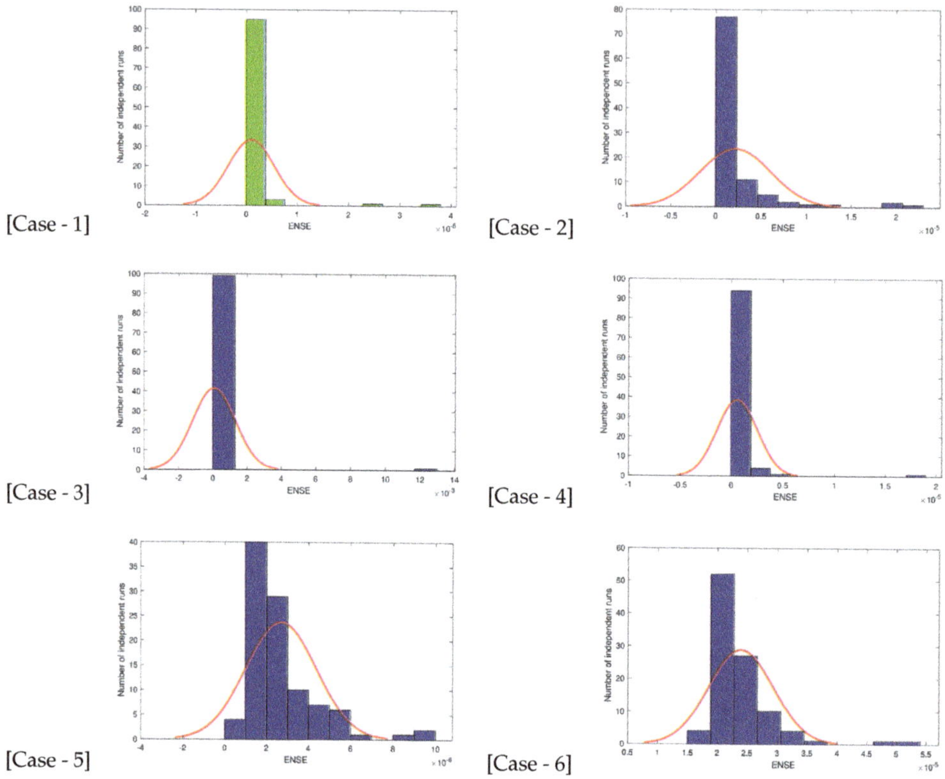

Figure 11. Normal plots of ENSE for different cases.

Table 5. Comparison of the min. values for the approximate function in different cases.

	Min Case 1		**Min Case 2**		**Min Case 3**	
t	**BHCS-ANN**	**FO-DPSO [54]**	**BHCS-ANN**	**FO-DPSO [54]**	**BHCS-ANN**	**FO-DPSO [54]**
0	4.04×10^{-12}	1.04×10^{-11}	3.88×10^{-13}	1.74×10^{-11}	2.09×10^{-14}	7.26×10^{-11}
0.1	1.03×10^{-11}	1.03×10^{-11}	1.09×10^{-12}	1.21×10^{-10}	5.51×10^{-14}	6.02×10^{-11}
0.2	1.18×10^{-13}	8.26×10^{-12}	1.28×10^{-13}	3.58×10^{-12}	2.09×10^{-14}	5.55×10^{-11}
0.3	2.08×10^{-12}	9.73×10^{-14}	3.91×10^{-13}	7.32×10^{-11}	1.10×10^{-14}	5.75×10^{-12}
0.4	7.19×10^{-13}	3.18×10^{-12}	6.67×10^{-13}	1.52×10^{-11}	7.49×10^{-14}	6.87×10^{-13}
0.5	1.44×10^{-13}	5.28×10^{-12}	2.91×10^{-14}	1.65×10^{-11}	1.41×10^{-14}	3.81×10^{-13}
0.6	4.93×10^{-13}	1.62×10^{-12}	4.71×10^{-13}	4.76×10^{-11}	3.81×10^{-14}	6.81×10^{-13}
0.7	4.19×10^{-14}	2.66×10^{-13}	7.29×10^{-13}	6.16×10^{-12}	1.21×10^{-13}	6.60×10^{-14}
0.8	3.17×10^{-14}	3.68×10^{-12}	5.00×10^{-15}	1.96×10^{-11}	8.68×10^{-15}	3.00×10^{-11}
0.9	5.76×10^{-15}	7.29×10^{-13}	1.52×10^{-12}	3.33×10^{-11}	1.30×10^{-13}	8.11×10^{-11}
1	2.10×10^{-15}	2.84×10^{-12}	3.48×10^{-13}	1.94×10^{-11}	1.26×10^{-14}	8.89×10^{-11}

Table 6. Comparison of the min. values for the approximate function in different cases.

t	Min Case 4		Min Case 5		Min Case 6	
	BHCS-ANN	**FO-DPSO [54]**	**BHCS-ANN**	**FO-DPSO [54]**	**BHCS-ANN**	**FO-DPSO [54]**
0	4.38×10^{-10}	7.61×10^{-10}	1.18×10^{-10}	1.21×10^{-10}	7.58×10^{-10}	4.40×10^{-10}
0.1	1.11×10^{-9}	8.83×10^{-10}	7.68×10^{-11}	7.74×10^{-11}	8.78×10^{-10}	1.06×10^{-9}
0.2	8.43×10^{-11}	6.64×10^{-10}	9.67×10^{-11}	9.70×10^{-11}	6.58×10^{-10}	8.38×10^{-11}
0.3	1.99×10^{-9}	1.26×10^{-12}	7.71×10^{-13}	7.66×10^{-13}	1.34×10^{-12}	2.00×10^{-9}
0.4	2.36×10^{-9}	3.49×10^{-10}	7.18×10^{-11}	7.23×10^{-11}	3.53×10^{-10}	2.40×10^{-9}
0.5	4.59×10^{-10}	5.09×10^{-10}	1.72×10^{-10}	1.68×10^{-10}	5.12×10^{-10}	4.62×10^{-10}
0.6	4.69×10^{-10}	1.32×10^{-10}	1.62×10^{-10}	1.59×10^{-10}	1.32×10^{-7}	4.72×10^{-10}
0.7	3.34×10^{-9}	3.23×10^{-11}	1.09×10^{-10}	1.12×10^{-10}	3.19×10^{-11}	3.35×10^{-9}
0.8	4.12×10^{-9}	2.94×10^{-10}	7.11×10^{-11}	7.08×10^{-11}	2.87×10^{-10}	4.18×10^{-9}
0.9	6.45×10^{-10}	1.64×10^{-10}	1.41×10^{-12}	1.36×10^{-12}	1.62×10^{-10}	6.54×10^{-10}
1	4.57×10^{-9}	1.45×10^{-10}	7.09×10^{-10}	7.11×10^{-10}	1.43×10^{-10}	4.60×10^{-9}

7. Conclusions

In this work, the BHCS-based neural network is applied for the first time to the CS model. The results are presented in the form of figures and tables, where Adam's method is taken as a reference method. We observed the following on the basis of our analysis.

- This approach effectively minimized the fitness function and provided the best approximation of the solution to the problem.
- The proposed approach demonstrated efficacy in all CSM scenarios and identified the optimum approximation for the CSM geometry in all scenarios.
- In figures, the results were compared with Adam's numerical solution, where the BHCS-ANN showed a better trend.
- The statistical evaluations such as MAD, TIC, and ENSE were evaluated in 100 different runs, and the results showed that the proposed approach outperformed the current state of the art.
- The obtained results for the minimum approximated functions were compared with the FO-DPSO algorithm, where BHCS-ANN performed better in all the cases.

Author Contributions: Conceptualization, W. and A.U.; methodology, A.U. and F.A.A.; software, A.U. and W.; validation, E.A.A.I., A.U. and W.; formal analysis, A.U. and W.; investigation, A.U. and E.A.A.I.; resources, W. and A.U.; data curation, F.A.A. and A.U.; writing—original draft preparation, A.U., E.A.A.I. and F.A.A.; visualization, A.U., W. and F.A.A.; supervision, A.U. and W. All authors have read and agreed to the published version of the manuscript.

Funding: Researchers Supporting Project number (RSPD2023R1060), King Saud University, Riyadh, Saudi Arabia.

Data Availability Statement: No data are used in this study.

Acknowledgments: Researchers Supporting Project number (RSPD2023R1060), King Saud University, Riyadh, Saudi Arabia.

Conflicts of Interest: The authors declare no conflict of interest.

References

1. Corsato, C.; De Coster, C.; Omari, P. The Dirichlet problem for a prescribed anisotropic mean curvature equation: Existence, uniqueness and regularity of solutions. *J. Differ. Equ.* **2016**, *260*, 4572–4618. [CrossRef]
2. Okrasiński, W.; Płociniczak, Ł. A nonlinear mathematical model of the corneal shape. *Nonlinear Anal. Real World Appl.* **2012**, *13*, 1498–1505. [CrossRef]
3. Coelho, I.; Corsato, C.; Omari, P. A one-dimensional prescribed curvature equation modeling the corneal shape. *Bound. Value Probl.* **2014**, *2014*, 127. [CrossRef]
4. Komai, Y.; Ushiki, T. The three-dimensional organization of collagen fibrils in the human cornea and sclera. *Investig. Ophthalmol. Vis. Sci.* **1991**, *32*, 2244–2258.
5. Peh, G.S.; Beuerman, R.W.; Colman, A.; Tan, D.T.; Mehta, J.S. Human corneal endothelial cell expansion for corneal endothelium transplantation: An overview. *Transplantation* **2011**, *91*, 811–819. [CrossRef] [PubMed]

6. Almubrad, T.; Akhtar, S. Structure of corneal layers, collagen fibrils, and proteoglycans of tree shrew cornea. *Mol. Vis.* **2011**, *17*, 2283.
7. Płociniczak, Ł.; Okrasiński, W.; Nieto, J.J.; Dominguez, O. On a nonlinear boundary value problem modeling corneal shape. *J. Math. Anal. Appl.* **2014**, *414*, 461–471. [CrossRef]
8. He, J.H. A remark on "A nonlinear mathematical model of the corneal shape". *Nonlinear Anal. Real World Appl.* **2012**, *13*, 2863–2865. [CrossRef]
9. Chen, C.L.; Liu, Y. Solution of two-point boundary-value problems using the differential transformation method. *J. Optim. Theory Appl.* **1998**, *99*, 23. [CrossRef]
10. Abukhaled, M.; Khuri, S.; Sayfy, A. A numerical approach for solving a class of singular boundary value problems arising in physiology. *Int. J. Numer. Anal. Model.* **2011**, *8*, 353–363.
11. Lu, J. Variational iteration method for solving two-point boundary value problems. *J. Comput. Appl. Math.* **2007**, *207*, 92–95. [CrossRef]
12. Malekzadeh, P.; Golbahar Haghighi, M.; Atashi, M. Free vibration analysis of elastically supported functionally graded annular plates subjected to thermal environment. *Meccanica* **2011**, *46*, 893–913. [CrossRef]
13. Płociniczak, Ł.; Griffiths, G.W.; Schiesser, W.E. ODE/PDE analysis of corneal curvature. *Comput. Biol. Med.* **2014**, *53*, 30–41. [CrossRef] [PubMed]
14. Griffiths, G.W.; Płociniczak, Ł.; Schiesser, W. Analysis of cornea curvature using radial basis functions–Part I: Methodology. *Comput. Biol. Med.* **2016**, *77*, 274–284. [CrossRef]
15. Abukhaled, M.; Khuri, S. A semi-analytical solution of amperometric enzymatic reactions based on Green's functions and fixed point iterative schemes. *J. Electroanal. Chem.* **2017**, *792*, 66–71. [CrossRef]
16. Abukhaled, M. Green's function iterative method for solving a class of boundary value problems arising in heat transfer. *Appl. Math. Inf. Sci* **2017**, *11*, 229–234. [CrossRef]
17. Kafri, H.; Khuri, S.A. Bratu's problem: A novel approach using fixed-point iterations and Green's functions. *Comput. Phys. Commun* **2016**, *198*, 97–104. [CrossRef]
18. Żur, K. Green's function approach to frequency analysis of thin circular plates. *Bull. Pol. Acad. Sciences. Tech. Sci.* **2016**, *64*. [CrossRef]
19. Żur, K.K. Free vibration analysis of elastically supported functionally graded annular plates via quasi-Green's function method. *Compos. Part B Eng.* **2018**, *144*, 37–55. [CrossRef]
20. Żur, K.K. Quasi-Green's function approach to free vibration analysis of elastically supported functionally graded circular plates. *Compos. Struct.* **2018**, *183*, 600–610. [CrossRef]
21. Andrade, F.M. Exact Green's function for rectangular potentials and its application to quasi-bound states. *Phys. Lett. A* **2014**, *378*, 1461–1468. [CrossRef]
22. Ahyoune, S.; Sieiro, J.; Carrasco, T.; Vidal, N.; Lopez-Villegas, J.M.; Roca, E.; Fernández, F.V. Quasi-static PEEC planar solver using a weighted combination of 2D and 3D analytical Green's functions and a predictive meshing generator. *Integration* **2018**, *63*, 332–341. [CrossRef]
23. Abukhaled, M. Green's function iterative approach for solving strongly nonlinear oscillators. *J. Comput. Nonlinear Dyn.* **2017**, *12*, 051021. [CrossRef]
24. Mehdi, H.M.; Azeem, M.K.; Ahmad, I. Artificial intelligence based nonlinear control of hybrid DC microgrid for dynamic stability and bidirectional power flow. *J. Energy Storage* **2023**, *58*, 106333. [CrossRef]
25. Raja, M.A.Z.; Mehmood, A.; Niazi, S.A.; Shah, S.M. Computational intelligence methodology for the analysis of RC circuit modelled with nonlinear differential order system. *Neural Comput. Appl.* **2018**, *30*, 1905–1924. [CrossRef]
26. Khan, J.A.; Raja, M.A.Z.; Rashidi, M.M.; Syam, M.I.; Wazwaz, A.M. Nature-inspired computing approach for solving non-linear singular Emden–Fowler problem arising in electromagnetic theory. *Connect. Sci.* **2015**, *27*, 377–396. [CrossRef]
27. Raja, M.A.Z. Solution of the one-dimensional Bratu equation arising in the fuel ignition model using ANN optimised with PSO and SQP. *Connect. Sci.* **2014**, *26*, 195–214. [CrossRef]
28. Ahmad, I.; Ahmad, F.; Raja, M.A.Z.; Ilyas, H.; Anwar, N.; Azad, Z. Intelligent computing to solve fifth-order boundary value problem arising in induction motor models. *Neural Comput. Appl.* **2018**, *29*, 449–466. [CrossRef]
29. Sabir, Z.; Manzar, M.A.; Raja, M.A.Z.; Sheraz, M.; Wazwaz, A.M. Neuro-heuristics for nonlinear singular Thomas-Fermi systems. *Appl. Soft Comput.* **2018**, *65*, 152–169. [CrossRef]
30. Silva, G.A. A new frontier: The convergence of nanotechnology, brain machine interfaces, and artificial intelligence. *Front. Neurosci.* **2018**, *12*, 843. [CrossRef] [PubMed]
31. Raja, M.A.Z.; Khan, M.A.R.; Mahmood, T.; Farooq, U.; Chaudhary, N.I. Design of bio-inspired computing technique for nanofluidics based on nonlinear Jeffery–Hamel flow equations. *Can. J. Phys.* **2016**, *94*, 474–489. [CrossRef]
32. Umar, M.; Sabir, Z.; Raja, M.A.Z. Intelligent computing for numerical treatment of nonlinear prey–predator models. *Appl. Soft Comput.* **2019**, *80*, 506–524. [CrossRef]
33. Raja, M.A.Z.; Sabir, Z.; Mehmood, N.; Al-Aidarous, E.S.; Khan, J.A. Design of stochastic solvers based on genetic algorithms for solving nonlinear equations. *Neural Comput. Appl.* **2015**, *26*, 1–23. [CrossRef]
34. Raja, M.A.Z. Stochastic numerical treatment for solving Troesch's problem. *Inf. Sci.* **2014**, *279*, 860–873. [CrossRef]

35. Motyl, J. Upper separated multifunctions in deterministic and stochastic optimal control. *Appl. Math. Nonlinear Sci.* **2017**, *2*, 479–484. [CrossRef]
36. Azad, A.K.; Wang, L.; Guo, N.; Tam, H.Y.; Lu, C. Signal processing using artificial neural network for BOTDA sensor system. *Opt. Express* **2016**, *24*, 6769–6782. [CrossRef]
37. Edelen, A.L.; Biedron, S.; Chase, B.; Edstrom, D.; Milton, S.; Stabile, P. Neural networks for modeling and control of particle accelerators. *IEEE Trans. Nucl. Sci.* **2016**, *63*, 878–897. [CrossRef]
38. Pinsky, P.M.; Datye, D.V. A microstructurally-based finite element model of the incised human cornea. *J. Biomech.* **1991**, *24*, 907–922. [CrossRef]
39. Pandolfi, A.; Manganiello, F. A model for the human cornea: Constitutive formulation and numerical analysis. *Biomech. Model. Mechanobiol.* **2006**, *5*, 237–246. [CrossRef]
40. Ahmad, I.; Raja, M.A.Z.; Ramos, H.; Bilal, M.; Shoaib, M. Integrated neuro-evolution-based computing solver for dynamics of nonlinear corneal shape model numerically. *Neural Comput. Appl.* **2021**, *33*, 5753–5769. [CrossRef]
41. Płociniczak, Ł.; Okrasiński, W. Nonlinear parameter identification in a corneal geometry model. *Inverse Probl. Sci. Eng.* **2015**, *23*, 443–456. [CrossRef]
42. Erturk, V.S.; Ahmadkhanlu, A.; Kumar, P.; Govindaraj, V. Some novel mathematical analysis on a corneal shape model by using Caputo fractional derivative. *Optik* **2022**, *261*, 169086. [CrossRef]
43. Sáez-Gutiérrez, F.L.; Velázquez, J.S.; del Barrio, J.A.; Alio, J.L.; Cavas, F. Novel Multivariable Evolutionary Algorithm-Based Method for Modal Reconstruction of the Corneal Surface from Sparse and Incomplete Point Clouds. *Bioengineering* **2023**, *10*, 989. [CrossRef] [PubMed]
44. Jawad, K.; Mahto, R.; Das, A.; Ahmed, S.U.; Aziz, R.M.; Kumar, P. Novel Cuckoo Search-Based Metaheuristic Approach for Deep Learning Prediction of Depression. *Appl. Sci.* **2023**, *13*, 5322. [CrossRef]
45. Aziz, R.M.; Desai, N.P.; Baluch, M.F. Computer vision model with novel cuckoo search based deep learning approach for classification of fish image. *Multimed. Tools Appl.* **2023**, *82*, 3677–3696. [CrossRef]
46. Sahu, B.; Das, P.K.; Kumar, R. A modified cuckoo search algorithm implemented with SCA and PSO for multi-robot cooperation and path planning. *Cogn. Syst. Res.* **2023**, *79*, 24–42. [CrossRef]
47. Liu, C.; Wang, J.; Zhou, L.; Rezaeipanah, A. Solving the multi-objective problem of IoT service placement in fog computing using cuckoo search algorithm. *Neural Process. Lett.* **2022**, *54*, 1823–1854. [CrossRef]
48. Yang, Q.; Huang, H.; Zhang, J.; Gao, H.; Liu, P. A collaborative cuckoo search algorithm with modified operation mode. *Eng. Appl. Artif. Intell.* **2023**, *121*, 106006. [CrossRef]
49. Figueiredo Camargo, R.; Chiacchio, A.O.; Capelas de Oliveira, E. Differentiation to fractional orders and the fractional telegraph equation. *J. Math. Phys.* **2008**, *49*, 033505. [CrossRef]
50. Tenreiro Machado, J.; Silva, M.F.; Barbosa, R.S.; Jesus, I.S.; Reis, C.M.; Marcos, M.G.; Galhano, A.F. Some applications of fractional calculus in engineering. *Math. Probl. Eng.* **2010**, *2010*, 639801. [CrossRef]
51. Podlubny, I. *Fractional Differential Equations, Mathematics in Science and Engineering*; Academic Press: San Diego, CA, USA, 1999.
52. Ding, X.; Xu, Z.; Cheung, N.J.; Liu, X. Parameter estimation of Takagi–Sugeno fuzzy system using heterogeneous cuckoo search algorithm. *Neurocomputing* **2015**, *151*, 1332–1342. [CrossRef]
53. Cheung, N.J.; Ding, X.M.; Shen, H.B. A nonhomogeneous cuckoo search algorithm based on quantum mechanism for real parameter optimization. *IEEE Trans. Cybern.* **2016**, *47*, 391–402. [CrossRef] [PubMed]
54. Waseem, W.; Sulaiman, M.; Alhindi, A.; Alhakami, H. A soft computing approach based on fractional order DPSO algorithm designed to solve the corneal model for eye surgery. *IEEE Access* **2020**, *8*, 61576–61592. [CrossRef]

fractal and fractional

MDPI

Article

Efficient Analysis of Large-Size Bio-Signals Based on Orthogonal Generalized Laguerre Moments of Fractional Orders and Schwarz–Rutishauser Algorithm

Eman Abdullah Aldakheel [1], Doaa Sami Khafaga [1], Islam S. Fathi [2], Khalid M. Hosny [3,*] and Gaber Hassan [4]

1 Department of Computer Sciences, College of Computer and Information Sciences, Princess Nourah bint Abdulrahman University, P.O. Box 84428, Riyadh 11671, Saudi Arabia; eaaldakheel@pnu.edu.sa (E.A.A.); dskhafga@pnu.edu.sa (D.S.K.)

2 Department of Information Systems, Al Alson Higher Institute, Cairo 11762, Egypt; i_said76@yahoo.com

3 Department of Information Technology, Faculty of Computers and Informatics, Zagazig University, Zagazig 44519, Egypt

4 Department of Computer Science, Obour High Institute for Management & Informatics, Obour 11848, Egypt; gh_mcs86@yahoo.com

* Correspondence: k_hosny@yahoo.com or k_hosny@zu.edu.eg

Abstract: Orthogonal generalized Laguerre moments of fractional orders (FrGLMs) are signal and image descriptors. The utilization of the FrGLMs in the analysis of big-size signals encounters three challenges. First, calculating the high-order moments is a time-consuming process. Second, accumulating numerical errors leads to numerical instability and degrades the reconstructed signals' quality. Third, the QR decomposition technique is needed to preserve the orthogonality of the higher-order moments. In this paper, the authors derived a new recurrence formula for calculating the FrGLMs, significantly reducing the computational CPU times. We used the Schwarz–Rutishauser algorithm as an alternative to the QR decomposition technique. The proposed method for computing FrGLMs for big-size signals is accurate, simple, and fast. The proposed algorithm has been tested using the MIT-BIH arrhythmia benchmark dataset. The results show the proposed method's superiority over existing methods in terms of processing time and reconstruction capability. Concerning the reconstructed capability, it has achieved superiority with average values of 25.3233 and 15.6507 with the two metrics PSNR and MSE, respectively. Concerning the elapsed reconstruction time, it also achieved high superiority with an efficiency gain of 0.8. The proposed method is suitable for utilization in the Internet of Healthcare Things.

Keywords: bio-medical signals; signal reconstruction; fractional Laguerre moments; Schwarz–Rutishauser; internet of healthcare things; EEG; ECG; EMG

1. Introduction

The study of moments as a mathematical tool for describing 1-D, 2-D, and 3-D objects has become the focus of attention of many researchers since the middle of the previous century. Mathematically, the moments represent the projection of the object function onto certain functions called basis functions. This projection results in some statistical quantities representing significant features of the object [1]. One important type of moment is the Orthogonal Moments (OMs) set, where the basis functions are orthogonal. According to the object's coordinate space type, OMs exist in Continuous Orthogonal Moments (COMs) and Discrete Orthogonal Moments (DOMs) moments.

The first set of DOMs was discrete Tchebichef moments, which were introduced in 2001 by Mukundan et al. [2]. Later, many sets of DOMs were introduced, such as Krawtchouk moments, Hahn moments, Dual Hahn moments, Charlier moments, and Racah moments [3–7]. The different sets of DOMs are widely used in many signal and image processing applications, such as image reconstruction [8], image retrieval [9,10], image compression [11,12], image steganography [13], and image watermarking [14]. DOMs reveal high-efficiency concerns representing different bio-medical signals: ECG, EEG, and EMG. Hosny et al. [15] suggested an efficient Algorithm for the compression of different types of bio-medical signals based on discrete Tchebichef moments and the Artificial Bee Colony (ABC). Fathi et al. [16–18] introduced different algorithms based on different types of DOMs for the efficient energy compression of bio-medical signals: ECG and FPCG. Such algorithms reveal high superiority concerning remote healthcare monitoring systems. In Cardiovascular Diseases (CVDs), continuous patient monitoring is very important for better diagnosis; healthcare systems that use ECG signals need long-term monitoring. As such, the size of the ECG signal collected by sensors to use in heart diagnosis is large. Concerning large-size bio-signals, Daoui et al. [19,20] suggested different approaches for reconstructing and compressing such signals. The presented approaches are based on Tchebichef moments and Meixner moments, respectively.

The successful utilization of DOMs with 2-D objects (i.e., images) motivates researchers to use these DOMs with 1-D objects (i.e., signals). Many studies used the DOMs as a feature descriptor for signals such as signal reconstruction and compression [15–17,21] and signal watermarking [22,23]. Other sets of moments are called complex moments. It is used basically in solving eigenvalue problems and has been used in image reconstruction applications. In the image reconstruction application, a formulation is shown to obtain an estimated original image from the degraded image moments and the blur parameter [24,25]. Complex Moments (CMs) were initially proposed as a straightforward and uncomplicated approach to reconstruction images. Still, the kernel functions of CMs lack orthogonality, which complicates reconstructing an image from its CMs.

Previous studies show that orthogonal moments of fractional orders outperformed their corresponding integer orthogonal moments of integer orders [26,27]. Orthogonal Moments of fractional orders are used to analyze medical signals, especially those characterized by their large size [19,20,28,29]. Despite the superiority of fractional versions of DOMs in many applications, some common problems occur when deriving the polynomial values: first, numerical instability results from the large increase (i.e., fluctuation) of the basis function values that occurs while increasing the moments' order. Secondly, a high computational time is required when calculating the polynomial values with the classical form of the polynomial equation. Thirdly, there is the propagation and accumulation of numerical errors, especially at higher orders, with large signals. These drawbacks cause the loss of the polynomial's orthogonality.

To overcome the previous problems, researchers used the weighted form of the fractional Chebychev polynomials, resulting in more numerical stability during calculations of polynomial values. Also, to overcome the highly time-consuming problem, they used a recurrence formula based on a normalization factor. The third problem vanished using the most common QR decomposition algorithms: the Gram–Schmidt Method (GSM), Householder Method (HM), and Given Rotations Method (GRM) [18].

In the current study, we introduced an efficient algorithm for large-size bio-signal signal reconstruction and analysis. The importance of this proposed algorithm lies in its high ability to compress the electrocardiogram (ECG) biomedical signals and transmit them over long distances in a short time. Also, due to this compression, the IoHT can transmit the ECG signals through a small bandwidth; hence, there is low energy consumption. The proposed algorithm depends on the set fractional-order generalized Laguerre moments (FrGLMs) and the Schwarz–Rutishauser approach. Through the current study, we derived three three-term second-order recurrence formulas for the normalized form of the FrGLMs. An important term when computing the normalized form of FrGLMs is the squared norm $h_k^{(\alpha,\lambda)}$. By using the simple recursive formula of the gamma function, we deduced a recursive formula for evaluating the squared norm $h_k^{(\alpha,\lambda)}$. The derived three-term recurrence formula with the recursive formula of the squared norm $h_k^{(\alpha,\lambda)}$ has great benefits in saving computation time.

The utilization of the Schwarz–Rutishauser algorithm [30,31] is another contribution of this study, where the Schwarz–Rutishauser algorithm is used to preserve the orthogonality property when analyzing the large-sized bio-signals using high-order moments. The researchers are accustomed to using classical QR decomposition methods: the Gram–Schmidt Method (GSM), Householder Method (HM), and Given Rotations Method (GRM), but the empirical experiments reveal that the use of these leads to a significant increase in signal processing time, which leads to a lack of efficiency in both IoHT devices and real-time applications with the use of Schwarz–Rutishauser, which is an adaptation of the classical Gram–Schmidt. The complexity of the Schwarz–Rutishauser algorithm is ($\boldsymbol{mn^2}$), which is ($\boldsymbol{n}$)-times less than the complexity of the classical QR decomposition methods: GSM, HM, and GRM, which motivated us to use it in the proposed algorithm, which obtains better results concerning complexity and numerical stability. Uwe et al. [32] proved the efficiency of the Schwarz–Rutishauser algorithm concerning real-time fetal ECG monitoring systems, and it helped in raising the efficiency of the proposed system in terms of improving the system performance and energy consumption rate. To confirm the robustness of the FrGLMs with Schwarz–Rutishauser, samples of ECG bio-medical signal are used. These samples have been obtained from a benchmark dataset called MIT-BIH arrhythmia. An empirical experiment was carried out with the ECG bio-medical signals and revealed high superiority.

The contributions of this study are:

- A three-term second-order recurrence formula for the normalized form of FrGLMs has been derived.
- A recursive formula for the squared norm $h_k^{(\propto,\lambda)}$ has been derived.
- A novel QR-decomposition approach called Schwarz–Rutishauser gives more numerical stability and less processing time than the classical approaches.

The rest of this paper is: Section 2 briefly reviews the FrGLMs. Section 3 presents the proposed computations of the fractional generalized Laguerre polynomial (FrGLP). In Section 4, we introduce the proposed Schwarz–Rutishauser. The proposed algorithm of the FrGLMs based on the three-term second-order recurrence formula of the normalized FrGLP and the Schwarz–Rutishauser is discussed in detail in Section 5. The results are figured out and discussed in Sections 6 and 7, Respectively. The conclusions of this study are presented in Section 8.

2. Fractional-Order Generalized Laguerre Orthogonal Moments

The one-dimensional (1D) fractional-order generalized Laguerre orthogonal moments. $\mathrm{F_r\hat{L}M_i}$ with the order, i can be defined by the fractional-order generalized Laguerre polynomials $\mathrm{F_r\tilde{L}_i}^{(\propto,\lambda)}$ as follows:

$$\mathrm{F_r\hat{L}M}_i = \sum_{x=0}^{N-1} \mathrm{F_r\tilde{L}_i}^{(\propto,\lambda)} s(x), \quad i = 0,1,2,\ldots,N-1. \tag{1}$$

where $s(x)$ is a $(1 \times N)$ signal.

From the inverse transformation of fractional Laguerre moments, the original signal S(x) is reconstructed as follows:

$$S(x) = \sum_{i=0}^{i_{max}} \mathrm{F_r\hat{L}M}_i \mathrm{F_r\tilde{L}_i}^{(\propto,\lambda)}, \quad x = 0,1,2,\ldots,N-1. \tag{2}$$

where $F_r\hat{L}M_i$ *and* $F_r\tilde{L}_i^{(\propto,\lambda)}$ are the fractional-order Laguerre moments and polynomials, respectively.

3. Proposed Computation of Fractional Laguerre Orthogonal Polynomials

The fractional-order generalized Laguerre polynomials (FGLPs) can be generated rapidly according to the following three-term recurrence formula [31]:

$$F_rL_{i+1}^{(\propto,\lambda)}(x) = \frac{1}{i+1}\left[\left(2i+\propto+1-x^{\lambda}\right)F_rL_i^{(\propto,\lambda)}(x) - (i+\propto)F_rL_{i-1}^{(\propto,\lambda)}(x)\right],\ \ i = 1,2,\ldots,N \quad (3)$$

with the two initial conditions:

$$F_rL_0^{(\propto,\lambda)}(x) = 1 \text{ and } F_rL_1^{(\propto,\lambda)}(x) = 1+\propto-x^{\lambda}.$$

Also, the analytical form of $F_rL_i^{(\propto,\lambda)}(x)$ of the fractional degree $i\lambda$ can be obtained as:

$$F_rL_i^{(\propto,\lambda)}(x) = \sum_{k=0}^{i}(-1)^k\frac{\Gamma(i+\propto+1)}{\Gamma(k+\propto+1)(i-k)!k!}x^{\lambda k},\ \ i = 0,1,\ldots$$

The orthogonality property for FGLPs is also satisfied according to the following:

$$\int_0^{\infty} F_rL_j^{(\propto,\lambda)}(x)F_rL_k^{(\propto,\lambda)}(x)w^{(\propto,\lambda)}(x)dx = h_k,$$

where $w^{(\propto,\lambda)}(x)$ is the weight function, defined as follows:

$$w^{(\propto,\lambda)}(x) = \lambda x^{(\propto+1)\lambda-1}e^{-x^{\lambda}},$$

Also, the squared norm h_k is defined as follows:

$$h_k^{(\propto,\lambda)} = \begin{cases} \frac{\Gamma(i+\propto+1)}{k!} & j = k, \\ 0, & j \neq k. \end{cases} \quad (4)$$

The normalized form of fractional-order generalized Laguerre polynomials (FGLPs) can obtained in terms of the weight and squared norm functions as follows:

$$\tilde{F_rL_i}^{(\propto,\lambda)}(x) = \sqrt{\frac{w^{(\propto,\lambda)}(x)}{h_k}}F_rL_i^{(\propto,\lambda)}(x), \quad (5)$$

Figure 1a,b illustrate the values of polynomials for normalized fractional Laguerre and the values of polynomials for fractional Laguerre for N = 100 and n = 0, 1, 2, 3, 4, and 5.

$$\alpha = 1,\ \lambda = 1.1.$$

The three-term recurrence relation of the normalized FGLPs ($\tilde{F_rL_i}^{(\propto,\lambda)}(x)$) can be deduced as follows.

At first, the two initial conditions can be obtained as the follows.

From Equations (3) and (5), one can deduce the following:

$$\tilde{F_rL_0}^{(\propto,\lambda)}(x) = \sqrt{\frac{w^{(\propto,\lambda)}(x)}{h_0}}F_rL_0^{(\propto,\lambda)}(x) = \sqrt{\frac{w^{(\propto,\lambda)}(x)0!}{\Gamma(0+\propto+1)}}F_rL_0^{(\propto,\lambda)}(x) = \sqrt{\frac{w^{(\propto,\lambda)}(x)}{\Gamma(\propto+1)}}, \quad (6)$$

and

$$\tilde{F_rL_1}^{(\propto,\lambda)}(x) = \sqrt{\frac{w^{(\propto,\lambda)}(x)}{h_1}}F_rL_1^{(\propto,\lambda)}(x) = \sqrt{\frac{w^{(\propto,\lambda)}(x)1!}{\Gamma(1+\propto+1)}}F_rL_1^{(\propto,\lambda)}(x) = \left(1+\propto-x^{\lambda}\right)\sqrt{\frac{w^{(\propto,\lambda)}(x)}{\Gamma(\propto+2)}}. \quad (7)$$

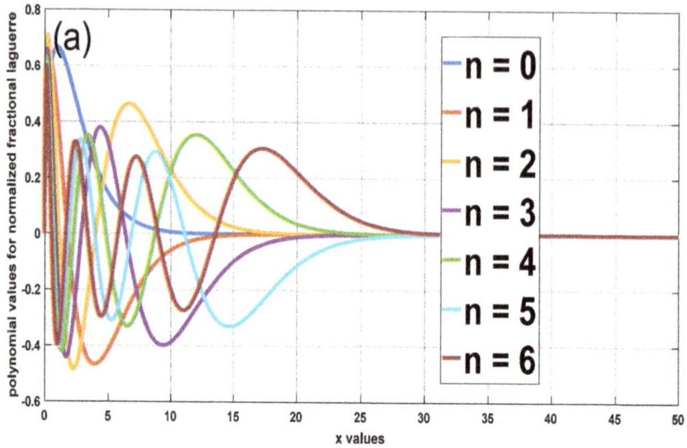

(a)

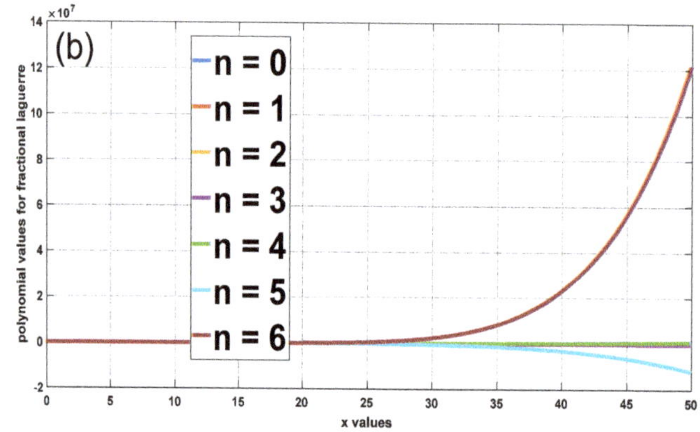

(b)

Figure 1. Plots of (**a**) $\widetilde{F_rL_i}^{(\alpha,\lambda)}(x)$ and (**b**) $F_rL_{i+1}^{(\alpha,\lambda)}(x)$ for the first even orders with parameter values.

Secondly, the recurrence formula can be obtained as follows.

Based on the three-term recurrence relation of Equations (5) and (6), we can deduce the following:

$$\begin{gathered}\sqrt{\frac{h_{i+1}}{w^{(\alpha,\lambda)}(x)}}\widetilde{F_rL_{i+1}}^{(\alpha,\lambda)}(x)=\frac{1}{i+1}\left[(2i+\alpha+1-x^{\lambda})\sqrt{\frac{h_1}{w^{(\alpha,\lambda)}(x)}}\widetilde{F_rL_i}^{(\alpha,\lambda)}(x)-(i+\alpha)\sqrt{\frac{h_{i-1}}{w^{(\alpha,\lambda)}(x)}}\widetilde{F_rL_{i-1}}^{(\alpha,\lambda)}(x)\right],i=1,2,\ldots\\ \sqrt{h_{i+1}}\widetilde{F_rL_{i+1}}^{(\alpha,\lambda)}(x)=\frac{1}{i+1}\left[(2i+\alpha+1-x^{\lambda})\sqrt{h_i}\widetilde{F_rL_i}^{(\alpha,\lambda)}(x)-(i+\alpha)\sqrt{h_{i-1}}\widetilde{F_rL_{i-1}}^{(\alpha,\lambda)}(x)\right].\end{gathered} \tag{8}$$

By using the recursive formula of the gamma function, one can deduce the following:

$$\Gamma(k+\alpha+1)=(k+\alpha)\Gamma(k+\alpha), \tag{9}$$

by substituting from Equation (9) into Equation (4):

$$\begin{aligned}h_k^{(\alpha,\lambda)}&=\frac{\Gamma(\alpha+k+1)}{k!}=\frac{(k+\alpha)\Gamma(k+\alpha)}{k(k-1)!}=\frac{(k+\alpha)}{k}\frac{\Gamma(k+\alpha)}{(k-1)!}=\frac{(k+\alpha)}{k}h_{k-1}^{(\alpha,\lambda)},\\ h_k^{(\alpha,\lambda)}&=\frac{(k+\alpha)}{k}h_{k-1}^{(\alpha,\lambda)}.\end{aligned} \tag{10}$$

Equation (10) represents a recursive formula for evaluating the squared norm $h_k^{(\propto,\lambda)}$. This formula has great benefits in saving computation time.

From Equation (10), we can deduce the following:

$$h_k^{(\propto,\lambda)} = \frac{(k+\propto)}{k} h_{k-1}^{(\propto,\lambda)} = \frac{(k+\propto)}{k}\frac{(k+\propto-1)}{k-1} h_{k-2}^{(\propto,\lambda)}, \tag{11}$$

$$h_{k+1}^{(\propto,\lambda)} = \frac{(k+\propto+1)}{k+1} h_k^{(\propto,\lambda)} = \frac{(k+\propto+1)}{k+1}\frac{(k+\propto)}{k}\frac{(k+\propto-1)}{k-1} h_{k-2}^{(\propto,\lambda)}, \tag{12}$$

$$h_{k-1}^{(\propto,\lambda)} = \frac{(k+\propto-1)}{k-1} h_{k-2}^{(\propto,\lambda)}. \tag{13}$$

Equation (8) can be rewritten as follows:

$$\tilde{F_rL}_{i+1}^{(\propto,\lambda)}(x) = \frac{1}{i+1}\left[\left(2i+\propto+1-x^{\lambda}\right)\frac{\sqrt{h_i}}{\sqrt{h_{i+1}}}\tilde{F_rL}_i^{(\propto,\lambda)}(x) - (i+\propto)\frac{\sqrt{h_{i-1}}}{\sqrt{h_{i+1}}}\tilde{F_rL}_{i-1}^{(\propto,\lambda)}(x)\right], \tag{14}$$

from Equations (11)–(13):

$$\frac{\sqrt{h_k}}{\sqrt{h_{k+1}}} = \sqrt{\frac{(k+1)}{(\propto+k+1)}}, \tag{15}$$

$$\frac{\sqrt{h_{k-1}}}{\sqrt{h_{k+1}}} = \sqrt{\frac{k(k+1)}{(\propto+k+1)(\propto+k)}}. \tag{16}$$

By substituting from Equations (15) and (16) into Equation (14):

$$\tilde{F_rL}_{i+1}^{(\propto,\lambda)}(x) = \frac{(2i+\propto+1-x^{\lambda})}{(i+1)}\sqrt{\frac{(i+1)}{(\propto+i+1)}}\tilde{F_rL}_i^{(\propto,\lambda)}(x) - \frac{(i+\propto)}{(i+1)}\sqrt{\frac{i(i+1)}{(\propto+i+1)(\propto+i)}}\tilde{F_rL}_{i-1}^{(\propto,\lambda)}(x), \tag{17}$$

4. Schwarz–Rutishauser Algorithm

The Schwarz–Rutishauser algorithm adapts the classical Gram–Schmidt methods [30,33–35]. The Gram–Schmidt is a decomposition of matrix A as:

$$A = QR \tag{18}$$

where Q is an orthogonal matrix and R is an upper triangular matrix. The orthogonal matrix Q is produced based on the orthogonal projection. An orthogonal projection of a onto q is:

$$proj_{\vec{q}}\,\vec{a} = \frac{\langle \vec{q}, \vec{a} \rangle}{\langle \vec{q}, \vec{q} \rangle} \times \vec{q} = \frac{\langle \vec{q}, \vec{a} \rangle}{\left\| \vec{q} \right\|^2} \times \vec{q} \tag{19}$$

Each orthogonal vector q ∈ Q is determined by calculating the sum of projections and subtracting it from the corresponding vector a ∈ A. The entire Gram–Schmidt process yields an orthogonal matrix Q and can be expressed as:

$$\vec{q}_k = \vec{a}_k - \sum_{i=1}^{k-1} proj_{\vec{q}_i} \vec{a}_k, \tag{20}$$

$$\vec{q}_k = \frac{\vec{q}_k}{\left\| \vec{q}_k \right\|}. \tag{21}$$

The Gram–Schmidt method exhibits several drawbacks, including numerical instability and a significant increase in computational complexity for orthogonalizing matrices of a considerable size. The motivation behind the development of the Schwarz–Rutishauser algorithm stemmed from the objective of minimizing the computational complexity associated with the prevailing Gram–Schmidt projection-based approaches and improving their numerical stability.

Equation (21) can be simplified by removing the division by the squared norm from the sum of projections as follows:

$$\vec{q}_k = \vec{a}_k - \sum_{i=1}^{k-1} \left\langle \vec{q}_i^{\,T}, \vec{a}_k \right\rangle \times \vec{q}_i \tag{22}$$

We can easily find the i-th element of each column vector r by using the formula:

$$\vec{e}_k \mathrm{r}_{i,k} = \left\langle \vec{q}_i^{\,T}, \vec{a}_k \right\rangle \vec{e}_k \tag{23}$$

By substituting the Equation (23) in (22):

$$\vec{q}_k = \vec{a}_k - \sum_{i=1}^{k-1} \mathrm{r}_{k-1,k} \times \vec{q}_{k-1} \tag{24}$$

Based on Equations (23) and (24) above, this can be done recursively:

$$r_{i,k} = \left\langle \vec{q}_i^{\,T}, \vec{q}_k \right\rangle \tag{25}$$

$$\vec{q}_k = \vec{a}_k - \mathrm{r}_{k-1,k} \times \vec{q}_{k-1} \tag{26}$$

We subtract the product of the vector $q_i \in (k)$ and r_i from the vector q, which is the vector rejection of a. That is why the sum operator can be removed from Equation (24).

Besides the q, we compute the r kth diagonal element in R, as the norm $|q|$:

$$r_{k,k} = \left\| \vec{q}_k \right\| \tag{27}$$

5. Proposed Computation of Fractional Laguerre Orthogonal Moments Based on the Schwarz–Rutishauser Algorithm

Generally, the proposed signal analysis algorithm has two main methods: FrGLMs and Schwarz–Rutishauser. FrGLMs extract features from the signals and Schwarz–Rutishauser to preserve numerical stability with less complexity. The proposed algorithm is described as six steps. In step 1, set the maximum value (L) and (L_{max}) as the order of polynomials. Step 2 illustrates calculating the two initial conditions, $\tilde{F_rL}_0^{(\alpha,\lambda)}(x)$ and $\tilde{F_rL}_1^{(\alpha,\lambda)}(x)$, using the following equations:

$$\tilde{F_rL}_0^{(\alpha,\lambda)}(x) = \sqrt{\frac{w^{(\alpha,\lambda)}(x)}{\Gamma(\alpha+1)}},$$

$$\tilde{F_rL}_1^{(\alpha,\lambda)}(x) = (1+\alpha - x^{\lambda})\sqrt{\frac{w^{(\alpha,\lambda)}(x)}{\Gamma(\alpha+2)}}$$

In step 3, calculate the polynomials of order i depending on the initial conditions by the below equation:

$$\tilde{F_rL}_{i+1}^{(\alpha,\lambda)}(x) = \frac{(2i+\alpha+1-x^{\lambda})}{(i+1)}\sqrt{\frac{(i+1)}{(\alpha+i+1)}}\tilde{F_rL}_i^{(\alpha,\lambda)}(x) - \frac{(i+\alpha)}{(i+1)}\sqrt{\frac{i(i+1)}{(\alpha+i+1)(\alpha+i)}}\tilde{F_rL}_{i-1}^{(\alpha,\lambda)}(x)$$

After computing Laguerre polynomials of orders i, in step 4, we use the Schwarz–Rutishauser to obtain the orthogonal matrix Q and normalize Q by dividing it by its norm using the following equations:

$$r_{n,m} = \left\langle \overrightarrow{Q}_{1:L,n}^{T}, \overrightarrow{Q}_{1:L,m} \right\rangle,$$
$$Q_{1:L,m} = Q_{1:L,m} - r_{n,m} \times Q_{1:L,n},$$
$$Q_{1:L,m} = Q_{1:L,m} / \|Q_{1:L,m}\|.$$

In step 5, the fractional-order generalized Laguerre moments are applied on matrix Q to get the features from the signal using the following equation:

$$\mathrm{F_r\hat{L}M_i} = \sum_{x=0}^{N-1} \mathrm{F_r\tilde{L}_i}^{(\propto,\lambda)} \mathrm{s(x)}, \quad \mathrm{i} = 0, 1, 2, \ldots, \mathrm{N}-1$$

Then, apply the inverse of the fractional Laguerre moments to get the reconstructed signal $\mathrm{S(x)}$ based on the below equation:

$$\mathrm{S(x)} = \sum_{i=0}^{i_{max}} \mathrm{F_r\hat{L}M_i F_r\tilde{L}_i}^{(\propto,\lambda)}, \quad \mathrm{x} = 0, 1, 2, \ldots, \mathrm{N}-1.$$

An Algorithm of the Proposed Method

The algorithm's pseudo code is presented in Algorithm 1.

Algorithm 1. The algorithm's pseudo-code

{—— Step 1: Determine the value L and $\mathbf{L_{max}}$——}
Input the original signal $\boldsymbol{s(x)}$
Set the highest value (L) of variable x.
Set a polynomial's order ($\boldsymbol{L_{max}}$).
{——Step 2: Calculate the initial conditions of the polynomials——}
for x←0 to L-1 do
Calculate $\boldsymbol{F_r\tilde{L}_0}^{(\propto,\lambda)}(\boldsymbol{x})$ using Equation (6).
Calculate $\boldsymbol{F_r\tilde{L}_1}^{(\propto,\lambda)}(\boldsymbol{x})$ using Equation (7).
{—— Step 3: Calculate the polynomials of order i ——}
for $\boldsymbol{i} \leftarrow \mathbf{2}$ to $\boldsymbol{L_{max}} - \mathbf{1}$ do
Calculate $\boldsymbol{F_r\tilde{L}_i}^{(\propto,\lambda)}(\boldsymbol{x})$ using Equation (17).
end for
{—— Step 4: Obtain the orthogonal matrix Q using the Schwarz-Rutishauser ——}
$\boldsymbol{FL} = \boldsymbol{F_r\tilde{L}_i}^{(\propto,\lambda)}(\boldsymbol{x})$
For n ← **1** to L do
$\boldsymbol{Q_{1:N,n}} = \boldsymbol{FL_{1:N,n}}$
for $\boldsymbol{m} \leftarrow \mathbf{0}$ to $\mathbf{n}-\mathbf{1}$ do
$\boldsymbol{r_{n,m}} = \left\langle \overrightarrow{\boldsymbol{Q}}_{1:L,n}^{T}, \overrightarrow{\boldsymbol{Q}}_{1:L,m} \right\rangle$
$\boldsymbol{Q_{1:L,m}} = \boldsymbol{Q_{1:L,m}} - \boldsymbol{r_{n,m}} \times \boldsymbol{Q_{1:L,n}}$
end for
$\boldsymbol{Q_{1:L,m}} = \boldsymbol{Q_{1:L,m}} / \|\boldsymbol{Q_{1:L,m}}\|$
end for
end for
{——Step 5: Get the features of the input signal using Fractional Laguerre moments ——}
Apply fractional Laguerre moments ($\mathbf{F_r\hat{L}M}_{\boldsymbol{i}}$) using Equation (1).
{—— Step 6: return the reconstructed signal ——}
Apply the inverse of fractional Laguerre moments to get the reconstructed signal $\boldsymbol{S(x)}$ using Equation (2).

6. Experiments and Discussion

We utilized some ECG signals from the MIT-BIH Arrhythmia Dataset in the experiments. The Mean Squared Error (MSE) and Peak Signal-to-Noise Ratio (PSNR) are utilized to evaluate the efficacy of the introduced algorithm [36].

- **Relative error (RelErr (%))**

The relative error is calculated by dividing the absolute error of the measurement by the value of the measurement itself:

$$\text{RelErr} = \left(\frac{stdev(f(x) - F(x))}{|f(x)|} \right) \times 100\% \tag{28}$$

- **Mean Squared Error (MSE)**

The Mean Squared Error (MSE) measures the average of the squares of the errors, that is, the average squared difference between the reconstructed signal $\text{F}(\text{x})$ and the original signal $\text{f}(\text{x})$:

$$\text{MSE} = \frac{1}{\text{N}} \sum_{\text{x}=0}^{\text{N}-1} \left(\text{f}(\text{x}) - \text{F}(\text{x}) \right)^2 \tag{29}$$

- **Peak Signal-to-Noise Ratio (PSNR)**

PSNR is a metric that quantifies the relationship between the maximum achievable signal power and the power of the noise that distorts it:

$$\text{SNR} = 20 \times \log_{10} \frac{max|f(x)|}{\sqrt{MSE}} \tag{30}$$

where $f(x)$ is the original signal, and $F(x)$ is a reconstructed signal.

Results

In this section, an experimental examination of the proposed algorithm is carried out to investigate and assess its performance in reconstructing the signals utilizing various scenarios. Table 1 presents the proposed algorithm's and FrGLMs' comparative results on some signals from the MIT-BIH Arrhythmia Dataset. The results illustrate the superiority of the proposed algorithm in reconstruction metrics (PSNR = 143.21, MSE = 0.01096, and RelErr (%) = 0.027) over using FrGLMs; this can also be seen in Figure 2.

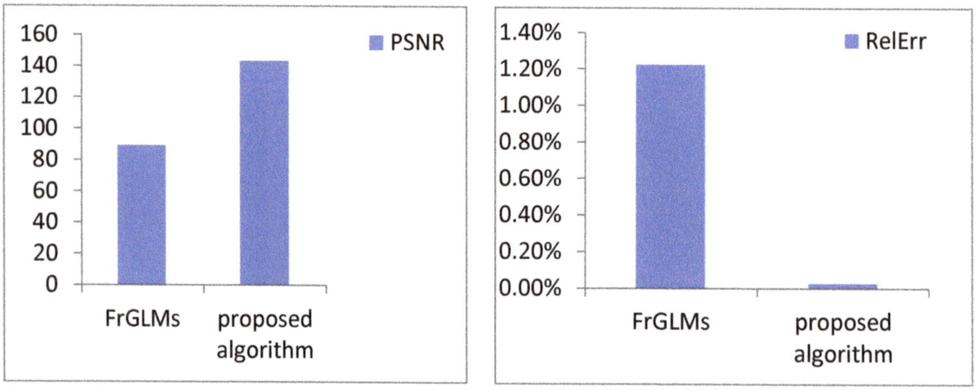

Figure 2. The average values of quality metrics (PSNR and RelErr (%)) for the introduced algorithm and FrGLMs.

Table 1. Empirical results of the introduced algorithm compared with FrGLMs.

Signal	FrGLMs			Proposed Algorithm		
	PSNR	MSE	RelErr (%)	PSNR	MSE	RelErr (%)
Rec. 101	84.61	0.23005	0.57	141.05	0.00992	0.025
Rec. 108	70.06	0.967	2.398	119.92	0.01496	0.037
Rec. 115	110.88	0.037	0.092	155.46	0.00328	0.008
Rec. 209	66.65	0.83865	2.079	135.82	0.00728	0.018
Rec. 214	80.83	0.60155	1.492	139.8	0.0304	0.075
Rec. 219	112.49	0.05465	0.136	163.2	0.00808	0.02
Rec. 230	78.05	0.722	1.79	151.41	0.00456	0.011
Rec. 234	74.11	0.49475	1.227	139.05	0.00936	0.023
Average	**89.21**	**0.4932**	**1.223**	**143.21**	**0.01096**	**0.027**

Table 2 shows the numerical results of the proposed algorithm against the algorithms that use GSM, HM, and GRM. The results in Table 1 demonstrate the advantage of the proposed algorithm over the other methods (GSM, HM, and GRM). The proposed algorithm achieves the best PSNR (143.21), MSE (0.01096), and RelErr (0.027%). Figure 3 depicts the average PSNR and RelErr of the proposed algorithm and other signal reconstruction algorithms employing GSM, HM, and GRM. It demonstrates that the introduced algorithm is superior in the reconstructed signal quality.

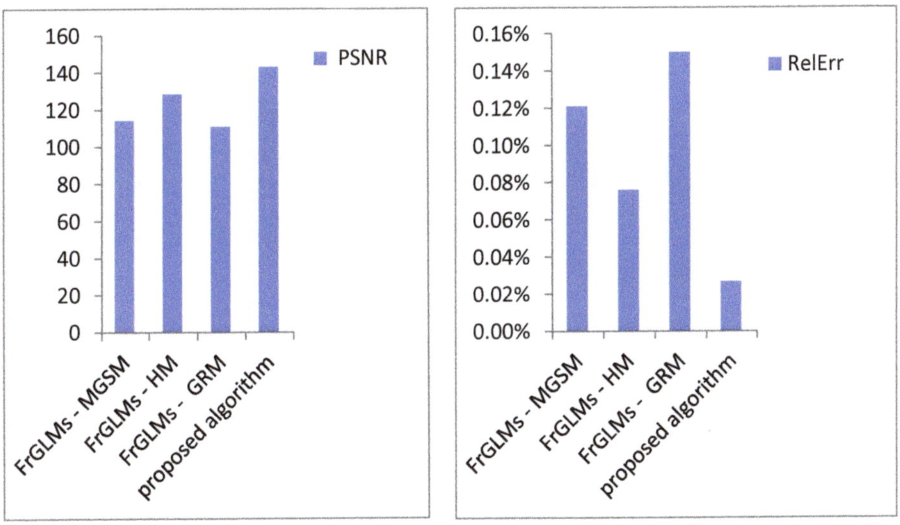

Figure 3. The average values of quality metrics (PSNR and RelErr (%)) for the introduced algorithm and FrGLMs—GSM, FrGLMs—HM, and FrGLMs—GRM.

Table 2. Comparative results of the introduced algorithm with FrGLMs—GSM, FrGLMs—HM, and FrGLMs—GRM.

Signal	FrGLMs—GSM			FrGLMs—HM			FrGLMs—GRM			Proposed Algorithm		
	PSNR	MSE	RelErr (%)	PSNR	MSE	RelErr (%)	PSNR	MSE	RelErr (%)	PSNR	MSE	RelErr (%)
Rec. 101	109.60	0.0359	0.089	128.22	0.01743	0.043	111.91	0.02548	0.063	141.05	0.00992	0.025
Rec. 108	93.022	0.2066	0.512	108.39	0.1064	0.264	88.38	0.2723	0.675	119.92	0.01496	0.037
Rec. 115	124.20	0.0203	0.050	139.72	0.01358	0.034	118.55	0.029792	0.074	155.46	0.00328	0.008

Table 2. *Cont.*

Signal	FrGLMs—GSM			FrGLMs—HM			FrGLMs—GRM			Proposed Algorithm		
	PSNR	MSE	RelErr (%)	PSNR	MSE	RelErr (%)	PSNR	MSE	RelErr (%)	PSNR	MSE	RelErr (%)
Rec. 209	109.06	0.0210	0.052	120.78	0.01967	0.049	104.73	0.029792	0.074	135.82	0.00728	0.018
Rec. 214	112.64	0.0508	0.126	124.86	0.04214	0.104	109.09	0.05985	0.148	139.80	0.0304	0.075
Rec. 219	129.54	0.0195	0.048	144.22	0.01491	0.037	128.10	0.02044	0.051	163.20	0.0080	0.020
Rec. 230	123.72	0.0142	0.035	135.56	0.01351	0.033	120.46	0.01631	0.040	151.41	0.00456	0.011
Rec. 234	112.09	0.0219	0.054	125.26	0.01652	0.041	107.287	0.02947	0.073	139.05	0.00936	0.023
Average	**114.23**	**0.0487**	**0.121**	**128.37**	**0.03052**	**0.076**	**111.06**	**0.06041**	**0.150**	**143.21**	**0.01096**	**0.027**

To confirm the superiority of the proposed algorithm in reconstruction quality, Figure 3 presents a set of reconstructed "Rec. 101" signal in terms of PSNR and RelErr for the introduced algorithm and FrGLMs—GSM, FrGLMs—HM, and FrGLMs—GRM. The results in Table 2 and Figures 3 and 4 demonstrate that the proposed algorithm has the best PSNR, MSE, and RelErr corresponding to all the used signals and the total average of PSNR, MSE, and RelErr.

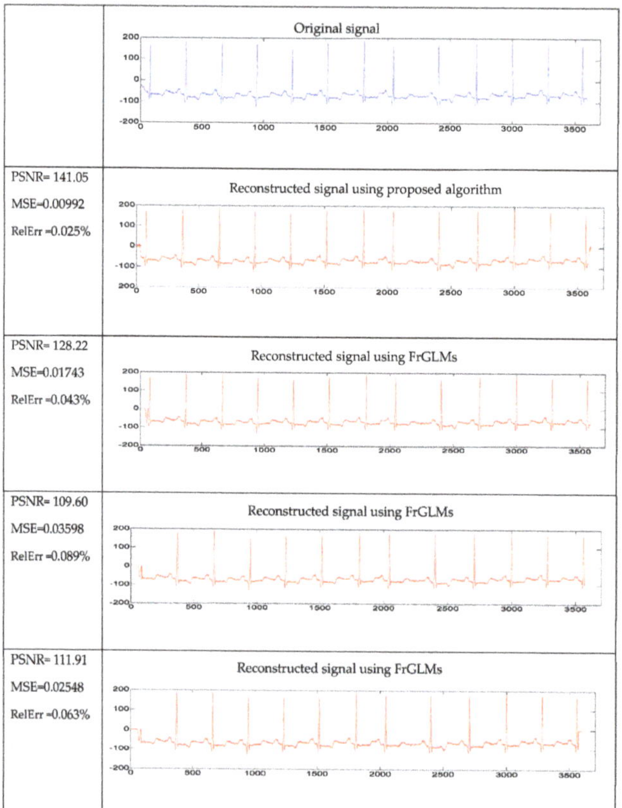

Figure 4. Set of reconstructed "Rec. 101" signal employing the introduced algorithm and FrGLMs—GSM, FrGLMs—HM, and FrGLMs—GRM.

A comparison is conducted between the proposed algorithm and FrGLMs—HM in reconstruction with orders from 50 and 500 to make the results more accurate. Table 3 presents the comparative results of the proposed algorithm and FrGLMs—HM in PSNR, MSE, and RelErr (%). The PSNR and MSE curves for the reconstructed signals (Rec. 101 and Rec. 219) at various orders from 50 to 500 are shown in Figures 5 and 6, respectively. As shown in Table 3 and Figure 5, the PSNR values increase proportionally as the number of moment orders increases, indicating an enhancement in the reconstructed signal quality. As shown in Table 3 and Figure 6, the best value of MSE is likewise obtained as the number of moment orders increases. The results also outperform the introduced algorithm compared to FrGLMs—HM at each order in terms of PSNR and MSE.

Table 3. Performance of introduced algorithm compared to FrGLMs—HM in various orders.

Signal	Order	FrGLMs—HM		Proposed Algorithm	
		PSNR	MSE	PSNR	MSE
Rec. 101	50	85.104	0.8541	88.104	0.3479
	100	90.658	0.3140	93.487	0.2011
	200	110.847	0.0220	119.639	0.0194
	300	116.014	0.0200	132.541	0.0148
	400	121.583	0.1984	137.965	0.0117
	500	128.22	0.01743	141.05	0.0099
Rec. 219	50	89.417	0.3851	105.487	0.1961
	100	101.541	0.2604	116.541	0.1358
	200	114.981	0.0833	129.574	0.0504
	300	125.635	0.0293	145.654	0.0117
	400	136.992	0.0199	157.541	0.0098
	500	144.22	0.0149	163.20	0.0080

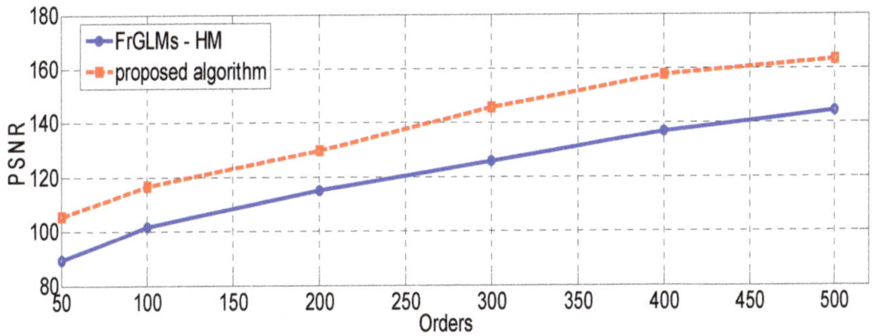

Figure 5. Values of PSNR for the reconstructed signal "Rec. 219" based on the proposed algorithm and FrGLMs—HM at different orders.

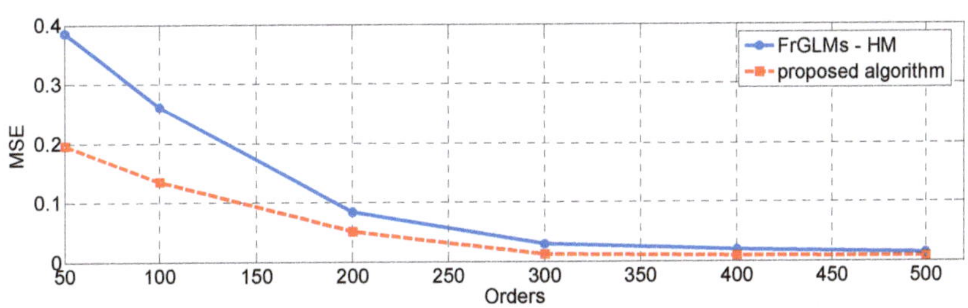

Figure 6. Values of MSE for the reconstructed signal "Rec. 219" based on the proposed algorithm and FrGLMs—HM at different orders.

A comparative investigation of other existing algorithms [8,18,20,36] in reconstruction quality is summarized in Table 4. Figures 7 and 8 display a graphic comparison of the introduced algorithm and other existing algorithms concerning PSNR and MSE, respectively. As shown in Table 4 and Figures 7 and 8, the proposed algorithm outperforms the existing algorithms, which have very high PSNR and the lowest MSE values.

Table 4. Comparative results of the introduced algorithm with other existing algorithms.

Techniques	MSE	PSNR
Charlier Moment—GSOP [8]	0.883	95.741
Krawtchouk—Householder [18]	0.0771	105.015
Meixner- MGS [20]	0.0948	85.654
Tchebichef–Householder [18]	0.0436	107.085
Hahn Moment Invariants (HMIs) [36]	0.0805	97.548
Proposed algorithm	0.0109	143.21

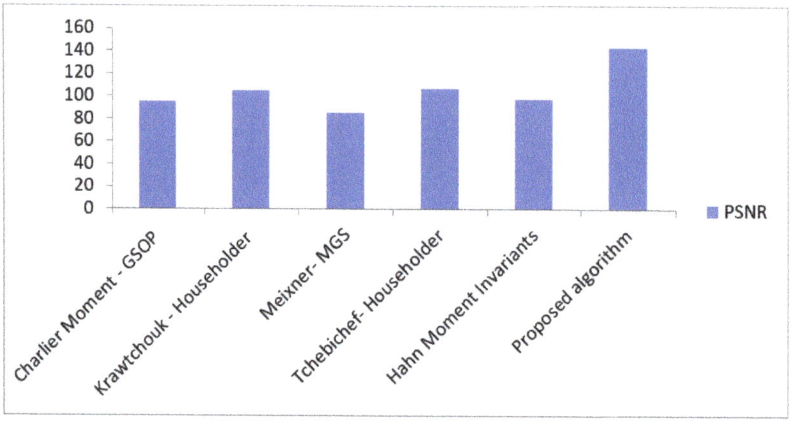

Figure 7. The average values of PSNR for the introduced algorithm compared with other existing algorithms.

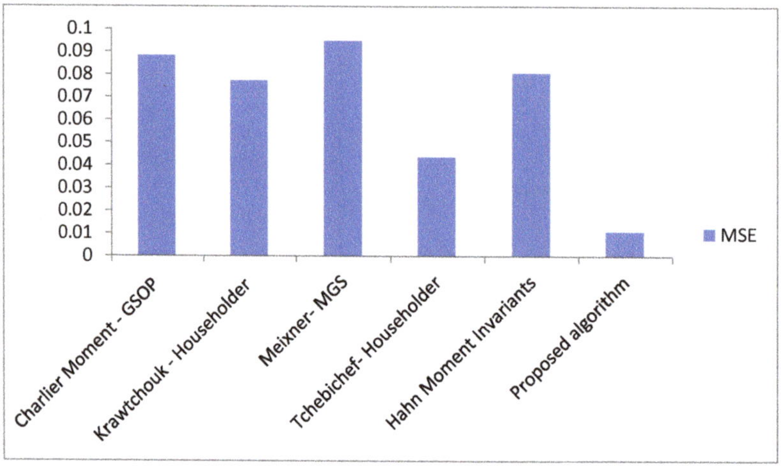

Figure 8. The average values of MSE for the introduced algorithm compared with other existing algorithms.

A comparative analysis is performed between the proposed algorithm and other existing algorithms in the context of reconstruction to ensure the accuracy of the proposed method. The analysis includes orders ranging from 50 to 500. Table 5 illustrates the comparison outcomes of the introduced and existing algorithms in terms of PSNR and MSE. Figures 9 and 10 display the PSNR and MSE curves corresponding to the reconstructed signal "Rec. 101" over different orders ranging from 50 to 500. The obtained results demonstrate the superior performance of the proposed method over the existing algorithms at every order, determined by PSNR and MSE.

Table 5. Performance of introduced algorithm compared to other existing algorithms in various orders.

Signal	Order	Tchebichef–Householder [18]		Krawtchouk—Householder [18]		Proposed Algorithm	
		PSNR	MSE	PSNR	MSE	PSNR	MSE
Rec. 101	50	75.232	0.949	73.048	1.2201	88.104	0.3479
	100	80.335	0.5273	77.213	0.7554	93.487	0.2011
	200	106.854	0.0249	104.067	0.0343	119.639	0.0194
	300	122.548	0.0201	118.474	0.03	132.541	0.0148
	400	129.198	0.0197	125.985	0.0284	137.965	0.0117
	500	132.017	0.0158	128.811	0.0203	141.05	0.0099

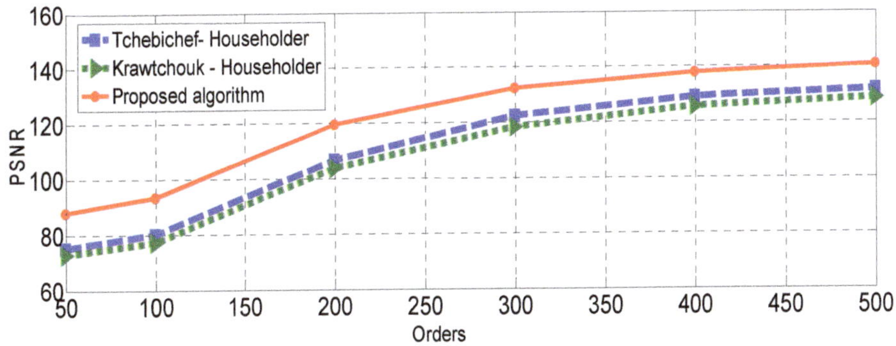

Figure 9. Values of PSNR of the reconstructed signal "Rec. 101" for the proposed algorithm and other existing algorithms at different orders.

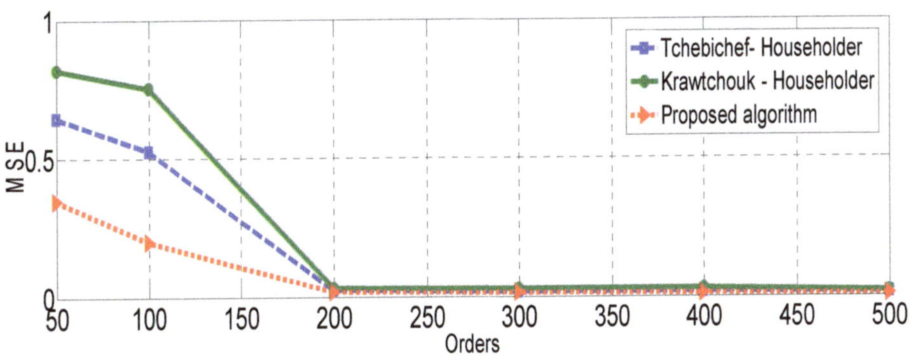

Figure 10. Values of MSE of the reconstructed signal "Rec. 101" for the proposed algorithm and other existing algorithms at different orders.

To investigate the complexity of the introduced algorithm, we compare the elapsed reconstruction time of the proposed algorithm and FrGLMs—GSM, FrGLMs—HM, and

FrGLMs—GRM. As shown in Figure 11, the proposed algorithm outperforms other algorithms in the elapsed reconstruction time at different orders. The visual inspection in Figure 11 shows that the introduced algorithm has less reconstruction time than FrGLMs—HM, FrGLMs—GRM, and FrGLMs—GSM. Table 6 and Figure 12 compare the introduced algorithm and the FrGLMs—HM algorithm in the elapsed reconstruction time and efficiency gain. The numerical results in Table 6 show that the elapsed reconstruction time of the proposed algorithm for the Rec. 101 signal is 0.7 s in contrast to 1.5 s for FrGLMs—HM. Also, concerning the Rec. 219 signal, the proposed algorithm elapses 0.9 s compared to 1.7 for FrGLMs—HM.

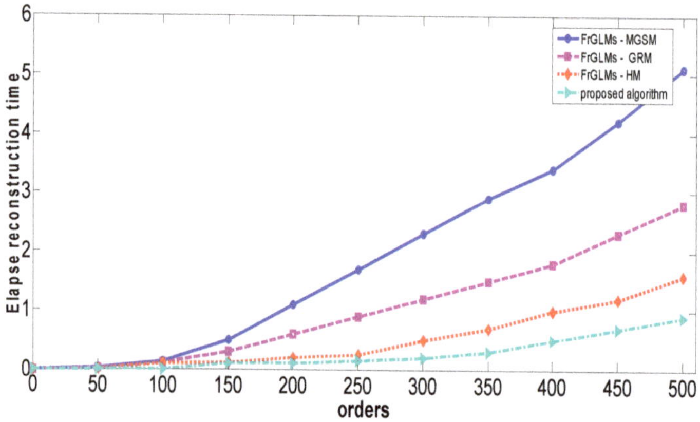

Figure 11. Elapsed reconstruction time for the proposed algorithm, FrGLMs—GSM, FrGLMs—HM, and FrGLMs—GRM at different orders.

Table 6. Elapsed reconstruction time of the proposed algorithm and FrGLMs—HM.

	Elapsed Reconstruction Time (s)	
	Rec. 101	**Rec. 219**
FrGLMs—HM	1.5	1.7
Proposed algorithm	0.7	0.9
Efficiency Gain	**0.8**	**0.8**

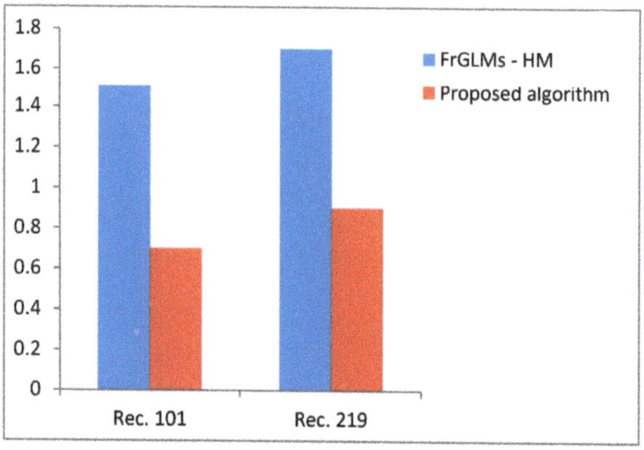

Figure 12. Comparison of elapsed reconstruction time between the proposed algorithm and FrGLMs—HM for "Rec. 101" and "Rec. 219" signals.

7. Discussion

This paper introduces a reconstruction algorithm based on FrGLMs and the Schwarz–Rutishauser algorithm. As seen previously and from the results of the comparative experiments, the proposed algorithm outperforms the algorithm that uses FrGLMs with GSM, HM, and GRM methods. The proposed algorithm was evaluated by assessing the quality of the reconstructed signal in terms of the elapsed time of reconstruction. The proposed method excelled in both aspects. The good results in quality reconstruction and elapsed reconstruction time go back to two main reasons. The first uses set fractional-order generalized Laguerre moments (FrGLMs), in which the term second-order recurrence formula is derived for the normalized form of the FrGLMs. Also, using the simple recursive formula of the gamma function, we deduced a recursive formula for evaluating the squared norm $h_k^{(\alpha,\lambda)}$. It has great benefits in saving computation time. The second reason is using the Schwarz–Rutishauser algorithm to preserve the orthogonality property. The empirical experiments reveal that using the Schwarz–Rutishauser algorithm with FrGLMs takes less elapse time in reconstruction. In contrast to using the GSM, HM, and GRM methods with FrGLMs, due to its complexity, the Schwarz–Rutishauser algorithm is ($\boldsymbol{mn}^2$), which is ($\boldsymbol{n}$)-times less than GSM.

8. Conclusions

In conclusion, we would like to point out that we have provided an ideal approach for large-size bio-signals. The proposed approach is based on an ultramodern set of DOMs called FrGLMs. For more fast and accurate calculations, we derived a term second-order recurrence formula for the normalized form of FrGLMs. Also, we used a novel QR decomposition method called Schwarz–Rutishauser, which gives more accurate and stable calculations, especially at higher orders of FrGLMs. The MIT-BIH Arrhythmia Dataset analyzed the proposed algorithm's performance concerning MSE, PSNR, and elapsed reconstruction time. The empirical results reveal superiority in favor of the proposed algorithm (i.e., FrGLMs with the Schwarz–Rutishauser algorithm) when compared with FrGLMs with the classical QR decomposition techniques (i.e., GSM, HM, and GRM). Regarding the PSNR metric, the proposed algorithm gives average efficiency gain with values of 28.98, 14.84, and 32.15 when compared with FrGLMs—MGSM, FrGLMs—HM, and FrGLMs—GRM, respectively. The MSE metric gives average efficiency gain with values of 0.03784, 14.84, and 32.15 when compared with FrGLMs—MGSM, FrGLMs—HM, and FrGLMs—GRM, respectively. The proposed approach also achieves high superiority concerning the elapsed reconstruction time.

Author Contributions: Conceptualization, G.H., I.S.F. and K.M.H.; methodology, G.H., I.S.F. and K.M.H.; software, G.H., I.S.F. and K.M.H.; validation, G.H., I.S.F., K.M.H., D.S.K. and E.A.A.; formal analysis, G.H., I.S.F., K.M.H., D.S.K. and E.A.A.; investigation, D.S.K.; resources, D.S.K., E.A.A. and I.S.F.; data curation, G.H., I.S.F., D.S.K. and E.A.A.; writing—original draft preparation, G.H. and I.S.F.; writing—review and editing, K.M.H.; visualization, G.H., I.S.F., K.M.H., D.S.K. and E.A.A.; supervision, K.M.H.; project administration, D.S.K. and E.A.A.; funding acquisition, D.S.K. and E.A.A. All authors have read and agreed to the published version of the manuscript.

Funding: Princess Nourah bint Abdulrahman University Researchers Supporting Project number (PNURSP2023R409), Princess Nourah bint Abdulrahman University, Riyadh, Saudi Arabia.

Data Availability Statement: Data will be available open a responsible request.

Conflicts of Interest: The authors declare no conflict of interest to report regarding the present study.

References

1. Flusser, J.; Suk, T.; Zitová, B. *Moments and Moment Invariants in Pattern Recognition*, 1st ed.; Wiley Online Library: London, UK, 2009; pp. 18–20.
2. Mukundan, R.; Ong, S.H.; Lee, P.A. Image analysis by Tchebichef moments. *IEEE Trans. Image Process.* **2001**, *10*, 1357–1364. [CrossRef] [PubMed]

3. Yap, P.T.; Paramesran, R.; Ong, S.H. Image analysis by Krawtchouk moments. *IEEE Trans. Image Process.* **2003**, *12*, 1367–1377. [PubMed]
4. Yap, P.T.; Paramesran, R.; Ong, S.H. Image analysis using Hahn moments. *IEEE Trans. Pattern Anal. Mach. Intell.* **2007**, *29*, 2057–2062. [CrossRef] [PubMed]
5. Zhu, H.; Shu, H.; Zhou, J.; Luo, L.; Coatrieux, J. Image analysis by discrete orthogonal dual Hahn moments. *Pattern Recognit. Lett.* **2007**, *28*, 1688–1704. [CrossRef]
6. Zhu, H.; Shu, H.; Liang, J.; Luo, L.; Coatrieux, J.-L. Image analysis by discrete orthogonal Racah moments. *Signal Process.* **2007**, *87*, 687–708. [CrossRef]
7. Xiao, B.; Luo, J.; Bi, X.; Li, W.; Chen, B. Fractional discrete Tchebyshev moments and their applications in image encryption and watermarking. *Inf. Sci.* **2020**, *516*, 545–559. [CrossRef]
8. Daoui, A.; Yamni, M.; Elogri, O.; Karmouni, H.; Sayyouri, M.; Qjidaa, H. Stable computation of higher order Charlier moments for signal and image reconstruction. *Inf. Sci.* **2020**, *521*, 251–276. [CrossRef]
9. Hassan, G.; Hosny, K.M.; Farouk, R.M.; Alzohairy, A.M. An efficient retrieval system for biomedical images based on radial associated Laguerre moments. *IEEE Access* **2020**, *8*, 175669–175687. [CrossRef]
10. Wu, H.; Yan, S. Computing invariants of Tchebichef moments for shape based image retrieval. *Neurocomputing* **2016**, *215*, 110–117. [CrossRef]
11. Ernawan, F.; Kabir, N.; Zamli, K.Z. An efficient image compression technique using Tchebichef bit allocation. *Optik* **2017**, *148*, 106–119. [CrossRef]
12. Xiao, B.; Lu, G.; Zhang, Y.; Li, W.; Wang, G. Lossless image compression based on integer Discrete Tchebichef Transform. *Neurocomputing* **2016**, *214*, 587–593. [CrossRef]
13. Liao, X.; Yu, Y.; Li, B.; Li, Z.; Qin, Z. A New Payload Partition Strategy in Color Image Steganography. *IEEE Trans. Circuits Syst. Video Technol.* **2019**, *30*, 685–696. [CrossRef]
14. Hosny, K.M.; Darwish, M.M. New geometrically invariant multiple zero-watermarking algorithm for color medical images. *Biomed. Signal Process. Control* **2021**, *70*, 103007. [CrossRef]
15. Hosny, K.M.; Khalid, A.M.; Mohamed, E.R. Efficient compression of bio-signals by using Tchebichef moments and Artificial Bee Colony. *Biocybern. Biomed. Eng.* **2018**, *38*, 385–398. [CrossRef]
16. Fathi, I.S.; Makhlouf, M.A.A.; Osman, E.; Ahmed, M.A. An Energy-Efficient Compression Algorithm of ECG Signals in Remote Healthcare Monitoring Systems. *IEEE Access* **2022**, *10*, 39129–39144. [CrossRef]
17. Fathi, I.S.; Ahmed, M.A.; Makhlouf, M.A. An efficient compression technique for Foetal phonocardiogram signals in remote healthcare monitoring systems. *Multimed. Tools Appl.* **2023**, *82*, 19993–20014. [CrossRef]
18. Fathi, I.S.; Ahmed, M.A.; Makhlouf, M.A. An efficient computation of discrete orthogonal moments for bio-signals reconstruction. *EURASIP J. Adv. Signal Process.* **2021**, *2022*, 107854. [CrossRef]
19. Daoui, A.; Yamni, M.; Karmouni, H.; El Ogri, O.; Sayyouri, M.; Qjidaa, H. Efficient Reconstruction and Compression of Large Size ECG Signal by Tchebichef Moments. In Proceedings of the 2020 International Conference on Intelligent Systems and Computer Vision (ISCV), Fez, Morocco, 9–11 June 2020.
20. Daoui, A.; Sayyouri, M.; Qjidaa, H. Efficient computation of high-order Meixner moments for large-size signals and images analysis. *Multimed. Tools Appl.* **2021**, *80*, 1641–1670. [CrossRef]
21. Mahmmod, B.M.; bin Ramli, A.R.; Abdulhussain, S.H.; Jassim, W.A.; Al-Haddad, S.A.R. Signal compression and enhancement using a new orthogonal-polynomial-based discrete transform. *IET Signal Process.* **2018**, *12*, 129–142. [CrossRef]
22. Kumar, A.; Ranganatham, R.; Singh, S.; Komaragiri, R.; Kumar, M. A robust digital ECG signal watermarking and compression using biorthogonal wavelet transform. *Res. Biomed. Eng.* **2021**, *37*, 79–85. [CrossRef]
23. Khaldi, A.; Kafi, M.R.; Meghni, B. Electrocardiogram signal security by digital watermarking. *J. Ambient. Intell. Humaniz. Comput.* **2022**, *14*, 13901–13913. [CrossRef]
24. Honarvar, B.; Paramesran, R.; Lim, C.-L. Image reconstruction from a complete set of geometric and complex moments. *Signal Process.* **2014**, *98*, 224–232. [CrossRef]
25. Imakura, A.; Morikuni, K.; Takayasu, A. Complex moment-based methods for differential eigenvalue problems. *Numer. Algorithms* **2023**, *92*, 693–721. [CrossRef]
26. Hosny, K.M.; Darwish, M.M.; Eltoukhy, M.M. Novel Multi-Channel Fractional-Order Radial Harmonic Fourier Moments for Color Image Analysis. *IEEE Access* **2020**, *8*, 40732–40743. [CrossRef]
27. Hosny, K.M.; Darwish, M.M.; Aboelenen, T. Novel fractional-order generic Jacobi-Fourier moments for image analysis. *Signal Process.* **2020**, *172*, 107545. [CrossRef]
28. Yamni, M.; Daoui, A.; El Ogri, O.; Karmouni, H.; Sayyouri, M.; Qjidaa, H.; Flusser, J. Fractional Charlier moments for image reconstruction and image watermarking. *Signal Process.* **2020**, *171*, 107509. [CrossRef]
29. Daoui, A.; Yamni, M.; Karmouni, H.; Sayyouri, M.; Qjidaa, H. Biomedical signals reconstruction and zero-watermarking using separable fractional order Charlier–Krawtchouk transformation and Sine Cosine Algorithm. *Signal Process.* **2020**, *180*, 107854. [CrossRef]
30. Gander, W. Algorithms for the QR decomposition. *Res. Rep.* **1980**, *80*, 1251–1268.

31. Bhrawy, A.H.; Alhamed, Y.A.; Baleanu, D.; Al-Zahrani, A.A. New spectral techniques for systems of fractional differential equations using fractional-order generalized Laguerre orthogonal functions. *Fract. Calc. Appl. Anal.* **2014**, *17*, 1137–1157. [CrossRef]
32. Meyer-Baese, U.; Muddu, H.; Schinhaerl, S.; Kumm, M.; Zipf, P. Real-Time Fetal ECG System Design Using Embedded Microprocessors. *SPIE Commer.+Sci. Sens. Imaging* **2016**, *9871*, 43–56. [CrossRef]
33. Giraud, L.; Langou, J.; Rozložník, M.; Eshof, J.V.D. Rounding error analysis of the classical Gram-Schmidt orthogonalization process. *Numer. Math.* **2005**, *101*, 87–100. [CrossRef]
34. Kroonenberg, P.M.; Ten Berge, J.M.F.; Brouwer, P.; Kiers, H.A.L. Gram-Schmidt versus Bauer-Rutishauser in alternating least-squares algorithms for three-mode principal component analysis. *Comput. Stat. Q.* **1989**, *5*, 81–87.
35. Shanthini, C. Matrix theory on QR decomposition. *Malaya J. Mat.* **2020**, *9*, 4127–4130.
36. Daoui, A.; Karmouni, H.; Sayyouri, M.; Qjidaa, H. Fast and stable computation of higher-order Hahn polynomials and Hahn moment invariants for signal and image analysis. *Multimed. Tools Appl.* **2021**, *80*, 32947–32973. [CrossRef] [PubMed]

fractal and fractional

MDPI

Article

Fractal Dimension Analysis of the Tumor Microenvironment in Cutaneous Squamous Cell Carcinoma: Insights into Angiogenesis and Immune Cell Infiltration

Alexandra Buruiană [1], Mircea-Sebastian Șerbănescu [2,3,*], Bogdan Pop [1,4], Bogdan-Alexandru Gheban [5,6], Ioana-Andreea Gheban-Roșca [7], Raluca Maria Hendea [1], Carmen Georgiu [1,6], Doinița Crișan [1,6] and Maria Crișan [5,6]

[1] Department of Pathology, Iuliu Hațieganu University of Medicine and Pharmacy, 400012 Cluj-Napoca, Romania; buruiana.alexandra@umfcluj.ro (A.B.); bogdan.pop@umfcluj.ro (B.P.); maria.bungardean@elearn.umfcluj.ro (R.M.H.); cgeorgiu@umfcluj.ro (C.G.); dcrisan@umfcluj.ro (D.C.)

[2] Department of Medical Informatics and Biostatistics, University of Medicine and Pharmacy of Craiova, 200349 Craiova, Romania

[3] Department of Pathology, Philanthropy Municipal Clinical Hospital, 200143 Craiova, Romania

[4] Department of Pathology, "Prof. Dr. Ion Chiricuta" Oncology Institute, 400015 Cluj-Napoca, Romania

[5] Department of Histology, Iuliu Hațieganu University of Medicine and Pharmacy, 400012 Cluj-Napoca, Romania; gheban.bogdan@umfcluj.ro (B.-A.G.); maria.crisan@umfcluj.ro (M.C.)

[6] Emergency Clinical County Hospital, 400347 Cluj-Napoca, Romania

[7] Department of Medical Informatics and Biostatistics, Iuliu Hațieganu University of Medicine and Pharmacy, 400129 Cluj-Napoca, Romania; andreea.gheban-rosca@umfcluj.ro

* Correspondence: mircea_serbanescu@yahoo.com

Abstract: The global incidence of cutaneous squamous cell carcinoma (cSCC), a prevalent and aggressive skin cancer, has risen significantly, posing a substantial public health challenge. This study investigates the tumor microenvironment (TME) of cSCC by focusing on the spatial distribution patterns of immune and vascular markers (CD31, CD20, CD4, and CD8) using fractal dimension (FD) analysis. Our analysis encompassed 141 cases, including 100 invasive cSCCs and 41 specimens with pre-invasive lesions exclusively, and the rest were peripheral pre-invasive lesions from the invasive cSCC class. The FD values for each marker were computed and compared between pre-invasive and invasive lesion classes. The results revealed significant differences in FD values between the two classes for CD20 and CD31 markers, suggesting distinct alterations in B cell distribution and angiogenic activity during cSCC progression. However, CD4 and CD8 markers did not exhibit significant changes individually. Still, the CD4/CD8 ratio showed a significant difference, suggesting a potential shift in the balance between T helper and cytotoxic T cell responses, impacting the immune landscape as lesions progressed from pre-invasive to invasive stages. These findings underscore the complexity and heterogeneity of the TME in cSCC and highlight the potential of FD analysis as a quantitative tool for characterizing tumor progression. Further research is needed to elucidate the implications of these differences in the clinical management of cSCC.

Keywords: fractal dimension; cutaneous squamous cell carcinoma; digital image analysis; tumor microenvironment; angiogenesis; immune cells

1. Introduction

The incidence rate of cutaneous squamous cell carcinoma (cSCC), a malignant epithelial tumor originating from keratinocytes [1], has increased globally by approximately 36% between 1990 and 2019 [2]. This alarming rise in cSCC, the second most common type of skin cancer, represents a significant public health concern, with over 2.4 million new cases and more than 356,000 deaths attributed to it worldwide annually [2,3].

cSCC progresses through distinct stages, beginning with abnormal cell growth (dysplasia), as observed in actinic keratosis. It then develops into a pre-cancerous stage confined to the epidermis (carcinoma in situ or Bowen's disease), before ultimately transforming into invasive cancer that penetrates through the basement membrane into the dermis or deeper tissues [1].

The most common sites of cSCC development are sun-exposed areas, predominantly the head and neck, with the ears, lips, scalp, and face being the most frequently affected sites [1,4]. However, cSCC can also develop on the trunk and lower extremities, with the legs being a frequent site in women [4,5]. Risk factors associated with cSCC development, in addition to chronic sun exposure, include advanced age, with an increased incidence observed in individuals over 50 years, peaking over 70 [2]. Furthermore, immunosuppression, fair skin, chronic irritation, trauma (e.g., burn scars, chronic ulcers), and radiation exposure also contribute to an elevated risk of cSCC [1].

Histologically, cSCC is characterized by pleomorphic polygonal cells, exhibiting a degree of differentiation dependent on tumor grade [1]. These cells adhere together, forming nests or islands surrounded by tumor stroma, and may demonstrate variable keratin production [1]. The tumor stroma is a complex environment surrounding and interacting with the tumor cells [6]. It contains various cellular components, including immune cells [7,8], cancer-associated fibroblasts [9], and extracellular matrix components such as collagen [10] and blood vessels [11]. This composition of the tumor stroma can influence tumor progression, invasion, and metastasis [12].

Immune cells play a critical role in the tumor microenvironment (TME) [13]. CD8+ cytotoxic T cells can directly kill tumor cells, and their presence is associated with a better prognosis [14,15]. Tregs (CD4+ regulatory T cells), on the other hand, suppress the immune response [16] and their abundance is linked to poorer outcomes. The ratio of these two cell types within the TME can vary depending on factors like tumor stage and genetics [7]. Blood vessels are another vital component of the TME, supplying nutrients and oxygen to the tumor. Compared to basal cell carcinoma (BCC), in which the blood vessels are arranged at the periphery, cSCC lesions show a bigger vessel density with two vascular pedicles [17], indicating a possible involvement in the more aggressive tumor behavior.

Many natural objects have complex structures that stay complex across magnifications, and patterns repeat at different scales. This complexity and variation makes traditional measurements tricky, so fractal geometry can be used instead [18]. Fractal dimension measures how much space an object fills and can be estimated using image analysis [18]. It has been a helpful tool in biology for analyzing DNA, tumors, and understanding growth processes [18].

Benoît Mandelbrot, the visionary behind fractals, introduced fractal dimension, a tool to quantify the intricate patterns found in nature's seemingly irregular forms. From aiding in the diagnosis of tumors [19] and the analysis of brain scans [20] to providing insights into the intricacies of the circulatory system, the application of fractal dimension has emerged as a potent instrument in the ongoing exploration and comprehension of the human body's complexities [21].

In the realm of dermatology, fractal analysis has proven to be a valuable tool for characterizing various aspects of skin lesions. Notably, it was employed to evaluate the extent of field cancerization activity [22], a critical factor in understanding the progression of skin cancers. Additionally, fractal analysis aided in the investigation of melanoma and other pigmented lesions [23,24]. This investigation involved the analysis of both histopathological slides and dermatoscopic images [25], providing insights into the structural complexities of these lesions. Furthermore, researchers have utilized fractal dimensions to examine the vascularity of melanomas and their micrometastases [26], potentially contributing to the development of improved diagnostic and prognostic tools.

Our investigation centers on the TME of cutaneous squamous cell carcinoma (cSCC), with particular attention directed towards the spatial arrangement of CD20, CD31, CD4, and CD8 markers. By employing fractal dimension analysis, we seek to provide a quantitative characterization of the distributional patterns of these markers, stratified into two distinct categories (classes): pre-invasive and invasive lesions.

2. Materials and Methods

2.1. Material

The present research encompassed a total sample of 141 cases, comprising 100 consecutive cases of invasive cutaneous squamous cell carcinoma and an additional 41 cases characterized exclusively by the presence of pre-invasive lesions. In order to achieve a total number of 100 analyzed pre-invasive lesions, the sample was supplemented with pre-invasive lesions identified at the periphery within the class of 100 cSCC cases. The inclusion of pre-invasive lesions from the periphery of invasive cSCC cases was motivated by the recognition that invasive tumors frequently exhibit surrounding areas of pre-invasive changes, reflecting the stepwise progression of cSCC from pre-malignant to malignant stages. This approach aimed to enhance the representation of the pre-invasive spectrum within the study cohort, enabling a more comprehensive comparison between pre-invasive and invasive lesions, in terms of their tumor microenvironment characteristics and addressing the class imbalance at the same time. Ethical approval for this research was obtained from the Research Ethics Committee of the Emergency Clinical County Hospital, Cluj-Napoca, Romania (Approval No. 38789/13.09.2021), and the University of Medicine and Pharmacy "Iuliu Hatieganu" Cluj-Napoca (AVZ2/8.11.2021). In this study, lesions confined to the epidermis were classified as pre-invasive, while those infiltrating underlying structures were considered invasive.

Following standard histological processing and Hematoxylin-eosin (H&E) staining, additional sections were prepared from paraffin-embedded tissue blocks for immunohistochemical (IHC) analysis. IHC staining was performed using the BOND-MAX Fully Automated IHC and ISH Staining System (LEICA). The following antibodies and epitope retrieval solutions were utilized:

- **CD4:** Clone 4B12, mouse, ready-to-use (RTU), Leica. Antigen retrieval was achieved using Bond ER2 solution at an alkaline pH for 20 min.
- **CD8:** Clone 4B11, mouse, RTU, Leica. Antigen retrieval was conducted using Bond ER2 solution at an alkaline pH for 30 min.
- **CD20:** Clone L26, mouse, RTU, Leica. Antigen retrieval was performed using Bond ER1 solution at an alkaline pH for 20 min.
- **CD31:** Clone 1A10, mouse, RTU, Leica. Antigen retrieval was accomplished using Bond ER2 solution at an alkaline pH for 10 min.

The BOND-PRIME Polymer DAB Detection System kit was employed for signal detection, incorporating peroxide block, post-primary, polymer reagent, DAB chromogen, and hematoxylin counterstain. The staining protocol included a 5 min peroxide block, followed by three washes, 15 min of primary antibody incubation, three washes, 8 min of post-primary incubation, three washes, 8 min of polymer incubation, two washes, and a distilled water wash. Subsequently, slides were immersed in DAB Refine for 5 min (repeated twice), washed three times with distilled water, and counterstained with hematoxylin for 5 min. Finally, all slides (H&E and IHC) were digitally scanned using a Pannoramic SCAN II slide scanner (3DHISTECH, Budapest, Hungary) equipped with a 40× objective. Figure 1 shows the control stains for each antibody used on a sample of lingual tonsil tissue.

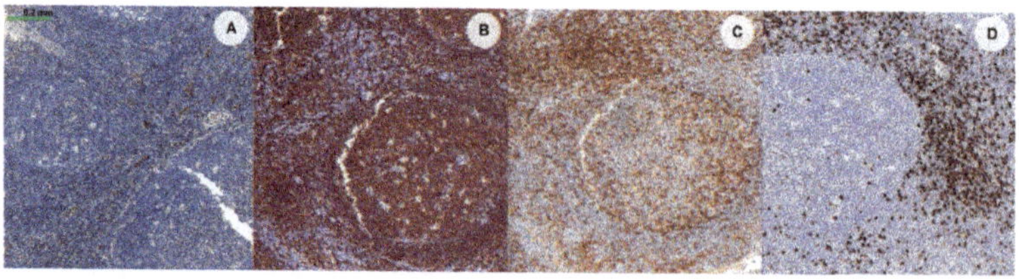

Figure 1. Internal stain control for CD31 (**A**), CD20 (**B**), CD 4 (**C**), and CD8 (**D**) was performed on a sample of lingual tonsil tissue.

2.2. Image Selection

Trained dermatopathologists selected and cropped five images for each case. Hematoxylin and eosin (H&E) staining was used as the reference standard to identify and outline squamous cell carcinoma (SCC) and pre-invasive lesions. The other immunohistochemical stainings (CD31, CD20, CD4, and CD8) were manually aligned to match the corresponding H&E images. Figure 2 shows a sample of images from both pre-invasive and invasive classes. The images were cropped to a resolution of 1024 $\times$ 1024 pixels, captured at a magnification equivalent to a 20$\times$ objective, with a spatial resolution of 5 microns per pixel.

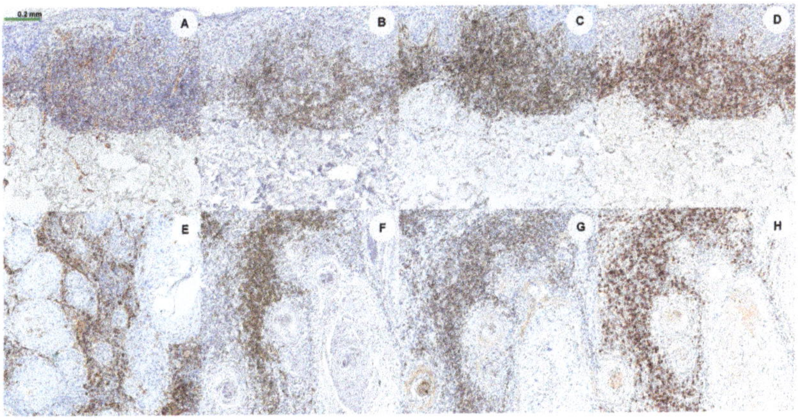

Figure 2. Dataset sample: pre-invasive CD31 (**A**), CD20 (**B**), CD 4 (**C**), and CD8 (**D**), and invasive CD31 (**E**), CD20 (**F**), CD 4 (**G**), and CD8 (**H**).

2.3. Algorithm

The images underwent preprocessing to correct variations in staining, as the staining process could not be performed simultaneously due to the large number of slides. To standardize the stainings, a color transfer method was applied. For each staining type, an image with a well-balanced color distribution was empirically selected as the reference (target). All other images of the same staining type were adjusted to match the color profile of this target image. This normalization was performed in the LAB color space using an algorithm proposed by Reinhard et al. [27], which adjusts the mean and standard deviation of each color channel to align with those of the target image. While a hardware-based marker could have provided more consistent results [28], this action was not feasible at the current stage.

Next, each immunohistochemical stained image was segmented into three distinct masks using a channel-splitting algorithm suggested by Reyes-Aldasoro C.C. The mask for marked structures encompasses regions stained positively with the specific antibody used for immunohistochemistry. It represents the cellular structures expressing the target protein, such as the cytoplasm and membrane of immune cells or endothelial cells, depending on the marker being investigated. The mask for unmarked structures comprises areas that remain unstained by the specific antibody but exhibit basophilic staining. These regions typically correspond to cellular structures rich in nucleic acids, such as the nuclei of tumor cells or other cells that were not targeted by IHC within the tumor microenvironment. The mask for the background encompasses the remaining areas of the image, excluding both marked and unmarked structures. It theoretically represents the stromal compartment and non-cellular spaces within the tumor microenvironment. Figure 3 shows examples of these segmented masks for both pre-invasive and invasive lesions.

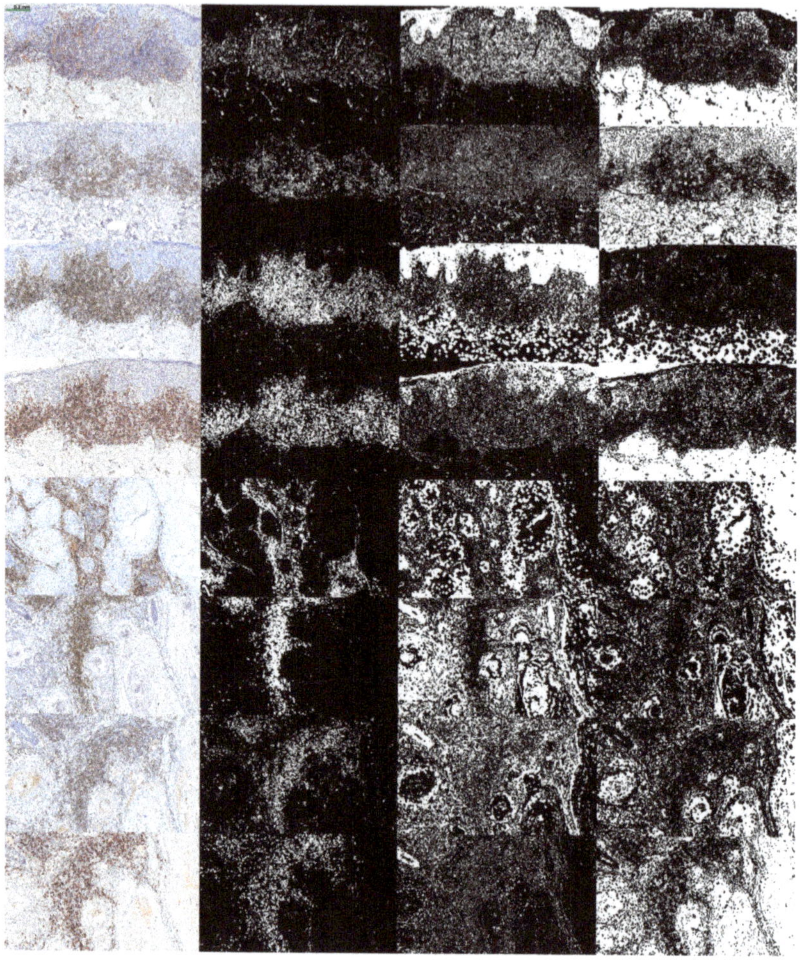

Figure 3. IHC channel split. First column—IHC image, second column—marked structures, third column—unmarked structures, and fourth column—background. Rows, from top to bottom: pre-invasive CD31, CD20, CD4, CD8, and invasive CD31, CD20, CD4, CD8.

Following segmentation, a box-counting algorithm was employed to estimate the fractal dimension of each mask, quantifying its complexity by analyzing how detail in the pattern changes with scale. The algorithm involves covering the object with grids of boxes (squares) of varying sizes, in powers of 2, and counting how many of these boxes contain part of the object. The fractal dimension is estimated by plotting the logarithm of the number of occupied boxes against the logarithm of the inverse box size and calculating the slope of the resulting line. The exact implementation of this algorithm is described in a previous paper [29]. For other applications, we proposed a faster box-counting method based on integral images [30], but this action was not necessary here due to the relatively small number of images.

For each of the four immunohistochemical stained images, of each case, we computed three fractal dimension component values: one for the marked structures, one for the unmarked structures, and one for the remaining background.

We compared the mean FD values of each component between the classes. Furthermore, we compared different component ratios between the classes, like CD4/CD8 and (CD4 + CD8)/CD20.

2.4. Statistical Assessment

All fractal dimension (FD) values were logged, and for each staining and component, values between the first and third quartiles were retained, resulting in a sample of 50 for each component, staining, and class. Data normality within each class was evaluated using the Shapiro–Wilk and Kolmogorov–Smirnov tests. Since all variables followed a normal distribution, comparisons between different values were made using the parametric Student's *t*-test. A *p*-value <0.05 was considered significant.

3. Results

The results, presented as the mean ± standard deviation (SD) of the computed FD for the marked structures for each of the four stainings and each class, are shown in Table 1. Similarly, the results for the unmarked structures are shown in Table 2, while the background results are presented in Table 3. Visual representations of these values are presented as boxplots in Figures 4–6.

Table 1. FD on the marked structures. Mean and SD of the computed FD.

	CD31	CD20	CD4	CD8
Pre-invasive n = 100	1.645 ± 0.024	1.321 ± 0.104	1.623 ± 0.041	1.530 ± 0.041
Invasive n = 100	1.661 ± 0.035	1.220 ± 0.102	1.610 ± 0.046	1.527 ± 0.053
p, *t*-test	0.010	**<0.001**	0.133	0.738

Table 2. FD on the unmarked structures. Mean and SD of the computed FD.

	CD31	CD20	CD4	CD8
Pre-invasive n = 100	1.827 ± 0.019	1.827 ± 0.006	1.835 ± 0.020	1.774 ± 0.019
Invasive n = 100	1.876 ± 0.012	1.827 ± 0.009	1.875 ± 0.021	1.783 ± 0.014
p, *t*-test	**<0.001**	0.619	**<0.001**	**0.007**

Table 3. FD on the background. Mean and SD of the computed FD.

	CD31	CD20	CD4	CD8
Pre-invasive n = 100	1.926 ± 0.011	1.966 ± 0.002	1.934 ± 0.015	1.967 ± 0.004
Invasive n = 100	1.906 ± 0.011	1.973 ± 0.001	1.922 ± 0.017	1.969 ± 0.004
p, *t*-test	**<0.001**	**<0.001**	**<0.001**	0.019

The individual levels of CD4 and CD8 did not differ significantly between the two classes. However, CD20 levels did show a significant difference. When we calculated the CD4/CD8 ratio, we observed a statistically significant difference between the classes, as shown in Table 4. A similar significant difference was also found when analyzing the ratio of CD4 + CD8 to CD20.

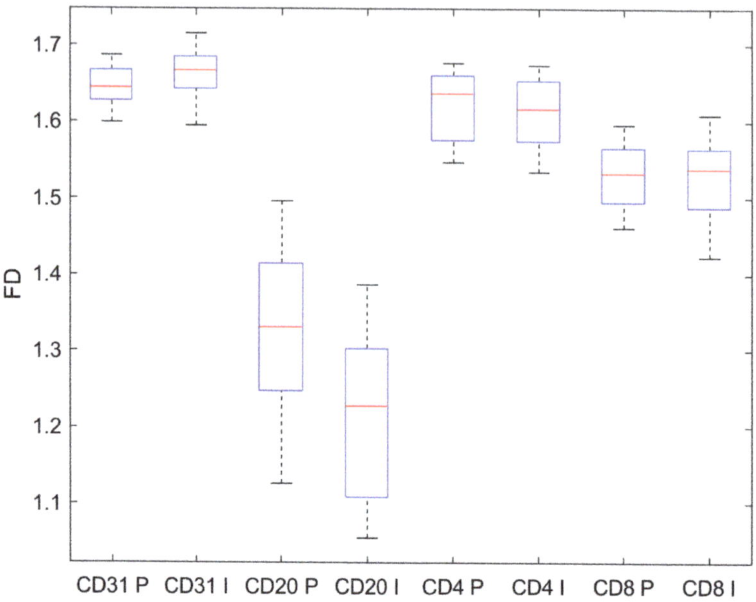

Figure 4. FD on the marked structures. CD31 and CD20 show statistically different values, while CD4 and CD8 do not. P (n = 100) stands for pre-invasive, while I (n = 100) stands for invasive. Red line marking the median, a blue box representing the range between the first quartile (Q1) and third quartile (Q3), and black lines (whiskers) indicating the minimum and maximum values.

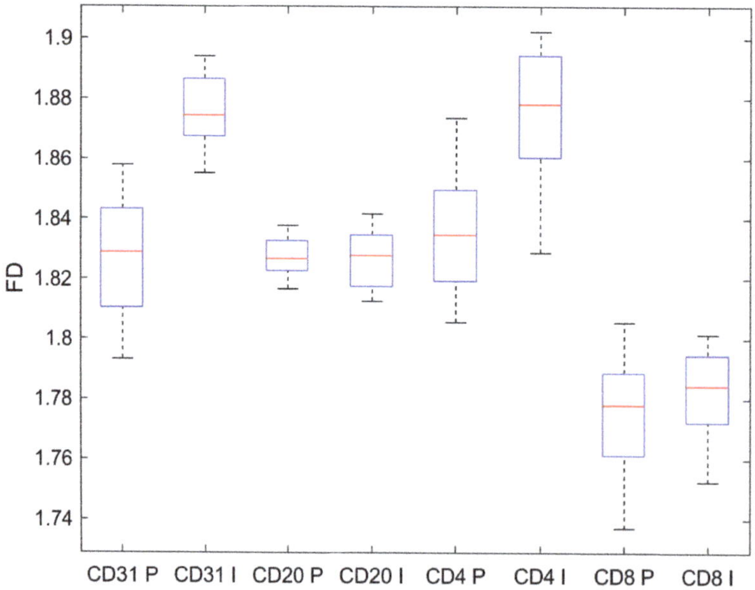

Figure 5. FD on the unmarked structures. CD31, CD4, and CD8 show statistically different values, while CD20 does not. P (n = 100) stands for pre-invasive, while I (n = 100) stands for invasive. Red line marking the median, a blue box representing the range between the first quartile (Q1) and third quartile (Q3), and black lines (whiskers) indicating the minimum and maximum values.

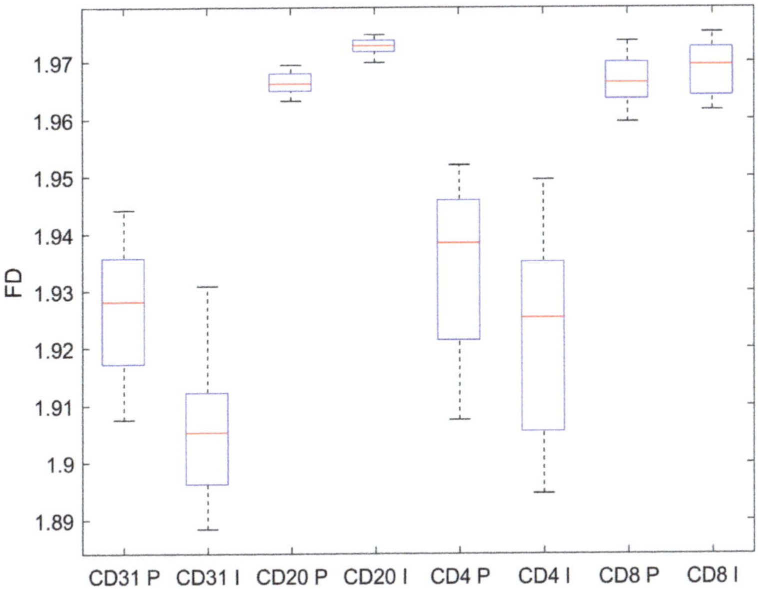

Figure 6. FD on the background. All immunohistochemical staining exhibit statistically different FD values. P (n = 100) stands for pre-invasive, while I (n = 100) stands for invasive. Red line marking the median, a blue box representing the range between the first quartile (Q1) and third quartile (Q3), and black lines (whiskers) indicating the minimum and maximum values.

Table 4. FD on the marked structures. Mean and SD of the computed FD ratios.

	CD4/CD8	CD4 + CD8	(CD4 + CD8)/CD20
Pre-invasive n = 100	1.061 ± 0.006	3.153 ± 0.082	2.397 ± 0.132
Invasive n = 100	1.055 ± 0.009	3.136 ± 0.099	2.581 ± 0.136
p, *t*-test	0.010	0.368	**<0.001**

4. Discussion

The present study employed an innovative approach to investigate the TME in cSCC by utilizing FD analysis on several IHC stains (specifically CD31, CD20, CD4, and CD8). The findings revealed intriguing insights into the complexity and heterogeneity of the TME, particularly highlighting differences between two important classes of tumors: pre-invasive and invasive cSCC lesions.

Our previous research concentrated on characterizing the TME across various tumor types. Specifically, in the context of prostate adenocarcinoma, we investigated correlations between the intratumoral interstitial fibrillary network and tumor architecture [31], as well as between the intratumoral vascular network and tumor architecture [32]. We also explored the relationships between the intratumoral interstitial fibrillary and vascular network [33]. This line of inquiry was further advanced by employing FD analysis to study the components of tumor architecture in prostate adenocarcinoma [29]. In colorectal cancer research, we identified predictive markers for primary tumors [34] and evaluated potential markers of colorectal cancer stem cells [35]. Moving closer to cutaneous pathology, we demonstrated that nodular and micronodular subtypes of basal cell carcinoma are distinct entities, based not only on their morphological architecture but also on their TME [36]. Additionally, in the study of palate squamous cell carcinomas, we described the distribution and expression of certain tumor invasiveness markers [37], providing a foundation for our current work on squamous cell carcinoma at a different site. This body of previous research, including direct studies on squamous cell carcinoma at varying sites, laid the groundwork for the findings presented in our current study.

CD31, also known as Platelet Endothelial Cell Adhesion Molecule-1 (PECAM-1) [38], is a protein primarily expressed on the surface of endothelial cells [38], which line blood vessels, as well as on platelets, certain leukocytes, and a subset of macrophages [39]. CD31 plays a critical role in several physiological processes of the vascular and immune systems. Particularly, CD31 has numerous functions in the formation and maintenance of the endothelial barrier [40], angiogenesis [41], transmigration of leukocytes across the endothelial layer [42], and platelet activation and aggregation [43]. Having all these functions, one could suspect that, as part of the TME, the CD31 pattern evolves with the tumors. This idea is also reinforced by our previous studies on other tumor types. The current study shows that CD31 marking has significantly different FD values between pre-invasive and invasive classes, with a lower value in the former, as seen in Table 1 and Figure 4. This difference indicates a possible differentiation between the two classes and could lead to further investigations as the vessels are subjected to analysis with non-invasive imaging techniques, and in turn, this action could bring useful information in the clinical decision.

CD20 is a protein found on the surface of B cells, which are a type of white blood cell involved in the immune system. The CD20 molecule plays a key role in B cell development, differentiation, and activation [44]. It is not present on early B cells or plasma cells, but it is expressed on mature B cells. B cells exhibiting CD20, are present in different diseases like leukemia, lymphoma [45], and autoimmune diseases [46] and are used for targeted therapy, showing their role in the immune intervention. The current study shows that CD20 marking has significantly different FD values between pre-invasive invasive classes, with a lower value in the latest, as seen in Table 1 and Figure 4. This difference indicates a possible differentiation between the two classes and could lead to further investigations.

CD4 is a glycoprotein expressed on the surface of certain immune cells, including T helper cells [47], monocytes, macrophages [48], and dendritic cells [49]. CD4 is a co-receptor that plays a crucial role in the immune system by aiding in the activation and coordination of the immune response [47]. Particularly, CD4 has numerous functions like orchestrating the immune response by helping to activate other immune cells, including B cells (which produce antibodies) [47], cytotoxic T cells (which kill infected cells) [50], and macrophages [48] (which engulf and destroy pathogens). It also has a role in immune regulation, where CD4+ T cells are involved in regulating the immune response, ensuring that it is appropriately robust to fight infections but also controlled to prevent excessive inflammation or autoimmune reactions [47]. CD4+ T cells can play a role in both pro-inflammatory and anti-inflammatory responses. The type of response depends on the specific subtype of CD4+ T cell involved and the signals it receives [51]. When these CD4+ T cells recognize a foreign antigen presented by other immune cells, they can initiate a variety of immune responses, including pro-inflammatory ones [52]. The current study shows that CD4 marking has no significantly different FD values between pre-invasive and invasive classes, as seen in Table 1 and Figure 4. This observation could indicate that CD4-expressing cells are highly involved in both pre-invasive and invasive lesions.

CD8 is a glycoprotein found on the surface of certain immune cells, primarily cytotoxic T cells (also known as CD8+ T cells) [53]. It serves as a co-receptor that is crucial in the immune system, particularly in the identification and elimination of infected or cancerous cells [54]. CD8+ T cells have the ability to directly kill cells that are infected with viruses or other intracellular pathogens, as well as cells that are cancerous or otherwise abnormal [55]. They accomplish this action by releasing cytotoxic molecules like perforin and granzymes, which induce apoptosis (programmed cell death) in the target cell [55]. CD8+ T cells interact with MHC class I molecules, which are present on almost all nucleated cells [55]. This interaction allows them to survey cells for signs of infection or transformation. The current study shows that CD8 expression (as measured by FD values) does not differ significantly between pre-invasive and invasive classes, as seen in Table 1 and Figure 4. Similar with the CD4 expression, this lack of significant difference could indicate that CD8 expressing cells are highly involved in both pre-invasive and invasive lesions.

Following Table 1 and Figure 4, we found that CD4 and CD8 do not exhibit significant changes in the FD within the pre-invasive and invasive classes. However, when we computed the CD4 to CD8 ratio of the obtained FD ratio, we found it shows a significant difference, as seen in Table 4. The invasive class has a lower overall FD ratio. Since the individual values of CD4 and CD8 showed no statistical difference, we were forced to take into consideration both the influence of the denominator and numerator without being able to point out the one that changes.

Following a similar approach when aiming to see the T to B FD ratio, we computed (CD4 + C8)/CD20 and found out that the FD ratio is statistically different between the two classes, as pointed out in Table 4. With CD20 itself showing statistically different values between classes, and with the CD4 + CD8 showing no statistical difference, it is unclear if the CD4 + CD8 has a contribution in this matter.

We focused on marked structures for three reasons: (1) they directly represent the spatial distribution of the specific immune cells that we are interested in (CD4+, CD8+, and CD20+ cells), allowing us to analyze their arrangement; (2) the CD4/CD8 and (CD4 + CD8)/CD20 ratios are relevant in other cancers, like breast cancer [56], and using FD values helps quantify the spatial distribution of these cells; and (3) unmarked structures and the background are different from the marked immune cells and could confuse our interpretation of the results.

The analysis of FD values in unmarked structures—areas not stained for specific markers but showing high basophilic staining—revealed significant differences between pre-invasive and invasive cSCC in the CD31, CD4, and CD8 images. Invasive cSCC showed higher FD values in unmarked structures across all three markers, as illustrated in Table 2 and Figure 5. However, FD values for unmarked structures in CD20 images did not differ between the two classes. The underlying causes for these insignificant FD differences in the T line cells, as well as the significant differences in unmarked structures, remain unclear. The phenomena are opposite in the B cell line. This observation is particularly intriguing because it suggests a mirroring effect: when marked structures show significant differences, the unmarked structures do not, and vice versa.

The background mask was created by excluding both marked and unmarked structures, theoretically representing the stroma and non-cellular spaces. For the average FD, all components showed statistically significant differences between the classes, as detailed in Table 3 and Figure 6. Higher FD values were observed in the non-invasive class for CD31 and CD4, while CD8 and CD20 showed higher values in the invasive class. Given that at least one statistically significant difference was found in the combination of marked and unmarked structures for all four stainings—CD31 showing differences in both—it is challenging to interpret these findings at this stage. However, this observation may be useful for future studies aimed at identifying correlations.

The presence of CD4+ and CD8+ T cells is generally associated with anti-tumor immune responses [57], and their increased complexity in invasive cSCC could reflect an ongoing immune response against the tumor or a more complex interplay between different T cell subsets. It should be noted that, in other studies, a decrease in T reg CD4+, also evaluated by digital image analysis, was observed in invasive cSCC lesions compared to premalignant lesions [7]. On the other hand, the same study [7] stated that there is a progressive increase in CD8 T cells in cSCC carcinogenesis.

Furthermore, the analysis of FD values on background regions, representing areas not occupied by cells, also showed significant differences between pre-invasive and invasive cSCC for all four IHC markers. The decrease in FD values for CD31 observed in invasive cSCC suggests a reduction in background complexity, potentially indicating alterations in the extracellular matrix or stromal components surrounding the tumor cells (such as blood vessels). These changes in the background could impact cell–cell interactions, signaling pathways, and overall TME dynamics, potentially contributing to tumor progression and invasion [58].

While individual levels of CD4 and CD8 T cells did not show significant differences between pre-invasive and invasive classes, the ratio of CD4 to CD8 was significantly lower in the invasive class. This lower ratio suggests a potential shift in the balance of T cell subsets during progression to invasive disease. Additionally, CD20 levels were significantly different between classes, and the ratio of combined CD4 and CD8 T cells to CD20 was also significantly lower in the invasive classes. This ratio may indicate alterations in the interplay between T cells and B cells (CD20+) in the TME as the disease advances. These findings highlight the potential importance of T cell and B cell ratios as biomarkers or therapeutic targets in cSCC.

The observed shift in the CD4/CD8 ratio, indicative of a potential recalibration between T helper and cytotoxic T cell populations, may hold significant implications for the clinical management of cSCC. As highlighted in a previous review article [58], the TME exerts a profound influence on cancer progression and therapeutic response. The intricate interplay between immune cells, stromal elements, and angiogenic factors within the TME significantly shapes tumor behavior and its susceptibility to various treatment modalities. Our findings, revealing a significant alteration in the CD4/CD8 ratio during cSCC progression, suggest a potential shift in the balance of immune responses within the TME. This could impact the efficacy of immunotherapeutic strategies, such as immune checkpoint inhibitors, which hinge on a robust T cell response for effective tumor targeting and elimination.

Moreover, the observed changes in CD31 expression, a well-established marker of angiogenesis, underscore the dynamic nature of the tumor vasculature during cSCC progression. This observation reinforces the potential of anti-angiogenic therapies, designed to disrupt neovascularization, as a viable therapeutic strategy in cSCC [59]. Furthermore, our results align with the growing recognition of inter-patient variability in TME composition, even among individuals presenting with similar disease stages [58]. This heterogeneity underscores the necessity for personalized therapeutic approaches in cSCC, as the specific TME profile, including immune cell composition and angiogenic patterns, can significantly influence treatment responses [60]. By characterizing the unique TME of each patient's tumor, clinicians could potentially tailor treatment strategies to optimize efficacy and minimize adverse events [58]. Our study not only deepens our understanding of the dynamic TME in cSCC but also lays the foundation for future investigations into the clinical implications of these findings. The integration of FD analysis with other imaging and molecular techniques could further refine our ability to characterize the TME, paving the way for the development of personalized therapeutic strategies that target both the malignant cells and their supportive microenvironment.

So far, the literature about the use of fractal dimension in cutaneous squamous cell carcinoma is limited. The only study that we found applied nuclear FD to describe and compare morphometric aspects and the expression of factors related to apoptosis and cell proliferation in actinic keratosis (AK), in both photoexposed and photoprotected epidermis [22].

However, the FD was used in the study of the tumor stroma of oral squamous cell carcinoma by assessing the nuclear FD of lymphocytes present in the stroma, showing that high nuclear FDs are associated with an increased number of lymphocytes in the tumor stroma [61]. In our study, unlike Bose et al.'s approach [61], which employed H&E staining, we opted for the enhanced specificity of IHC markers to more precisely identify and quantify the lymphocytes within the tumor microenvironment. Specifically, we utilized CD20 to identify B lymphocytes, CD4 for helper T lymphocytes (TCD4+), and CD8 for cytotoxic T lymphocytes (TCD8+). In a separate investigation pertaining to oral carcinomas, Goutzanis et al. [62] proposed that the FD can serve as a dependable indicator for assessing angiogenic activity within oral squamous cell carcinoma. A distinct study from Margaritescu et al. [63] shows that fractal analysis demonstrated a rise in lymphatic network complexity as oral mucosal lesions progressed from normal to premalignant, offering supplementary prognostic insights into oral malignancies.

In the context of non-melanoma skin cancer (NMSC), the fractal dimension (FD) was also butilized by Capasso et al. [64] to analyze the stroma of basal cell carcinoma (BCC) in patients with kidney transplants. They employed WSIs with H&E and Trichrome staining. Their findings indicated that the microenvironment of BCC in kidney transplant patients exhibited a higher density of inflammatory cells in comparison to the control group [64]. Similarly, in our research, using immunohistochemical markers for B cells and T cells, we observed a tendency towards decreased structural complexity and irregularities in invasive lesions when compared to pre-invasive ones.

It would be valuable to further investigate how these immune cell aggregates differ in complexity between invasive cutaneous squamous cell carcinoma and premalignant lesions in comparison to BCC. Additionally, examining the complexity of blood vessels in cSCC and BCC is warranted, as previous research showed that, unlike BCC, where blood vessels are located at the periphery, cSCC lesions display a higher vessel density with two vascular pedicles [17], potentially contributing to their more aggressive tumor behavior. Our current findings, which demonstrate significantly different CD31 marking FD values between pre-invasive and invasive classes—with lower values observed in the former—further emphasize the need for future investigations. These studies should aim to establish a direct link between our observations regarding CD31 expression, a marker of angiogenesis, and the more aggressive clinical behavior of cSCC in comparison to BCC. Such a connection could offer a deeper understanding of the role of angiogenesis in cSCC progression and potentially pave the way for the development of novel therapeutic strategies targeting tumor vascularization. As we show in previous studies researching the vascular network architecture with the help of FD, we have observed that the complexity of the vascular architecture tends to get lower in poorly differentiated patterns of prostatic adenocarcinoma, with a more linear type arrangement [29].

Integrating FD analysis with complementary imaging modalities (e.g., high-resolution microscopy, multiphoton microscopy, optical coherence tomography, confocal microscopy, and skin sonography [17]) could provide a more comprehensive understanding of the tumor microenvironment, potentially revealing subtle alterations in tissue architecture, cellular interactions, and vascular networks. Furthermore, combining FD analysis with molecular profiling techniques (e.g., gene expression analysis and proteomics [65]) could uncover correlations between spatial patterns and molecular aberrations, facilitating the identification of novel biomarkers or therapeutic targets. Integrating FD values with clinical and molecular data could also enable the development of predictive models for disease progression and treatment response, aiding in personalized treatment strategies. Finally, the real-time application of FD analysis during image-guided surgery or targeted drug delivery could enhance precision and therapeutic efficacy.

Given the dynamic and intricate nature of the TME, it is imperative to extend the application of FD analysis beyond the scope of immune and vascular markers. The TME comprises a complex network of cellular and extracellular components, each playing an essential role in tumor progression [58]. Therefore, future research should delve into the FD analysis of other key players within the TME, such as fibroblasts, as well as extracellular matrix components like collagen. By quantifying the structural complexity and spatial organization of these elements, we can gain a more comprehensive understanding of their interplay and contribution to cSCC development.

In light of the pivotal role of cancer-associated fibroblasts (CAFs) in tumor progression and therapeutic resistance, future research should extend the application of FD analysis to encompass these important stromal cells. By quantifying the complexity and spatial distribution of CAFs, we can gain deeper insights into their dynamic interactions within the tumor microenvironment. This benefit could potentially enable the identification of distinct FD patterns associated with specific CAF subtypes, such as immunomodulatory or matrix-remodeling CAFs [9] and their correlation with clinical outcomes. Furthermore, investigating the relationship between CAF FD and the FD of other TME components, such as immune cells and blood vessels, could unveil intricate communication networks and their impact on cSCC progression. Ultimately, integrating FD analysis of CAFs into future studies holds promise for uncovering novel prognostic biomarkers and therapeutic targets, thereby contributing to the development of more effective treatment strategies for cSCC.

CAFs exert a multifaceted inhibitory influence on both CD8+ and CD4+ T cell responses within the tumor microenvironment, significantly hindering anti-tumor immunity [66]. CAFs not only create physical and chemical barriers that impede T cell infiltration and access to cancer cells but also actively suppress T cell function through the secretion of inhibitory factors [66] and the upregulation of co-inhibitory receptors, leading to T cell exhaustion and reduced cytotoxic activity [67,68]. Furthermore, the impact of CAFs on CD4+ T cell differentiation and function remains complex and context-dependent, with evidence suggesting both the promotion of immunosuppressive regulatory T cell (Treg) differentiation and the inhibition of effector and memory T cell development [66]. The multifaceted suppressive mechanisms employed by CAFs contribute to an immunosuppressive tumor microenvironment, ultimately promoting tumor growth and progression [66]. Understanding the intricate interplay between CAFs and T cell responses is crucial for developing effective therapeutic strategies aimed at overcoming CAF-mediated immunosuppression and enhancing anti-tumor immunity.

The current investigation possesses certain limitations that merit acknowledgment. First, the data originate from a single center and encompass a relatively restricted sample size. This limitation potentially hinders the ability to fully capture the spectrum of variability in immune cell and angiogenic patterns associated with cSCC and may also constrain the statistical power and generalizability of the findings. Future research endeavors should prioritize expanding this study to include a larger, multi-center cohort. Such an approach would not only enhance the robustness of the results but also account for potential geographical and demographic influences on cSCC presentation and its microenvironment. Second, the manual alignment of IHC images to the corresponding H&E images, although performed meticulously, might introduce minor registration errors that could affect FD calculations. Last, but maybe the most important, is that the invasive class lacks subclass stratification; as one would expect, there are differences between poorly, moderated, and high-grade subclasses. However, due to the sample size, this problem could not be resolved within this iteration.

5. Conclusions

This study introduced a novel approach by applying FD analysis to IHC images to investigate the tumor TME in cSCC. The results demonstrated significant differences in structural complexity and heterogeneity between the two classes taken into consideration: pre-invasive and invasive lesions, with notable changes observed in blood vessel distribution, immune cell infiltration, and overall background complexity.

Specifically, the FD values of CD20 and CD31-marked structures differed significantly between pre-invasive and invasive classes. Similarly, unmarked structures associated with CD31, CD4, and CD8 showed statistically significant differences in FD values. Additionally, the background, which was defined by excluding both marked and unmarked structures, revealed statistically significant differences in the computed FD across all four IHC stainings.

These findings enhance our understanding of the dynamic nature of the TME in cSCC and could potentially inform the development of new diagnostic and therapeutic strategies targeting the TME to improve patient outcomes. Further research with larger sample sizes and more advanced image analysis techniques is needed to explore the complex relationship between the TME and cSCC progression.

Author Contributions: Conceptualization, A.B. and M.-S.Ș.; methodology, A.B. and M.-S.Ș.; software, M.-S.Ș.; validation, C.G., D.C. and M.C.; formal analysis, M.-S.Ș.; investigation, A.B.; resources, A.B., D.C., B.-A.G., I.-A.G.-R. and B.P.; data curation, A.B. and M.-S.Ș.; writing—original draft preparation, A.B.; writing—review and editing, A.B., R.M.H. and M.-S.Ș.; visualization, A.B. and M.-S.Ș.; supervision, M.C.; project administration, M.C. All authors have read and agreed to the published version of the manuscript.

Funding: This research received no external funding.

Institutional Review Board Statement: This study was conducted in accordance with the Declaration of Helsinki and was approved by the Institutional Research Ethics Committee of the Emergency Clinical County Hospital, Cluj-Napoca, Romania (Approval No. 38789/ 13.09.2021), and of the University of Medicine and Pharmacy "Iuliu Hatieganu" Cluj-Napoca (AVZ2/8.11.2021).

Informed Consent Statement: Written informed consent was obtained, according to hospital protocol, from the patients to publish this paper.

Data Availability Statement: The data used in the present study can be shared upon reasonable request.

Conflicts of Interest: The authors declare no conflicts of interest.

References

1. Scolyer, R.A.; Messina, J.; Brenn, T.; Calonje, J.E.; Rongioletti, F. Keratinocytic/Epidermal Tumours. In *WHO Classification of Tumours Editorial Board. Skin Tumours*; International Agency for Research on Cancer (IACR): Lyon, France, 2023; Volume 12.
2. Guo, A.; Liu, X.; Li, H.; Cheng, W.; Song, Y. The Global, Regional, National Burden of Cutaneous Squamous Cell Carcinoma (1990–2019) and Predictions to 2035. *Eur. J. Cancer Care* **2023**, *2023*, e5484597. [CrossRef]
3. Caudill, J.; Thomas, J.E.; Burkhart, C.G. The Risk of Metastases from Squamous Cell Carcinoma of the Skin. *Int. J. Dermatol.* **2023**, *62*, 483–486. [CrossRef] [PubMed]
4. Fijałkowska, M.; Koziej, M.; Antoszewski, B. Detailed Head Localization and Incidence of Skin Cancers. *Sci. Rep.* **2021**, *11*, 12391. [CrossRef]
5. Tokez, S.; Wakkee, M.; Louwman, M.; Noels, E.; Nijsten, T.; Hollestein, L. Assessment of Cutaneous Squamous Cell Carcinoma (cSCC) In Situ Incidence and the Risk of Developing Invasive cSCC in Patients with Prior cSCC In Situ vs the General Population in the Netherlands, 1989–2017. *JAMA Dermatol.* **2020**, *156*, 973–981. [CrossRef]
6. Guo, S.; Deng, C.-X. Effect of Stromal Cells in Tumor Microenvironment on Metastasis Initiation. *Int. J. Biol. Sci.* **2018**, *14*, 2083–2093. [CrossRef]
7. Stravodimou, A.; Tzelepi, V.; Papadaki, H.; Mouzaki, A.; Georgiou, S.; Melachrinou, M.; Kourea, E.P. Evaluation of T-Lymphocyte Subpopulations in Actinic Keratosis, in Situ and Invasive Squamous Cell Carcinoma of the Skin. *J. Cutan. Pathol.* **2018**, *45*, 337–347. [CrossRef]
8. Nishida, H.; Kondo, Y.; Kusaba, T.; Kawamura, K.; Oyama, Y.; Daa, T. CD8/PD-L1 Immunohistochemical Reactivity and Gene Alterations in Cutaneous Squamous Cell Carcinoma. *PLoS ONE* **2023**, *18*, e0281647. [CrossRef]
9. Schütz, S.; Solé-Boldo, L.; Lucena-Porcel, C.; Hoffmann, J.; Brobeil, A.; Lonsdorf, A.S.; Rodríguez-Paredes, M.; Lyko, F. Functionally Distinct Cancer-Associated Fibroblast Subpopulations Establish a Tumor Promoting Environment in Squamous Cell Carcinoma. *Nat. Commun.* **2023**, *14*, 5413. [CrossRef] [PubMed]
10. van Kempen, L.C.L.T.; Rijntjes, J.; Claes, A.; Blokx, W.A.M.; Gerritsen, M.-J.P.; Ruiter, D.J.; van Muijen, G.N.P. Type I Collagen Synthesis Parallels the Conversion of Keratinocytic Intraepidermal Neoplasia to Cutaneous Squamous Cell Carcinoma. *J. Pathol.* **2004**, *204*, 333–339. [CrossRef]
11. Tzoutzos, K.; Batistatou, A.; Kitsos, G.; Liasko, R.; Stefanou, D. Study of Microvascular Density and Expression of Vascular Endothelial Growth Factor and Its Receptors in Cancerous and Precancerous Lesions of the Eyelids. *Anticancer Res.* **2014**, *34*, 4977–4983.
12. Bussard, K.M.; Mutkus, L.; Stumpf, K.; Gomez-Manzano, C.; Marini, F.C. Tumor-Associated Stromal Cells as Key Contributors to the Tumor Microenvironment. *Breast Cancer Res.* **2016**, *18*, 84. [CrossRef] [PubMed]
13. Saeidi, V.; Doudican, N.; Carucci, J.A. Understanding the Squamous Cell Carcinoma Immune Microenvironment. *Front. Immunol.* **2023**, *14*, 1084873. [CrossRef] [PubMed]
14. Xie, Q.; Ding, J.; Chen, Y. Role of $CD8^+$ T Lymphocyte Cells: Interplay with Stromal Cells in Tumor Microenvironment. *Acta Pharm. Sin. B* **2021**, *11*, 1365–1378. [CrossRef] [PubMed]
15. Rosa, M.L.; Reinert, T.; Pauletto, M.M.; Sartori, G.; Graudenz, M.; Barrios, C.H. Implications of Tumor-Infiltrating Lymphocytes in Early-Stage Triple-Negative Breast Cancer: Clinical Oncologist Perspectives. *Transl. Breast Cancer Res.* **2024**, *5*. [CrossRef] [PubMed]
16. Dwivedi, M.; Tiwari, S.; Kemp, E.H.; Begum, R. Implications of Regulatory T Cells in Anti-Cancer Immunity: From Pathogenesis to Therapeutics. *Heliyon* **2022**, *8*, e10450. [CrossRef]
17. Bungărdean, R.-M.; Stoia, M.-A.; Pop, B.; Crişan, M. Morphological Aspects of Basal Cell Carcinoma Vascularization. *Rom. J. Morphol. Embryol.* **2023**, *64*, 15–23. [CrossRef]

18. Cross, S.S. Fractals in Pathology. *J. Pathol.* **1997**, *182*, 1–8. [CrossRef]
19. da Silva, L.G.; da Silva Monteiro, W.R.S.; de Aguiar Moreira, T.M.; Rabelo, M.A.E.; de Assis, E.A.C.P.; de Souza, G.T. Fractal Dimension Analysis as an Easy Computational Approach to Improve Breast Cancer Histopathological Diagnosis. *Appl. Microsc.* **2021**, *51*, 6. [CrossRef]
20. Di Ieva, A. Fractal Analysis in Clinical Neurosciences: An Overview. *Adv. Neurobiol.* **2024**, *36*, 261–271. [CrossRef]
21. Di Ieva, A.; Al-Kadi, O.S. Computational Fractal-Based Analysis of Brain Tumor Microvascular Networks. *Adv. Neurobiol.* **2024**, *36*, 525–544. [CrossRef]
22. Miola, A.C.; Castilho, M.A.; Schmitt, J.V.; Marques, M.E.A.; Miot, H.A. Contribution to Characterization of Skin Field Cancerization Activity: Morphometric, Chromatin Texture, Proliferation, and Apoptosis Aspects. *An. Bras. Dermatol.* **2019**, *94*, 698–703. [CrossRef] [PubMed]
23. Bedin, V.; Adam, R.L.; de Sá, B.C.; Landman, G.; Metze, K. Fractal Dimension of Chromatin Is an Independent Prognostic Factor for Survival in Melanoma. *BMC Cancer* **2010**, *10*, 260. [CrossRef] [PubMed]
24. Piantanelli, A.; Maponi, P.; Scalise, L.; Serresi, S.; Cialabrini, A.; Basso, A. Fractal Characterisation of Boundary Irregularity in Skin Pigmented Lesions. *Med. Biol. Eng. Comput.* **2005**, *43*, 436–442. [CrossRef] [PubMed]
25. Popecki, P.; Kozakiewicz, M.; Ziętek, M.; Jurczyszyn, K. Fractal Dimension Analysis of Melanocytic Nevi and Melanomas in Normal and Polarized Light-A Preliminary Report. *Life* **2022**, *12*, 1008. [CrossRef]
26. Quatresooz, P.; Pierard-Franchimont, C.; Paquet, P.; Pierard, G.E. Angiogenic Fast-Growing Melanomas and Their Micrometastases. *Eur. J. Dermatol.* **2010**, *20*, 302–307. [CrossRef]
27. Reinhard, E.; Adhikhmin, M.; Gooch, B.; Shirley, P. Color Transfer between Images. *IEEE Comput. Graph. Appl.* **2001**, *21*, 34–41. [CrossRef]
28. Şerbănescu, M.S.; Pleşea, I.E. A Hardware Approach for Histological and Histopathological Digital Image Stain Normalization. *Rom. J. Morphol. Embryol.* **2015**, *56*, 735–741.
29. Pleşea, R.M.; Şerbănescu, M.S.; Ciovică, D.V.; Roşu, G.C.; Moldovan, V.T.; Bungărdean, R.M.; Popescu, N.A.; Pleşea, I.E. The Study of Tumor Architecture Components in Prostate Adenocarcinoma Using Fractal Dimension Analysis. *Rom. J. Morphol. Embryol.* **2019**, *60*, 501–519.
30. Șerbănescu, M.-S. Fractal Dimension Box-Counting Algorithm Optimization Through Integral Images. In Proceedings of the 7th International Conference on Advancements of Medicine and Health Care through Technology, Cluj-Napoca, Romania, 13–15 October 2020; Springer International Publishing: Cham, Switzerland, 2022; pp. 95–101.
31. Stoiculescu, A.; Pleşea, I.E.; Pop, O.T.; Alexandru, D.O.; Man, M.; Serbănescu, M.; Pleşea, R.M. Correlations between Intratumoral Interstitial Fibrillary Network and Tumoral Architecture in Prostatic Adenocarcinoma. *Rom. J. Morphol. Embryol.* **2012**, *53*, 941–950.
32. Pleşea, I.E.; Stoiculescu, A.; Serbănescu, M.; Alexandru, D.O.; Man, M.; Pop, O.T.; Pleşea, R.M. Correlations between Intratumoral Vascular Network and Tumoral Architecture in Prostatic Adenocarcinoma. *Rom. J. Morphol. Embryol.* **2013**, *54*, 299–308.
33. Mitroi, G.; Pleşea, R.M.; Pop, O.T.; Ciovică, D.V.; Şerbănescu, M.S.; Alexandru, D.O.; Stoiculescu, A.; Pleşea, I.E. Correlations between Intratumoral Interstitial Fibrillary Network and Vascular Network in Srigley Patterns of Prostate Adenocarcinoma. *Rom. J. Morphol. Embryol.* **2015**, *56*, 1319–1328. [PubMed]
34. Bărbălan, A.; Nicolaescu, A.C.; Măgăran, A.V.; Mercuţ, R.; Bălăşoiu, M.; Băncescu, G.; Şerbănescu, M.S.; Lazăr, O.F.; Săftoiu, A. Immunohistochemistry Predictive Markers for Primary Colorectal Cancer Tumors: Where Are We and Where Are We Going? *Rom. J. Morphol. Embryol.* **2018**, *59*, 29–42.
35. Harbiyeli, I.F.C.; Burtea, D.E.; Ivan, E.T.; Streață, I.; Nicoli, E.R.; Uscatu, D.; Șerbănescu, M.-S.; Ioana, M.; Vilmann, P.; Săftoiu, A. Assessing Putative Markers of Colorectal Cancer Stem Cells: From Colonoscopy to Gene Expression Profiling. *Diagnostics* **2022**, *12*, 2280. [CrossRef] [PubMed]
36. Șerbănescu, M.-S.; Bungărdean, R.M.; Georgiu, C.; Crișan, M. Nodular and Micronodular Basal Cell Carcinoma Subtypes Are Different Tumors Based on Their Morphological Architecture and Their Interaction with the Surrounding Stroma. *Diagnostics* **2022**, *12*, 1636. [CrossRef] [PubMed]
37. Pătru, A.; Şurlin, V.; Mărgăritescu, C.; Ciucă, E.M.; Matei, M.; Şerbănescu, M.S.; Camen, A. Analysis of the Distribution and Expression of Some Tumor Invasiveness Markers in Palate Squamous Cell Carcinomas. *Rom. J. Morphol. Embryol.* **2020**, *61*, 1259–1278. [CrossRef]
38. Lertkiatmongkol, P.; Liao, D.; Mei, H.; Hu, Y.; Newman, P.J. Endothelial Functions of Platelet/Endothelial Cell Adhesion Molecule-1 (CD31). *Curr. Opin. Hematol.* **2016**, *23*, 253–259. [CrossRef]
39. Newman, P.J. The Biology of PECAM-1. *J. Clin. Investig.* **1997**, *99*, 3–8. [CrossRef]
40. Mei, H.; Campbell, J.M.; Paddock, C.M.; Lertkiatmongkol, P.; Mosesson, M.W.; Albrecht, R.; Newman, P.J. Regulation of Endothelial Cell Barrier Function by Antibody-Driven Affinity Modulation of Platelet Endothelial Cell Adhesion Molecule-1 (PECAM-1)*. *J. Biol. Chem.* **2014**, *289*, 20836–20844. [CrossRef]
41. Cao, G.; O'Brien, C.D.; Zhou, Z.; Sanders, S.M.; Greenbaum, J.N.; Makrigiannakis, A.; DeLisser, H.M. Involvement of Human PECAM-1 in Angiogenesis and in Vitro Endothelial Cell Migration. *Am. J. Physiol. Cell Physiol.* **2002**, *282*, C1181–C1190. [CrossRef]

42. Andreata, F.; Clément, M.; Benson, R.A.; Hadchouel, J.; Procopio, E.; Even, G.; Vorbe, J.; Benadda, S.; Ollivier, V.; Ho-Tin-Noe, B.; et al. CD31 Signaling Promotes the Detachment at the Uropod of Extravasating Neutrophils Allowing Their Migration to Sites of Inflammation. *Elife* **2023**, *12*, e84752. [CrossRef]
43. Kuriri, F.A.; O'Malley, C.J.; Jackson, D.E. Molecular Mechanisms of Immunoreceptors in Platelets. *Thromb. Res.* **2019**, *176*, 108–114. [CrossRef] [PubMed]
44. Pavlasova, G.; Mraz, M. The Regulation and Function of CD20: An "Enigma" of B-Cell Biology and Targeted Therapy. *Haematologica* **2020**, *105*, 1494–1506. [CrossRef] [PubMed]
45. Casan, J.M.L.; Wong, J.; Northcott, M.J.; Opat, S. Anti-CD20 Monoclonal Antibodies: Reviewing a Revolution. *Hum. Vaccin. Immunother.* **2018**, *14*, 2820–2841. [CrossRef]
46. Carlson, A.K.; Amin, M.; Cohen, J.A. Drugs Targeting CD20 in Multiple Sclerosis: Pharmacology, Efficacy, Safety, and Tolerability. *Drugs* **2024**, *84*, 285–304. [CrossRef]
47. Sun, L.; Su, Y.; Jiao, A.; Wang, X.; Zhang, B. T Cells in Health and Disease. *Signal Transduct. Target. Ther.* **2023**, *8*, 235. [CrossRef] [PubMed]
48. Zhen, A.; Krutzik, S.R.; Levin, B.R.; Kasparian, S.; Zack, J.A.; Kitchen, S.G. CD4 Ligation on Human Blood Monocytes Triggers Macrophage Differentiation and Enhances HIV Infection. *J. Virol.* **2014**, *88*, 9934–9946. [CrossRef]
49. Jardine, L.; Barge, D.; Ames-Draycott, A.; Pagan, S.; Cookson, S.; Spickett, G.; Haniffa, M.; Collin, M.; Bigley, V. Rapid Detection of Dendritic Cell and Monocyte Disorders Using CD4 as a Lineage Marker of the Human Peripheral Blood Antigen-Presenting Cell Compartment. *Front. Immunol.* **2013**, *4*, 495. [CrossRef]
50. Chen, H.; Sameshima, J.; Yokomizo, S.; Sueyoshi, T.; Nagano, H.; Miyahara, Y.; Sakamoto, T.; Fujii, S.; Kiyoshima, T.; Guy, T.; et al. Expansion of CD4+ Cytotoxic T Lymphocytes with Specific Gene Expression Patterns May Contribute to Suppression of Tumor Immunity in Oral Squamous Cell Carcinoma: Single-Cell Analysis and in Vitro Experiments. *Front. Immunol.* **2023**, *14*, 1305783. [CrossRef]
51. Eizenberg-Magar, I.; Rimer, J.; Zaretsky, I.; Lara-Astiaso, D.; Reich-Zeliger, S.; Friedman, N. Diverse Continuum of $CD4^+$ T-Cell States Is Determined by Hierarchical Additive Integration of Cytokine Signals. *Proc. Natl. Acad. Sci. USA* **2017**, *114*, E6447–E6456. [CrossRef]
52. Kruse, B.; Buzzai, A.C.; Shridhar, N.; Braun, A.D.; Gellert, S.; Knauth, K.; Pozniak, J.; Peters, J.; Dittmann, P.; Mengoni, M.; et al. $CD4^+$ T Cell-Induced Inflammatory Cell Death Controls Immune-Evasive Tumours. *Nature* **2023**, *618*, 1033–1040. [CrossRef]
53. Janeway, C.A., Jr.; Travers, P.; Walport, M.; Shlomchik, M.J. T Cell-Mediated Cytotoxicity. In *Immunobiology: The Immune System in Health and Disease*, 5th ed.; Garland Science: New York, NY, USA, 2001.
54. Schmidt, M.E.; Varga, S.M. The CD8 T Cell Response to Respiratory Virus Infections. *Front. Immunol.* **2018**, *9*, 678. [CrossRef] [PubMed]
55. Koh, C.-H.; Lee, S.; Kwak, M.; Kim, B.-S.; Chung, Y. CD8 T-Cell Subsets: Heterogeneity, Functions, and Therapeutic Potential. *Exp. Mol. Med.* **2023**, *55*, 2287–2299. [CrossRef] [PubMed]
56. Wang, K.; Shen, T.; Siegal, G.P.; Wei, S. The CD4/CD8 Ratio of Tumor-Infiltrating Lymphocytes at the Tumor-Host Interface Has Prognostic Value in Triple-Negative Breast Cancer. *Hum. Pathol.* **2017**, *69*, 110–117. [CrossRef] [PubMed]
57. Brummel, K.; Eerkens, A.L.; de Bruyn, M.; Nijman, H.W. Tumour-Infiltrating Lymphocytes: From Prognosis to Treatment Selection. *Br. J. Cancer* **2023**, *128*, 451–458. [CrossRef]
58. Buruiană, A.; Gheban, B.-A.; Gheban-Roșca, I.-A.; Georgiu, C.; Crișan, D.; Crișan, M. The Tumor Stroma of Squamous Cell Carcinoma: A Complex Environment That Fuels Cancer Progression. *Cancers* **2024**, *16*, 1727. [CrossRef]
59. Liu, Z.-L.; Chen, H.-H.; Zheng, L.-L.; Sun, L.-P.; Shi, L. Angiogenic Signaling Pathways and Anti-Angiogenic Therapy for Cancer. *Signal Transduct. Target. Ther.* **2023**, *8*, 198. [CrossRef]
60. Fukumura, D.; Kloepper, J.; Amoozgar, Z.; Duda, D.G.; Jain, R.K. Enhancing Cancer Immunotherapy Using Antiangiogenics: Opportunities and Challenges. *Nat. Rev. Clin. Oncol.* **2018**, *15*, 325–340. [CrossRef]
61. Bose, P.; Brockton, N.T.; Guggisberg, K.; Nakoneshny, S.C.; Kornaga, E.; Klimowicz, A.C.; Tambasco, M.; Dort, J.C. Fractal Analysis of Nuclear Histology Integrates Tumor and Stromal Features into a Single Prognostic Factor of the Oral Cancer Microenvironment. *BMC Cancer* **2015**, *15*, 409. [CrossRef]
62. Goutzanis, L.P.; Papadogeorgakis, N.; Pavlopoulos, P.M.; Petsinis, V.; Plochoras, I.; Eleftheriadis, E.; Pantelidaki, A.; Patsouris, E.; Alexandridis, C. Vascular Fractal Dimension and Total Vascular Area in the Study of Oral Cancer. *Head. Neck* **2009**, *31*, 298–307. [CrossRef]
63. Margaritescu, C.; Raica, M.; Pirici, D.; Simionescu, C.; Mogoanta, L.; Stinga, A.C.; Stinga, A.S.; Ribatti, D. Podoplanin Expression in Tumor-Free Resection Margins of Oral Squamous Cell Carcinomas: An Immunohistochemical and Fractal Analysis Study. *Histol. Histopathol.* **2010**, *25*, 701–711. [CrossRef]
64. Capasso, A.; Viggiano, D.; Lee, M.W.; Palladino, G.; Bilancio, G.; Simeoni, M.; Capolongo, G.; Secondulfo, C.; Ronchi, A.; Caputo, A.; et al. Kidney Transplant Modifies the Architecture and Microenvironment of Basal Cell Carcinomas. *Kidney Blood Press. Res.* **2020**, *45*, 368–377. [CrossRef] [PubMed]
65. Lookian, P.P.; Chen, E.X.; Elhers, L.D.; Ellis, D.G.; Juneau, P.; Wagoner, J.; Aizenberg, M.R. The Association of Fractal Dimension with Vascularity and Clinical Outcomes in Glioblastoma. *World Neurosurg.* **2022**, *166*, e44–e51. [CrossRef] [PubMed]
66. Koppensteiner, L.; Mathieson, L.; O'Connor, R.A.; Akram, A.R. Cancer Associated Fibroblasts—An Impediment to Effective Anti-Cancer T Cell Immunity. *Front. Immunol.* **2022**, *13*, 887380. [CrossRef] [PubMed]

67. Gorchs, L.; Fernández Moro, C.; Bankhead, P.; Kern, K.P.; Sadeak, I.; Meng, Q.; Rangelova, E.; Kaipe, H. Human Pancreatic Carcinoma-Associated Fibroblasts Promote Expression of Co-Inhibitory Markers on $CD4^+$ and $CD8^+$ T-Cells. *Front. Immunol.* **2019**, *10*, 847. [CrossRef]
68. Ford, K.; Hanley, C.J.; Mellone, M.; Szyndralewiez, C.; Heitz, F.; Wiesel, P.; Wood, O.; Machado, M.; Lopez, M.-A.; Ganesan, A.-P.; et al. NOX4 Inhibition Potentiates Immunotherapy by Overcoming Cancer-Associated Fibroblast-Mediated CD8 T-Cell Exclusion from Tumors. *Cancer Res.* **2020**, *80*, 1846–1860. [CrossRef]

fractal and fractional

MDPI

Article

Fractional Electrodamage in A549 Human Lung Cancer Cells

Hilario Martines-Arano [1,*], Jose Alberto Arano-Martinez [2], Manuel Alejandro Mosso-Pani [3], Alejandra Valdivia-Flores [3], Martin Trejo-Valdez [4], Blanca Estela García-Pérez [3] and Carlos Torres-Torres [2,*]

1 Escuela Superior Tepeji del Río, Universidad Autónoma del Estado de Hidalgo, Tepeji del Río de Ocampo 42860, Mexico
2 Sección de Estudios de Posgrado e Investigación, Escuela Superior de Ingeniería Mecánica y Eléctrica Unidad Zacatenco, Instituto Politécnico Nacional, Ciudad de México 07738, Mexico
3 Departamento de Microbiología, Escuela Nacional de Ciencias Biológicas, Instituto Politécnico Nacional, Ciudad de México 11340, Mexico
4 Escuela Superior de Ingeniería Química e Industrias Extractivas, Instituto Politécnico Nacional, Ciudad de México 07738, Mexico
* Correspondence: hilario_martines@uaeh.edu.mx (H.M.-A.); ctorrest@ipn.mx (C.T.-T.)

Abstract: Fractional electrodamage in A549 human lung cancer cells was analyzed by introducing a non-integer order parameter to model the influence of electrical stimulation on cellular behavior. Numerical simulations were conducted to evaluate the conversion of electrical energy to heat within A549 cancer cells, emphasizing the electrocapacitive effects and electrical conductivity in modulating dielectric properties. Using the Riemann–Liouville fractional calculus framework, experimental results were accurately fitted, demonstrating the non-integer nature of electrodamage processes. The study identified a strong dependency of electrical behavior on frequency, revealing a critical role of fractional dynamics in the dielectric breakdown and susceptibility of A549 cells to voltage changes. These findings advance our understanding of cellular responses to electrical fields and provide insights into applications in cancer diagnostics, monitoring, and potential therapeutic treatments.

Keywords: A549 cells; fractional calculus; fractional electrodamage; biological cells capacitance; electrical tolerance threshold

1. Introduction

Important applications in the treatment of cancer can be addressed through the study of consequences of exceeding cancer cell membrane potentials [1]. The concept of electrical power dissipation in biological cells, leading to heat generation, has been explored as an alternative for cancer treatment.

Data from several studies suggest that at the beginning of this decade, lung, prostate, and breast cancer were a globally leading cause of death [2]. Among the most-encountered forms of lung cancer are non-small cell lung carcinomas [3]. Carcinoma human alveolar basal epithelial cells (A549 cancer cells) have emerged as a prominent in vitro model for studying cancer. The key characteristics of A549 cells that make them suitable for this study include their established use as an in vitro model for non-small cell lung carcinoma and their distinct electrochemical properties, such as membrane capacitance and resistance. These properties allow analysis of the interactions in cells with electrical stimuli, making them ideal for exploring electrocapacitive effects and fractional electrodamage mechanisms.

Apoptosis results when electrical pulses that are administered to cancer cells provoke thermal damage to internal structures and cell membranes [4]; it is known as inhibition of proliferation on biological cells [5]. Healthy cells that are in the surrounding media are less sensitive to applied electrical pulses, avoiding significant damage.

For the purpose of acquiring knowledge about the electrical properties and electrochemical behavior of A549 cancer cells, researchers have used electrochemical impedance spectroscopy (EIS) [6]. As a method for observing and determining how cells react to various stimuli in diverse disciplines, such as medicine [7] and biology [8], EIS is widely used in these disciplines. In the context of cancer research, EIS represents a prominent option for exploring electrical features of A549 cancer cells such as resistance [9] and membrane capacitance [10]. Cyclic voltammetry (CV) is commonly considered as an essential instrument in electrochemistry. This approach is often used to explore and evaluate electrode performance while also offering insights into electron transport mechanisms. Electrical impulse transmission over biological cells membranes is responsible for electrical signal movement that comes from outside [11]. External stimulation and signal transduction in cells are caused by electrical signal propagation over cells, resulting in a change in the electrical potential in the cell membrane [12]. A capacitive effect can be observed in cells, due to the existence of cell membranes, and they can be considered as natural capacitors [13], due to their composition. Proteins and lipids are the main components in cell membranes, and electrical charges on opposite sides are segregated by these membranes [14]. The cells membranes work as a natural energy store of an electrical charge on cells surface when a change on voltage exists. This dynamic electrical energy store is provoked by a capacitive effect on cell membranes. These capacitive features have an important role in biological processes such as cellular communication and neural excitability [15]. Cells response to an external electrical signal depends on the nature of stimulation, for instance, the response time of nervous cells is measured in the order of milliseconds [16], and it can be faster than other cells. Parameters such as propagation distance synaptic cell connectivity and ion channel density have an important relationship with the cellular response time and bioelectrical reactions [16]. A frequency-dependent electrical signal changes biological processes in cells and tissues in response to stimulation. Slow muscular contractions can be registered at low frequencies, whereas faster contractions can be observed at higher frequencies [17]. Signal transmission in neurons is influenced by frequency dependence and neurotransmitter release. It is known that frequency dependence can influence and contribute to biological functions but its ability to control cellular responses and physiological systems based on the electrical signals properties is still limited [17].

In this direction, anomalous replication of cancer cells can be described by fractional differential equations, since fractional modeling provides a more accurate description for representation of dynamic processes. Fractional calculus can be used for modeling complex interactions between cancer cells replication and the growth rate. Cellular proliferation can be described by fractional calculus and modeling anomalous diffusion and movements patterns in cancer cells. Localized damage due to light exposition in cancer cells can be described by fractional photodamage as a technique for determining it. Deeper knowledge about fractional photodamage in A549 cancer cells has prominent importance in several areas of health such as cancer treatment optimization. On the other hand, fractional electrodamage can be used as a therapeutic approach that uses electrical currents to selectively eliminate cancer cells. Fractional electrodamage refers to the analysis of electrical damage in biological cells using fractional calculus; it incorporates non-integer order parameters to model accurately dynamic processes. In comparison with conventional electrodamage approaches, fractional electrodamage considers the frequency-dependent and non-linear electrical behavior of cells, providing a representation of electrocapacitive effects and dielectric breakdown mechanisms.

It is remarkable that the electrical response of cells can be regulated by electrical pulse duration, repetition rate, and strength [18].

Figure 1 shows a roadmap of progress in the field of studies related to fractional electrodamage in A549 cancer cells. From Figure 1 can be seen chronological progression from the initial investigation of electric fields and cancer cell behavior to more refined techniques for characterizing cancer cells, ultimately culminating in the specialized study of cancerous cell differentiation based on their biophysical phenotype.

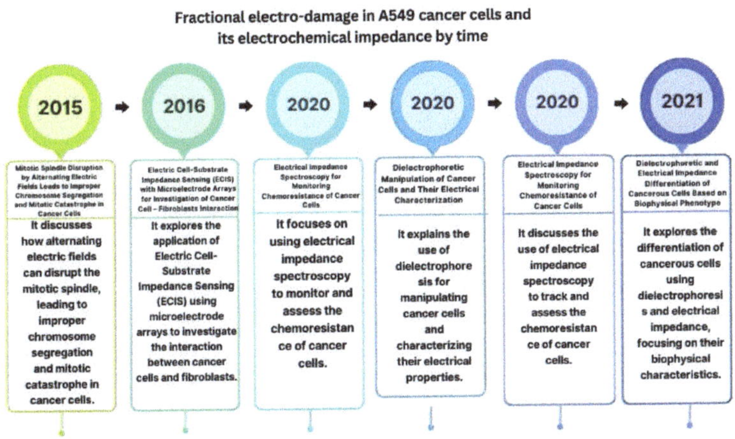

Figure 1. Roadmap describing the progress of the topic of study based on representative works. Refs. [19–24] for 2015–2021, respectively.

Past research has highlighted the role of material properties in enhancing therapeutic outcomes, particularly in targeting cancer cells while preserving healthy tissue [25]. These studies align with the present research by emphasizing the importance of precision and innovation in therapeutic approaches [26]. Incorporating these perspectives enriches the understanding of fractional electrodamage as a non-invasive, targeted method for cancer diagnostics and treatment, bridging materials science and biomedical applications. The present research surpasses prior studies by leveraging fractional calculus to model frequency-dependent dielectric breakdown mechanisms with unprecedented precision. It integrates experimental validation with the Riemann–Liouville framework, offering a significant advancement over conventional models in capturing the non-linear electrical behavior of A549 cancer cells.

In view of all these considerations, the main purpose of this study is to analyze physical mechanisms responsible for the fractional electrodamage exhibited by A549 cancer cells. The primary objective of studying fractional electrodamage in A549 human lung cancer cells is to analyze the physical mechanisms underlying the fractional dynamics of electrodamage induced by electrical stimulation. This has the purpose of enhancing the conception of the electrocapacitive properties of cancer cells and their susceptibility to voltage changes.

This study applies fractional calculus to model electrodamage in A549 lung cancer cells, emphasizing frequency-dependent dielectric breakdown. Using the Riemann–Liouville theory, it highlights the cancer cells' susceptibility to voltage changes and advances in non-invasive diagnostic and therapeutic methods, such as electrochemical hyperthermia.

We considered A549 cancer cell activities in the setting of lung carcinoma, underlying the response of these cells to electrical fields, enhancing the knowledge about electrocapacitive changes that can be related to cancer progression. It is considered that studies related to fractional electrodamage in cancer cells have prominent applications on biotechnology, drug delivery systems, and development of bioelectronic devices. It allows development of new therapeutic strategies such as pulsed electric current applications for inducing damage and inhibiting the growth of cancer cells. It highlighted the potential of monitoring cellular changes induced by electrical influence for assessing cancer cells response and different strategies in treatments.

2. Materials and Methods

2.1. Fractional Electrodamage in A549 Cancer Cells

With the purpose of calculating the impedance of the biological samples in a culture medium, we used the following equations [27]:

$$R_i = \rho_i \frac{l_i}{A}. \quad (1)$$

$$C_i = \frac{\varepsilon_0 \varepsilon_{ri} A}{l_i}. \quad (2)$$

where ρ_i is the resistivity of the material, ε_{ri} is the relative permittivity, ε_0 is the permittivity of the vacuum, A is the cross sectional area of the used Metrohm DS 220 AT electrode (the equipment was sourced from the Metrohm brand, Herisau, Switzerland), and the thickness of the culture medium drop is represented by l_i.

Considering that Z_i is the impedance of the drop and R_i is the resistance, we have [27]

$$Z_i = \frac{R_i(1 - j\omega C_i R_i)}{1 + \omega^2 C_i^2 R_i^2}. \quad (3)$$

where C_i is the capacitance in the system, j is the imaginary part, and ω is angular frequency.

On the other hand, with the purpose of modeling the numerical behavior of impedance and capacitance as a function of applied frequency for different concentration of cells we employed the Cole–Cole model. The total impedance can be expressed as follows [28]:

$$Z_T = R_s + \frac{R_p}{1 + (j\omega R_p C_p)^n}. \quad (4)$$

where R_p represents the resistance in the cells, C_p is the total capacitance on them, R_s denotes the total series resistance, and n represents the power order that most accurately fits the model obtained.

The numerical capacitance was calculated employing the Giaver theory. It describes the impedance between adherent cells and an electrode. The numerical capacitance can be considered as follows [29]:

$$C_{mem} = \frac{\varepsilon_0 \varepsilon_{ri}}{d_{mem}}. \quad (5)$$

where C_{mem} $\left[\mathrm{Fm}^{-2}\right]$ represents the capacitance of the cancer cells membrane per unit area. The permittivity of the vacuum is ε_0, ε_{mem} is the relative permittivity of the surrounding media, and d_{mem} represents the thickness of the cell membrane [29].

The imaginary part of the impedance can be described as follows [30]:

$$\lim_{\omega \to 0} [\omega \mathrm{Im}(Z)] = \frac{1}{C_{mem}}. \quad (6)$$

On the other hand, the real part was numerically calculated considering [30]:

$$\mathrm{Re}(Z) = \frac{\rho_i(0) L_{BULK}}{\rho_i l_i}. \quad (7)$$

where $\rho_i(0)$ denotes the resistivity at the center area of the cells, where the potential was applied, while L_{BULK} represents the distance half between two cancer cells [30].

With the intention of determining the electrodamage induced in A549 cancer cells, we used fractional calculus. To evaluate fractional electrodamage in A549 cancer cells, we introduce the concept of fractional calculus theory to effectively describe this phenomenon.

Fractional calculus and mathematical modeling techniques play a crucial role in this research because it provides a framework to describe the dynamic and non-linear behavior of A549 cancer cells under electrical stimulation. They enable simulations of electrical impedance and capacitance as functions of frequency, allowing for a better understanding of fractional electrodamage and its implications in cancer diagnostics and therapies.

Following the principles of the Riemann–Liouville fractional calculus operator theory, the integral of a function $f(t)$ of order α is defined as follows [31]:

$$\frac{d^{-\alpha}f(t)}{dt^{-\alpha}} = t_0D_t^{-\alpha}f(t) = \frac{1}{\Gamma(\alpha)}\int_{\alpha}^{t}(t-x)^{-\alpha-1}F(x)dx. \tag{8}$$

here, D in this context represents the antiderivative of α order, which is derived from the Cauchy formula. The parameter α signifies the order of the fractional derivative, and x indicates the elongation during the electrochemical changes in the A549 cancer cells. Additionally, t denotes the duration related to the experiment. For the purposes of this study, $\alpha = 0.8$ was selected as it provided the best fit to the experimental data.

In order to model interactions between historical and non-local properties in a process, we have employed the Caputo derivative formula. All these mathematical expressions are applied to calculate temperatures using a fractional approach, as explained in the Supplementary Material S1.

2.2. Cell Culture

A549 epithelial cells grown in culture bottles were detached using 2 mL of 0.05 g/L trypsin and 0.05 g/L EDTA solution (Sigma Aldrich, St. Louis, MO, USA). After, cell suspension was transferred to 15 mL conical tube and centrifuged at 1500 rpm during 5 min. The cell pellet was resuspended with 1 mL fresh culture medium and viable cells were quantified in a Neubauer chamber with 0.4% trypan blue solution. Then, the cell suspension was diluted with fresh medium to analyze three different concentrations of cells (125,000; 250,000; and 500,000 cells/60 µL). In order to observe the cells' morphology, the actin cytoskeleton was labeled with rhodamine-phalloidin, and nuclei were stained with DAPI (4′,6-diamidino-2-phenylindole). A confocal system coupled to an inverted microscope (LSM710 NLO Zeiss, Jena, Germany) was employed.

2.3. Electrochemical Impedance Analysis of A549 Cancer Cells: Frequency Response Study

Electrochemical investigations were carried out on biological samples of A549 cancer cells at a constant room temperature of 25 °C by triplicate. The cells contained in a drop of 60 µL were deposited in a Metrohm DS 220 AT electrode to measure their electrical response in an AUTOLAB 302N PGSTAT potentiostat (Metrohm, Herisau, Switzerland). An Ag/AgCl reference electrode and a platinum counter electrode were employed for experimentation [32]. The supporting electrolyte used was a 0.5 M KOH solution, which was pre-treated by degassing in an ultrasonic bath for 15 min and subsequent bubbling with nitrogen gas for 10 min. Data analyses were performed by using MATLAB software (R2023a) to extract meaningful information. From Figure 2a is possible to observe a representative photo of the studied A549 cancer cells located in the electrode. From

Figure 2b is possible to visualize the connections of the Metrohm DS 220 AT electrode: A Metrohm electrode, specifically the DS 220 AT model, was used.

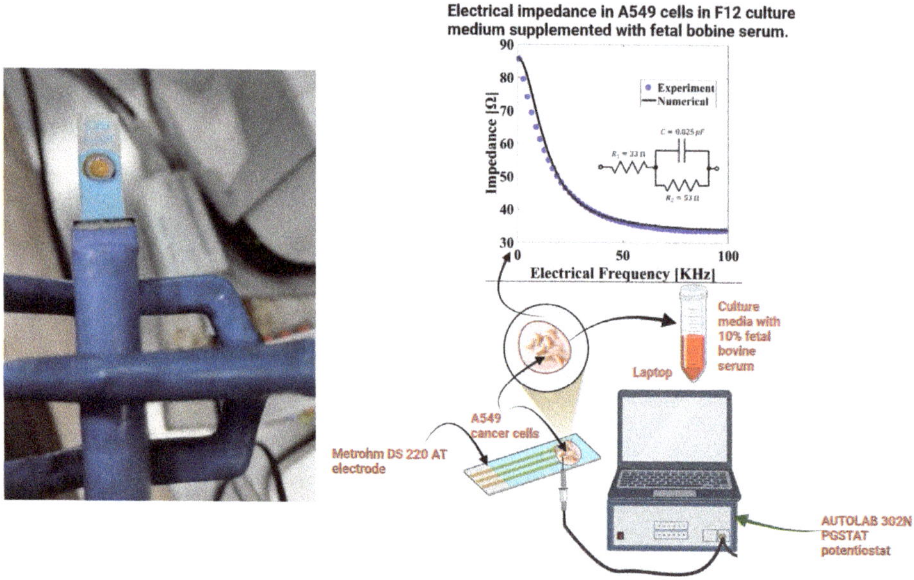

(a) (b)

Figure 2. (**a**) A549 cancer cells measured and deposited in the Metrohm DS 220 AT electrode; cancer cells were integrated into the drop using an electronic pipette, allowing precise control over the placement of cells. (**b**) Scheme of the experimental setup.

2.4. Apoptosis and Cell Viability in A549 Cells Through Electrical Stimulation and Flow Cytometry Analysis

Apoptosis and cell viability experiments were undertaken in order to guarantee changes in the cellular structure as part of the experimental procedure in our model. A549 cells were cultured in F-12 medium supplemented with 8% fetal bovine serum (FBS), 1% penicillin-streptomycin, and maintained at 37 °C in a humidified atmosphere containing 5% CO_2. Cells were subcultured every 3–4 days to maintain exponential growth. An electrical circuit for inducing electrical current in a suspension of 2.5×10^5 A549 cells prepared in a 96-well plate with 50 µL of culture media. The electrodamage stimulus was maintained for different time periods (0, 5, 10, 20, 30, 60, and 120 s). Following treatment, cells were immediately analyzed for membrane integrity and cell viability. Membrane integrity was evaluated using a trypan blue exclusion assay. Cells were mixed with an equal volume of 0.3% trypan blue solution and incubated for 5 min at room temperature. Cells with compromised membrane integrity were identified by their ability to uptake the trypan blue stain, whereas viable cells remained unstained. Photographs of stained cells were taken to document the results. Apoptosis and cell viability were assessed using flow cytometry with annexin V-FITC and propidium iodide (PI) staining. Following electrodamage treatment, cells were resuspended in annexin V binding buffer and stained with annexin V-FITC and PI according to the manufacturer's instructions (Cat. No. 640914, Biolegend, San Diego, CA, USA). The stained cells were then analyzed using a flow cytometer (FACSAria II, BD Bioscience, San Jose, CA, USA). Data were collected and analyzed using the FlowJo v.10 software to determine the percentage of live, early apoptotic, and necrotic cells. Live cells were identified as annexin V and PI negative (Q4), early apoptotic cells as annexin V positive and PI negative (Q1), and necrotic cells as annexin V and PI positive (Q2). The results are presented as the percentage of 10,000 cells collected. All experiments were performed in duplicate, and data were expressed as mean ± standard deviation. Comparisons between experimental conditions were performed using one-way ANOVA followed by Tukey's post hoc test. A p-value of <0.05 was considered statistically significant. GraphPad Prism software v.8 was used for all statistical analyses and graph generation.

To ensure the observed effects were specifically attributable to electrodamage, experiments were conducted with negative controls, including samples that did not receive electrical stimuli. These controls allowed for a baseline comparison, verifying those changes in cell viability, membrane integrity, and other parameters were a direct result of the applied electrical stimulation.

Figure 3 illustrates the sample in contact with the electrodes.

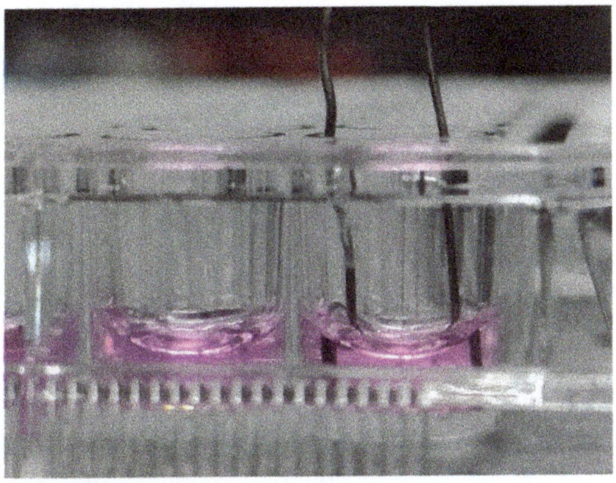

Figure 3. A549 cancer cells with an electrical current induced by metallic electrodes located along a diameter of the well.

3. Results

Figure 4 shows a confocal image of studied A549 cancer cells. From the images can be seen A549 cells with actin filaments distributed longitudinally in the cytoplasm. In order to contrast, the nuclei of cells were stained with DAPI (4′,6-diamidino-2-phenylindole) and were detected in blue emission. The purpose of using fluorescence was to observe the complex details and structure of the cellular components. Figure 5 combines red fluorescence for the actin cytoskeleton and blue fluorescence for the cell nuclei, providing a comprehensive and visually striking representation of the cellular morphology.

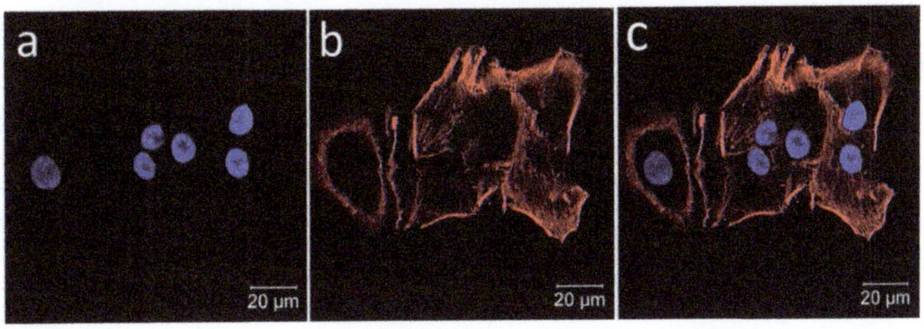

Figure 4. Confocal image of the representative A549 human lung epithelial cancer cells studied; (**a**) nuclei of individual cells in blue; (**b**) typical actin filaments were stained with rhodamine-phalloidin (red), and its longitudinal distributions are show; (**c**) merge of two tracks (red and blue). All figures at 40X.

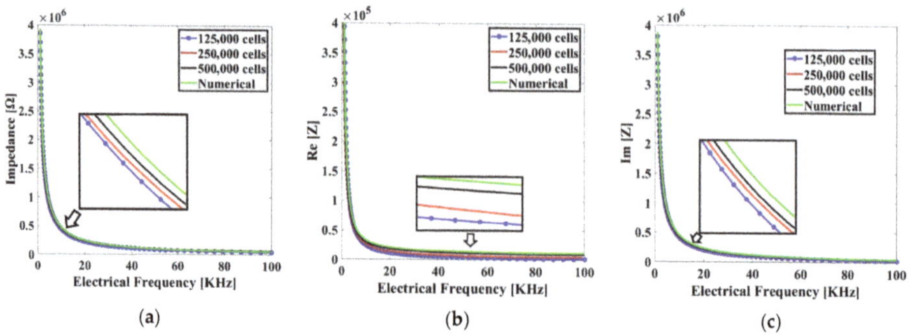

Figure 5. (**a**) Numerical and experimental results of electrical impedance as a function of frequency for varying cell concentrations in a drop, with clear labels highlighting the trends. (**b**) Real part of the measured electrical impedance with distinct legends emphasizing differences across frequencies. (**c**) Imaginary part of the measured electrical impedance, with annotations to aid in interpreting the observed variations.

For measuring the electrical response as a function of frequency in the A549 cancer cells, they were prepared under controlled conditions in order to ensure a uniform cell population. Later, the cells were exposed to electrical impulses. We induced a range of electric frequency parameters that were known to provoke electrodamage with voltage signals around 200 mV [33]. According to the literature it is sufficient to disrupt the cell membrane, inducing changes without causing cell death [33].

Figure 5a, represents the experimental impedance of A549 cancer cells for different cells concentrations. It must be mentioned that this measurement was conducted for three different cell concentrations: 126,000 cells, 250,000 cells, and 480,000 cells. Figure 5b,c presents the numerical and experimental calculation of the real and imaginary parts of impedance as a function of frequency of the samples; a numerical simulation for the ideal behavior is included. Using fractional calculus for the simulation of electrical impedance seems to be necessary for accurate modeling, it is well known that cells exhibit non-linear behavior that fractional models can solve effectively. On the other hand, fractional calculus allows a precise characterization of the frequency-dependent development of impedance and capacitance. Fractional calculus enables a better simulation of differences between different concentrations of cells, due to its better accuracy and reliability.

The real and imaginary parts of the impedance of A549 cancer cells at different electrical frequencies are plotted in Figure 5b,c, which suggests that the cells have capacitive properties, primarily associated with their cell membranes. Different fractional calculus theories, such as Riemann–Liouville, Caputo, and Grünwald–Letnikov, were considered with the purpose of determining the best fit with the experimental results. We used the Riemann–Liouville fractional-order derivative because it provides a precise framework for modeling the dynamic, non-linear, and frequency-dependent behavior of A549 cancer cells under electrical stimulation. It enables accurate fitting of experimental data, particularly in capturing the electrocapacitive effects and dielectric breakdown mechanisms, outperforming other fractional calculus theories.

MATLAB was used to perform all numerical simulations presented in the document, including those corresponding to Figure 5.

For further investigation of the electrochemical behavior of the cells, a sample was heuristically diluted in order to easily visualize the capacitive effect in the samples. Figure 6a shows electrical impedance measurements and Figure 6b shows the electrical capacitance. In Figure 6a the experimental determination of the impedance is represented by the black line. A numerical estimation was performed, depicted by the blue line. The fractional behavior was determined, and it is shown by the red dotted line at a value of $\alpha = 0.60$. We employed the Grünwald–Letnikov method, illustrated by the green dotted line with $\lambda = 0.75$. Additionally, the Riemann–Liouville (R-L) parameter was used, indicated by the yellow dot at $\hbar = 0.80$, and the Caputo parameter is shown by the brown dotted line. It was observed that the Riemann–Liouville fractional calculus theory provided the best fit to the experimental results. This implies that, among the considered fractional calculus approaches, the Riemann–Liouville theory most accurately describes the behavior of capacitance of A549 cancer cells based on the experimental data.

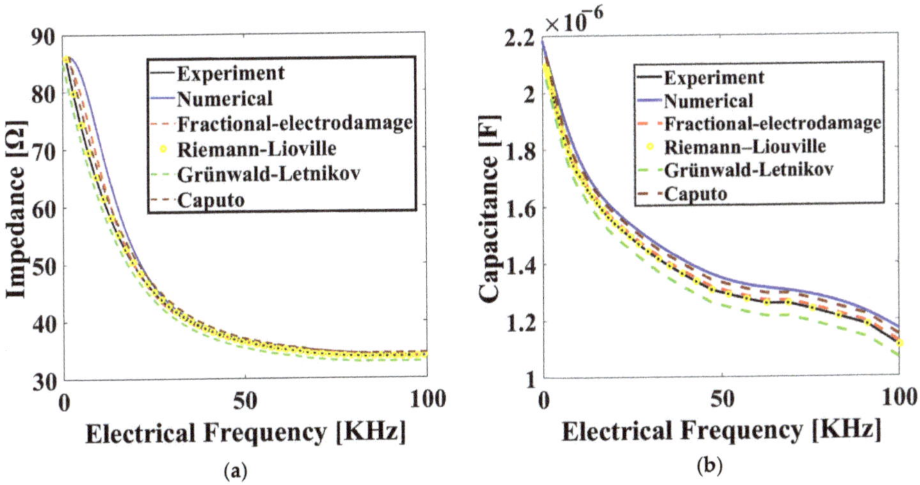

Figure 6. Comparison of experimental and numerical data for: (**a**) electrical impedance of the studied samples, and (**b**) capacitance of A549 cancer cells.

The changes in impedance and capacitance with varying cell concentrations are primarily due to the increased number of cell membranes acting as capacitive elements and the altered distribution for current flow in the suspension. A capacitance behavior is a measure related to the ability of a system to store electrical charge, and its decrease with electrical frequency. These effects are more pronounced as the concentration increases, showing a clear trend that can be explained by the cumulative impact of the cell's electrical properties and their interactions within the culture medium. For example, when the concentration of cancer cells was quadrupled to 500,000 cells, the close distribution of them reduced the resistance path making easier the current flow.

Experimentation indicates that damage to A549 human lung cancer cells by modulated voltage easily occurs at a higher frequency range since cells show an adverse response or suffer damage under voltage modulated applications. Identification of this fractional capacitive condition provides valuable information for understanding the frequency limits that affect the viability or behavior of A549 cells in the context of electrical experimentation.

The error in the numerical fit relative to the fractional fit to describe the electrical behavior of the sample refers to the discrepancies between the fractional model predictions and the actual values measured during experiments.

The challenges encountered in the study included ensuring the accuracy of experimental measurements and achieving reliable simulations of fractional electrodamage. These were addressed by using validated experimental setups, such as electrochemical impedance spectroscopy, and employing robust mathematical modeling techniques like the Riemann–Liouville fractional calculus theory. Additionally, repeated trials and statistical analyses ensured the reproducibility and reliability of the results.

The calculated error bar was ±2.5%, this shows the extent of the deviation between model predictions and experimental observations. As it can be considered, the percentage error is low; this indicates a close correspondence between the fractional model and the experimental data.

Figure 7 represents the heating induced by electrical signals in A549 cancer cells as a function of electrical frequency and voltage change for different cancer cells concentrations. The x-axis displays the electrical frequency ranging from 0 to 100 KHz, while the y-axis shows the voltage change from 100 mV to 200 mV. The color intensity in the heat map indicates the level of electrodamage, with darker colors representing higher damage levels and lighter colors indicating lower damage levels. The distribution of the electrodamage is linear, reflecting a proportional increase in damage with increasing frequency and voltage change. This visualization helps to identify the conditions under which the cells experience the most significant electrodamage.

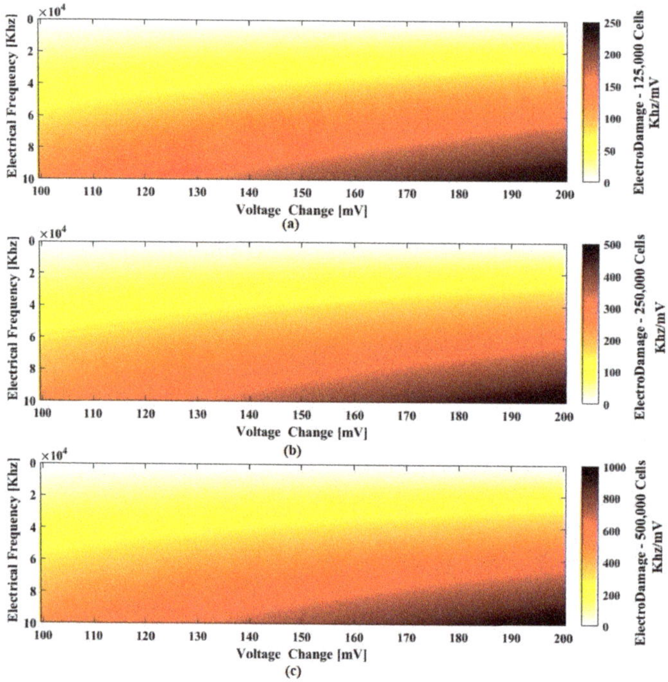

Figure 7. Heat map showing the electrodamage in A549 cancer cells as a function of electrical frequency (0–100 KHz) and voltage change (100–200 mV), for different cells concentration. The color intensity represents the level of electrodamage, with darker colors indicating higher damage levels. This linear distribution illustrates how electrodamage increases proportionally with higher frequencies and greater voltage changes. (**a**) Shows electrodamage as a function of applied voltage and electrical frequency, with a maximum electrodamage of 250 kHz/mV for 125,000 cells. (**b**) Displays a maximum electrodamage of 500 kHz/mV for 250,000 cells. (**c**) Exhibits a maximum electrodamage of 1000 kHz/mV for 500,000 cells.

In Figure 7, each subplot represents the relationship between electrical frequency (x-axis) and voltage change (y-axis) for a specific cell concentration. The z-axis represents the electrical damage caused. The color intensity on the surface of each subplot indicates the level of electrical damage. Each subplot is labeled with the corresponding cell concentration in the title, and the axes are labeled with the respective units.

Figure 8 provides a visual representation of how electrical frequency and voltage change affect the electrodamage for different cell concentrations. As the frequency increases, the membrane resistance decreases; it makes the cell more permeable to electrical currents. Higher frequencies and voltages both increase the electrodamage in cells.

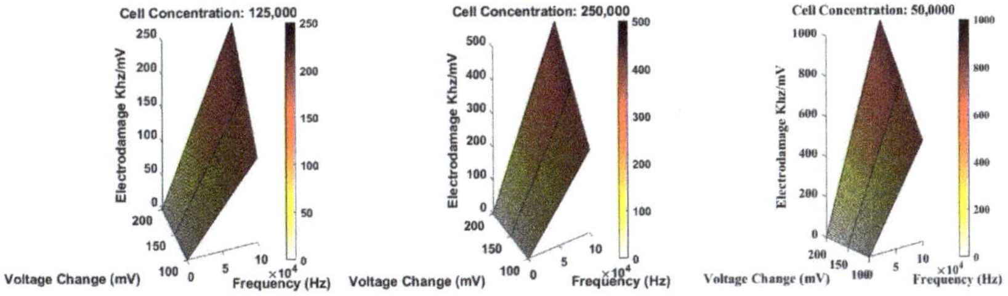

Figure 8. Variation in electrodamage as a function of electrical frequency and voltage change for different concentrations of cancerous cells.

Figure 9a represents the conversion of electrical energy to heat within cancer cells. For calculating the heat distribution within the A549 cancer cells and to evaluate processes in which electrical energy is converted into heat inside A549 cancer cells, we used the following formulas [34]:

$$Q = \int_0^{pw} \left(I_0 e^{\frac{-t}{RC}} \right)^2 R dt = \frac{CR^2 I_0^2}{2} \left(1 - e^{\frac{-2pw}{RC}} \right) = \frac{CV_0^2}{2} \left(1 - e^{\frac{-2pw}{RC}} \right). \tag{9}$$

$$Z = Z_0(1 + \varphi(T - T_0)). \tag{10}$$

where Q represents the heat generated in joules (J), t is the time exposition in seconds, R denotes the cancer cells' resistance at the experimental stage, pw is the electrical signal pulsed width, I_0 and V_0 are the peak current and voltage, C is the cancer cells capacitance, Z represents the cancer cells impedance, Z_0 denotes the cancer cells impedance at temperature T_0, φ is the temperature coefficient of resistivity in A549 cancer cells, and $(T - T_0)$ represents the change in temperature at the experiment stage. We decided to modify Equation (6), changing impedance instead of resistance, because electrical impedance was in function of electrical frequency.

Figure 9b describes the relationship between voltage applied and heat that originates inside cancer cells, which is governed by Joule law. The electrical resistance of the cells is considered. Where the change in voltage, $(T - T_0)$, was from 100 mV to 200 mV, the time, t, was considered from 0 to 30 s, the R resistance of A549 cells was 110 ohms, the capacitance C was 10 nanofarads, the peak current, I_0, was 3 mA, the pulsed width, pw, was considered as 10 milliseconds, the peak voltage, V_0, was 150 mV, and the temperature coefficient of resistivity, φ, was 0.0040 ohms [34].

The error bar associated with the measurement of the change in temperature and electrical conversion into heat in A549 cancer cells during the experimentation was calculated at about ±5%. It is important to mention that all the experiments reported in this article were performed 10 times, in order to guarantee repeatability and reliability in the measurements.

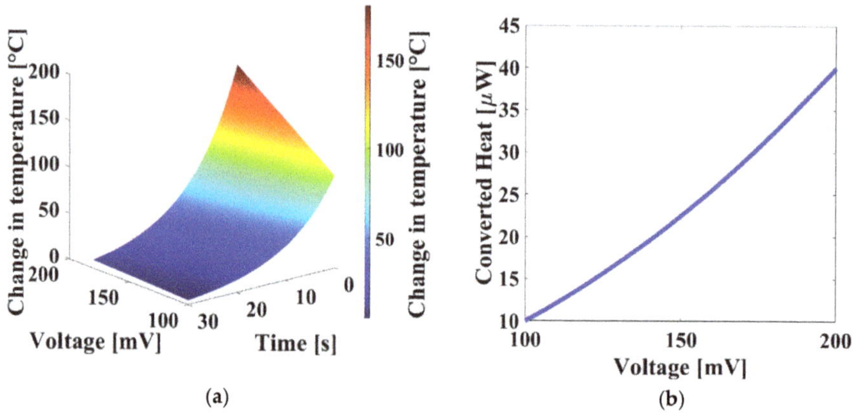

Figure 9. Change in temperature and electrical conversion into heat within A549 cancer cells. (**a**) Change in temperature representation inside A549 cancer cells. (**b**) Voltage and converted heat magnitude for electrical energy when it is converted into heat within biological cells.

In order to experimentally confirm the electrodamage effect on the membrane integrity and cell viability of A549 cells, cells in suspension were exposed to electrical current. Trypan blue staining allowed determination of the effect of stimulus on membrane integrity.

A significant reduction in membrane integrity was observed after 20 s of treatment, which was evidenced by the increase in the number of cells that were capable of uptaking the stain as can be observed in Figure 10.

Since a significant reduction in cell viability was noted after 30, 60, and 120 s of treatment, the fate of these cells was analyzed through an apoptosis assay, which identified apoptotic and necrotic cells.

The results are presented as the percentage of 10,000 cells collected in gate corresponding to A549 cells (Supplementary Material S2). This assay revealed a significant increase in apoptosis and cellular necrosis after 60 and 120 s, as can be observed in Figure 4, indicated that cell death was in progress. These findings highlight the impact of electrodamage on the viability and membrane integrity of A549 cells, with significant effects observed at specific time points, showing the induction of early apoptosis and the cell death by a necrosis process.

The observed effects of fractional electrodamage on A549 cells included significant reductions in cell viability, alterations in membrane integrity, and morphological changes indicative of apoptosis and necrosis. The experiments showed a strong dependence of electrodamage on electrical frequency and voltage, with higher frequencies and voltages causing more pronounced effects. These findings highlight the susceptibility of A549 cells to fractional electrodamage, providing critical insights into their metabolic and structural responses to electrical stimulation.

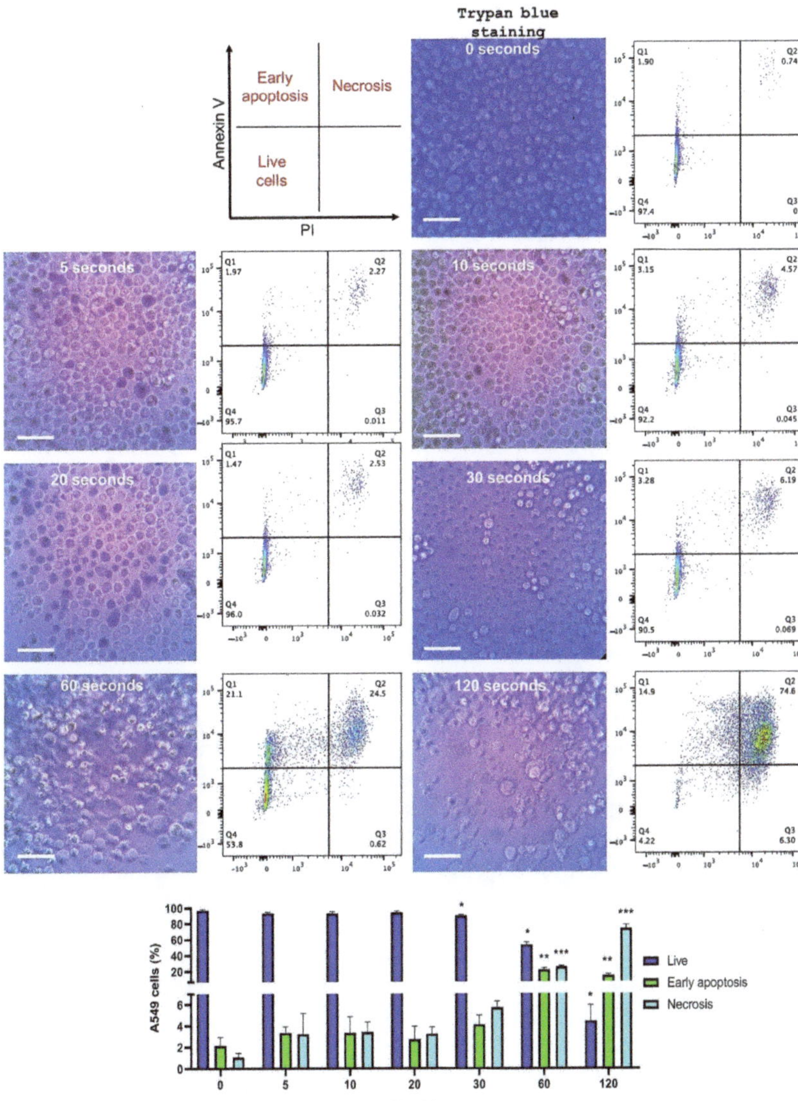

Figure 10. Effect of electrodamage on membrane integrity and viability of A549 cells. Blue cells in photographs represent the uptake of trypan blue staining by cells with compromised membrane integrity. Dot blots show the results for the apoptosis assay. The results are presented as the percentage of 10,000 cells. Live cells are found in quadrant 4 (Q4; Annexin V and PI negative), early apoptotic cells are indicated in Q1 (Annexin V positive and PI negative), dead cells by necrosis are demonstrated in Q2 (Annexin V and PI positive). The colors represent the collection of cells with the same intensity detected during flow cytometry, with blue representing low intensity (single cells) and red representing high intensity. Statistical analysis was conducted, with graphs representing the mean of two independent experiments with standard deviation. Comparisons between experimental conditions were performed using one-way ANOVA followed by Tukey's post hoc test (* indicates a p-value of <0.05 vs. time 0 living cells condition; ** indicates a p-value of <0.001 vs. time 0 early apoptosis condition; *** indicates a p-value of <0.001 vs. time 0 necrosis condition). Scale bars = 20 μm.

4. Discussion

Electrical behavior in suspended cells exhibits a clear frequency dependence, with reported capacitance inversely proportional to the applied frequency [35]. The cells can influence the ability of a biological system to store electrical charge due to their electrical and morphological properties [36]. The variation in capacitance at different frequencies reflects dynamic interactions between cancer cells and electrodes, offering a valuable perspective on their electrochemical behavior [37]. The culture medium influenced the electrical response. It affected electrical conductivity, dielectric properties, ionic composition, and the interaction between cells and the medium [38]. Changes in the medium due to cell growth, ion concentrations, and cell viability impacted the electrical response [39]. The potential impact of discovering the dominant fractional electrical response in cell measurements is significant. It enhanced our ability to monitor and assess the effects of different treatments or environmental conditions on cells [40]. The cells possess mechanisms to convert an electrical stimulus into a cellular response, involving substantial changes in the cell membrane. For example, allowing the entry of ions, such as sodium, which is responsible for changing the electrical potential in the region where the stimulus is received [41]. Various biological functions in cells are activated when the propagation of a voltage signal passes through their membrane [42]. An example of this is cell communication, which occurs when cells are able to transmit information through electrical signals to other cells that are around; this is essential for the coordination of functions in tissues and organs [43]. The permeability of cell membranes also facilitates ionic regulation, playing a crucial role in neurotransmitter secretion and cellular excitability [44]. Another event that occurs when an external voltage signal is applied to the cells is that it is responsible for using this signal to regulate the internal balance between ions and nutrients, thus, helping the control, cell survival, and adaptation of cells to their environment [45]. The maximum that a cell can withstand depends on the type of cell it is, as well as its physiological state. There is no single value that is applicable to all cells since they have different electrical properties and tolerances depending on the cell type. However, cell membrane potentials are of the order of 100 millivolts (mV), but if they exceed 200 mV, a dielectric breakdown within the biological cell could be reported, thus, forming arcs inside the cell [33]. In brain neurons, the resting membrane potential of these neurons usually registers in the range of −60 to −70 mV [46]. Drastic changes in voltage inside the cells could cause irreparable damage, such as undesirable cellular responses like apoptosis and cell lysis [47]. The electric current used to produce a killing effect on a cancer cell can be described by controlled application of electric current through electrodes placed near or within an affected tissue with cancer cells [48]. Electrochemical damage or electroporation involves cell membrane disruption caused by high voltage application [49]. It causes pores in the cell membrane and eventually cell death when the voltage is sufficiently high [49]. However, the electroporation can be reversible according to the magnitude and duration of the electrical stimulation in some cases when the voltage is moderate and a short exposition the damage is reversible [50]. On the other hand, prolonged exposures to high voltage cause an irreversible damage to cells, generating apoptosis [51]. Furthermore, this can be achieved by a pulsed electric current of low intensity and high frequency applied through the electrodes. The pulsed electric current causes a phenomenon called electroporation in the cell membrane of the cancer cell. During electroporation, pores in the cell membrane are temporarily opened, allowing molecules to enter that would not normally be able to enter [47]. The combination of the pulsed electric current and therapeutic agents inside the cancer cell can damage it and cause its death or inhibition of growth, thus, contributing to the destruction of the cancer. Electrical power dissipation in a cell occurs when an electrical current flows through the cell due to an applied potential difference. For instance, biological cells convert electrical energy into other types of energy such as heat during power dissipation [52]. It can be explained by the result of electrical resistance of structural components in cells such as ion channels and cell membranes. Because of the intrinsic resistance of the cell, a part of the electrical energy flowing through it is converted to heat [53]. Some other mechanisms for generation of heat in cells occur in the electrical signals propagated in nerve cells [54]. The voltage threshold for damage varies with frequency; at lower frequencies, higher voltage is required to provoke damage due to greater membrane resistance [55]. At lower frequency the cell membrane resists electrical current more, so it is necessary to have higher voltage application to provoke damage [55]. A critical frequency was identified around 90,000 Hz; here the membrane is susceptible to dielectric breakdown. In this study, the primary type of cellular damage observed is dielectric breakdown, where the cell membrane loses its integrity due to high voltage and frequency, leading to cell death [56,57]. Other potential types of damage include plasmolysis, which would require specific staining techniques and microscopy to identify [57]. To determine different types of damage, various assays such as live staining, electron microscopy, and biochemical markers for cell integrity and apoptosis would be needed [58]. In areas such as medicine, cells biology, and biotechnology, information that we have described is crucial for developing therapeutic approaches, diagnostics, and research.

This study advances existing work by focusing on the fractional electrodamage mechanism, explaining its frequency-dependent nature and the relevance of fractional modeling in predicting cellular responses to electrical stimulation. Different fractional calculus theories, such as Riemann–Liouville, Caputo, and Grünwald–Letnikov, were considered with the purpose of determining the best fit with the experimental results. It was observed that the Riemann–Liouville fractional calculus theory provided the best fit to the experimental data, suggesting a better fit in modeling the fractional electrodamage processes. This finding contrasts with past published studies where alternative approaches and tests were applied. Results did not achieve the same level of precision in capturing the frequency-dependent electrocapacitive behavior of A549 cancer cells.

The proposed exploration method leverages fractional calculus to model the electrodamage of A549 cancer cells, providing a better accuracy in capturing frequency-dependent and non-linear electrical behaviors. This method enables more precise simulations of electrocapacitive responses and dielectric breakdown, facilitating real-time monitoring.

The potential advantages of using fractional electrodamage over existing cancer treatment modalities include its ability to precisely target cancer cells by leveraging frequency-dependent electrical stimulation, minimizing damage to surrounding healthy tissue. The fractional approach enables a more accurate modeling of cellular responses. It offers real-time monitoring of cellular changes and provides a non-invasive platform for combining with other anticancer therapies.

The experiments were conducted at a fixed temperature of 25 °C and within specific voltage and frequency range to ensure controlled and reproducible conditions. While these parameters optimize experimental accuracy, they limit the direct applicability of findings to varied physiological or clinical environments where temperature and electrical conditions may fluctuate. Future studies should explore a broader range of conditions to enhance generalizability. In future research, nonlinearities in biological responses, such as thresholds for apoptosis or necrosis, will be considered to enhance the analysis of electrodamage. Although statistical tools like ANOVA were employed in this study to analyze experimental data, incorporating more robust statistical methods, such as effect size or regression analysis, could offer deeper insights into the relationships between voltage, frequency, and cellular damage. These approaches would enhance the interpretation of the results by quantifying the strength and nature of these interactions, providing a more comprehensive understanding of the underlying mechanisms.

To enhance its biological relevance, future analyses could explore how this heat generation correlates with known thermal thresholds for cancer cell death. Establishing these correlations would provide a clearer understanding of the role of heat in the electrodamage process.

This will address the current simplification of linear damage trends and provide a more accurate representation of the relationship between voltage, frequency, and biological outcomes.

5. Conclusions

This study demonstrates that fractional electrodamage effectively models the dynamic electrical behavior of A549 cancer cells, highlighting the frequency-dependent nature of dielectric breakdown. The use of the Riemann–Liouville fractional calculus theory offers unparalleled precision in simulating electrocapacitive responses, enabling the identification of key thresholds for cellular damage. These findings open new opportunities for advancing cancer diagnostics and therapies, particularly through non-invasive, targeted techniques such as electrochemical hyperthermia and electroporation. The integration of experimental data with robust mathematical modeling underscores the potential of fractional approaches to revolutionize cancer treatment by minimizing harm to healthy tissues while enhancing therapeutic efficacy. The novel aspects of this work include the application of fractional calculus to model electrodamage in A549 lung cancer cells, revealing a frequency-dependent dielectric breakdown mechanism. This study incorporates non-integer order mathematical modeling with experimental validations, pointing out the superior accuracy of the Riemann–Liouville theory compared to other fractional approaches. This work not only advances our understanding of cell–electrical interactions but also sets the stage for innovative applications in biotechnology and precision medicine.

Supplementary Materials: The following supporting information can be downloaded at: https://www.mdpi.com/article/10.3390/fractalfract9010034/s1. Supplementary Material S1: Fractional Description; Supplementary Material S2: Gating Strategy for the Apoptosis Assay. References [31,57,59] are cited in Supplementary Materials.

Author Contributions: H.M.-A.: writing—original draft, writing—review and editing, investigation; J.A.A.-M.: writing—review and editing, investigation; M.A.M.-P.: writing—review and editing, investigation; A.V.-F.: writing—review and editing, investigation; M.T.-V.: writing—review and editing, investigation; B.E.G.-P.: writing—review and editing, investigation; C.T.-T.: writing—review and editing, investigation, conceptualization. All authors have read and agreed to the published version of the manuscript.

Funding: Instituto Politécnico Nacional (SIP-2024) and Consejo Nacional de Humanidades Ciencias y Tecnologías CONAHCyT (CF-2023-I-2042) and through postdoctoral grant 2624226.

Data Availability Statement: Data and materials are available upon reasonable request to Carlos Torres-Torres (ctorrest@ipn.mx).

Acknowledgments: The authors kindly acknowledge to Instituto Politécnico Nacional, Universidad Autónoma del Estado de Hidalgo, Escuela Superior Tepeji del Río, and Consejo Nacional de Humanidades Ciencias y Tecnologías. The authors are also thankful to the Central Microscopy facilities of the CNMN-IPN.

Conflicts of Interest: The authors declare that they have no known competing financial interests or personal relationships that could have appeared to influence the work reported in this paper.

References

1. Akinlaja, J.; Sachs, F. The breakdown of cell membranes by electrical and mechanical stress. *Biophys. J.* **1998**, *75*, 247–254. [CrossRef] [PubMed]
2. Siegel, R.L.; Miller, K.D.; Jemal, A. Cancer statistics, 2020. *CA Cancer J. Clin.* **2020**, *70*, 7–30. [CrossRef] [PubMed]
3. Padinharayil, H.; Varghese, J.; John, M.C.; Rajanikant, G.K.; Wilson, C.M.; Al-Yozbaki, M.; Renu, K.; Dewanjee, S.; Sanyal, R.; Dey, A.; et al. Non-small cell lung carcinoma (NSCLC): Implications on molecular pathology and advances in early diagnostics and therapeutics. *Genes Dis.* **2023**, *10*, 960–989. [CrossRef]
4. Bhosale, P.B.; Kim, H.H.; Abusaliya, A.; Jeong, S.H.; Park, M.Y.; Kim, G.S. Inhibition of cell proliferation and cell death by apigetrin through death receptor-mediated pathway in hepatocellular cancer cells. *Biomolecules* **2023**, *13*, 1131. [CrossRef] [PubMed]
5. Perez-Fidalgo, J.A. Cell proliferation inhibitors and apoptosis promoters. *EJC Suppl.* **2020**, *15*, 73–76. [CrossRef] [PubMed]
6. Crowell, L.; Yakisich, J.; Aufderheide, B.; Adams, T. Electrical impedance spectroscopy for monitoring chemoresistance of cancer cells. *Micromachines* **2020**, *11*, 832. [CrossRef]
7. Chen, Z.-B.; Jin, H.-H.; Yang, Z.-G.; He, D.-P. Recent advances on bioreceptors and metal nanomaterials-based electrochemical impedance spectroscopy biosensors. *Rare Met.* **2023**, *42*, 1098–1117. [CrossRef]
8. Krukiewicz, K. Electrochemical impedance spectroscopy as a versatile tool for the characterization of neural tissue: A mini review. *Electrochem. Commun.* **2020**, *116*, 106742. [CrossRef]
9. Huerta-Nuñez, L.F.E.; Gutierrez-Iglesias, G.; Martinez-Cuazitl, A.; Mata-Miranda, M.M.; Golberg, A.; González-Díaz, C.A. A biosensor capable of identifying low quantities of breast cancer cells by electrical impedance spectroscopy. *Sci. Rep.* **2019**, *9*, 6419. [CrossRef]
10. Turcan, I.; Caras, I.; Schreiner, T.G.; Tucureanu, C.; Salageanu, A.; Olariu, M.A. Dielectrophoretic and electrical impedance differentiation of cancerous cells based on biophysical phenotype. *Biosensors* **2021**, *11*, 401. [CrossRef]
11. Elmslie, K.S. Passive propagation of electrical signals. In *eLS*; Wiley: Hoboken, NJ, USA, 2021; pp. 1–7.
12. Hagihara, T.; Toyota, M. Mechanical signaling in the sensitive plant *Mimosa pudica* L. *Plants* **2020**, *9*, 587. [CrossRef]
13. Brosseau, C.; Sabri, E. Resistor–capacitor modeling of the cell membrane: A multiphysics analysis. *J. Appl. Phys.* **2021**, *129*, 011101. [CrossRef]
14. Liang, W.; Zhao, Y.; Liu, L.; Wang, Y.; Li, W.J.; Lee, G.-B. Determination of cell membrane capacitance and conductance via optically induced electrokinetics. *Biophys. J.* **2017**, *113*, 1531–1539. [CrossRef] [PubMed]
15. Harris, M.P. Bioelectric signaling as a unique regulator of development and regeneration. *Development* **2021**, *148*, dev180794. [CrossRef]
16. Stratford, J.P.; Edwards, C.L.A.; Ghanshyam, M.J.; Malyshev, D.; Delise, M.A.; Asally, M. Electrically induced bacterial membrane-potential dynamics correspond to cellular proliferation capacity. *Proc. Natl. Acad. Sci. USA* **2019**, *116*, 9552–9557. [CrossRef] [PubMed]
17. Ladeynova, M.; Kuznetsova, D.; Mudrilov, M.; Vodeneev, V. Integration of electrical signals and phytohormones in the control of systemic response. *Int. J. Mol. Sci.* **2023**, *24*, 847. [CrossRef]
18. Jo, Y.; Sung, J.; Jeong, H.; Hong, S.; Jeong, Y.K.; Yoon, M. Effectiveness of a fractionated therapy scheme in tumor treating fields therapy. *Technol. Cancer Res. Treat.* **2019**, *18*, 1533033819845008. [CrossRef] [PubMed]
19. Giladi, M.; Schneiderman, R.S.; Voloshin, T.; Porat, Y.; Munster, M.; Palti, Y. Mitotic spindle disruption by alternating electric fields leads to improper chromosome segregation and mitotic catastrophe in cancer cells. *Sci. Rep.* **2015**, *5*, 18046. [CrossRef] [PubMed]
20. Tran, T.B.; Baek, C.; Min, J. Electric cell-substrate impedance sensing (ECIS) with microelectrode arrays for investigation of cancer cell–fibroblasts interaction. *PLoS ONE* **2016**, *11*, e0153813. [CrossRef]
21. Turcan, I.; Olariu, M.A. Dielectrophoretic manipulation of cancer cells and their electrical characterization. *ACS Comb. Sci.* **2020**, *22*, 554–578. [CrossRef]
22. Ghita, M.; Copot, D.; Ionescu, C.M. Lung cancer dynamics using fractional order impedance modeling on a mimicked lung tumor setup. *J. Adv. Res.* **2021**, *32*, 61–71. [CrossRef]
23. Chakraborty, A.; Dutta, P.; Wakankar, A.; RoyChaudhuri, C. Recent field effect transistors and electrical impedance spectroscopy based biosensing strategies for cancer biomarker screening: A mini review. *Biosens. Bioelectron. X* **2022**, *12*, 100253. [CrossRef]
24. Baidillah, M.R.; Riyanto, R.; Busono, P.; Karim, S.; Febryarto, R.; Taruno, W.P. Electrical impedance spectroscopy for skin layer assessment: A scoping review of electrode design, measurement methods, and post-processing techniques. *Measurement* **2024**, *226*, 114111. [CrossRef]
25. Yuan, Y.; Zhang, J.; Qi, X.; Li, S.; Liu, G.; Siddhanta, S.; Barman, I.; Song, X.; McMahon, M.T.; Bulte, J.W. Furin-mediated intracellular self-assembly of olsalazine nanoparticles for enhanced magnetic resonance imaging and tumour therapy. *Nat. Mater.* **2019**, *18*, 1376–1383. [CrossRef] [PubMed]
26. Qi, X.; Li, J.; Wei, W.; Zuo, G.; Su, T.; Pan, X.; Zhang, J.; Dong, W. Cationic Salecan-based hydrogels for release of 5-fluorouracil. *RSC Adv.* **2017**, *7*, 14337–14347. [CrossRef]

27. Meneses, J.; Fernandes, S.; Alves, N.; Pascoal-Faria, P.; Miranda, P.C. How to correctly estimate the electric field in capacitively coupled systems for tissue engineering: A comparative study. *Sci. Rep.* **2022**, *12*, 11049.
28. Gómez-Aguilar, F.; Rosales-García, J.; Guía-Calderón, M.; Bernal-Alvarado, J. Analysis of equivalent circuits for cells: A fractional calculus approach. *Ing. Investig. Tecnol.* **2012**, *13*, 375–384. [CrossRef]
29. Shiozawa, M.; Uno, S. An analytical formula for determining the electrical impedance between a single adherent cell and sensor substrate. *Jpn. J. Appl. Phys.* **2022**, *61*, 117001. [CrossRef]
30. López-García, J.J.; Horno, J.; Grosse, C. Impedance-frequency response of closed electrolytic cells. *Micromachines* **2023**, *14*, 368. [CrossRef] [PubMed]
31. Zhang, H.; Wang, P. Fractional calculus-based statistical damage model of unsaturated soil under the coupling effect of moistening and stress fields. *Appl. Sci.* **2023**, *13*, 9156. [CrossRef]
32. Bentley, C.L.; Perry, D.; Unwin, P.R. Stability and placement of Ag/AgCl quasi-reference counter electrodes in confined electrochemical cells. *Anal. Chem.* **2018**, *90*, 7700–7707. [CrossRef] [PubMed]
33. Wegner, L.H.; Flickinger, B.; Eing, C.; Berghöfer, T.; Hohenberger, P.; Nick, P. A patch clamp study on the electro-permeabilization of higher plant cells: Supra-physiological voltages induce a high-conductance, K+ selective state of the plasma membrane. *Biochim. Biophys. Acta Biomembr.* **2011**, *1808*, 1728–1736. [CrossRef]
34. Zhan, L.; Han, Z.; Shao, Q.; Etheridge, M.L.; Hays, T.; Bischof, J.C. Rapid Joule Heating Improves Vitrification Based Cryopreservation. *Nat. Commun.* **2022**, *13*, 6017. [CrossRef]
35. Bakhtiari, S.; Manshadi, M.K.D.; Candas, M.; Beskok, A. Changes in electrical capacitance of cell membrane reflect drug partitioning-induced alterations in lipid bilayer. *Micromachines* **2023**, *14*, 316. [CrossRef]
36. Baca, J.A.M.; Ortega, A.O.; Jiménez, A.A.; Principal, S.G. Cells electric charge analyses define specific properties for cancer cells activity. *Bioelectrochemistry* **2022**, *144*, 108028.
37. Di Gregorio, E.; Israel, S.; Staelens, M.; Tankel, G.; Shankar, K.; Tuszyński, J.A. The distinguishing electrical properties of cancer cells. *Phys. Life Rev.* **2022**, *43*, 139–188. [CrossRef]
38. Deivasigamani, R.; Mohd Maidin, N.N.; Abdul Nasir, N.S.; Abdulhameed, A.; Ahmad Kayani, A.B.; Mohamed, M.A.; Buyong, M.R. A correlation of conductivity medium and bioparticle viability on dielectrophoresis-based biomedical applications. *Electrophoresis* **2023**, *44*, 573–620. [CrossRef]
39. Silve, A.; Leray, I.; Poignard, C.; Mir, L.M. Impact of external medium conductivity on cell membrane electropermeabilization by microsecond and nanosecond electric pulses. *Sci. Rep.* **2016**, *6*, 19957. [CrossRef] [PubMed]
40. Reid, B.; Zhao, M. The electrical response to injury: Molecular mechanisms and wound healing. *Adv. Wound Care* **2014**, *3*, 184–201. [CrossRef] [PubMed]
41. Zhao, S.; Mehta, A.S.; Zhao, M. Biomedical applications of electrical stimulation. *Cell. Mol. Life Sci.* **2020**, *77*, 2681–2699. [CrossRef]
42. Klejchova, M.; Silva-Alvim, F.A.L.; Blatt, M.R.; Alvim, J.C. Membrane voltage as a dynamic platform for spatiotemporal signaling, physiological, and developmental regulation. *Plant Physiol.* **2021**, *185*, 1523–1541. [CrossRef] [PubMed]
43. Shindou, T.; Ochi-Shindou, M.; Murayama, T.; Saita, E.-I.; Momohara, Y.; Maruyama, I.N. Active propagation of dendritic electrical signals in *C. elegans*. *Sci. Rep.* **2019**, *9*, 3430. [CrossRef] [PubMed]
44. Chen, C.; Bai, X.; Ding, Y.; Lee, I.-S. Electrical stimulation as a novel tool for regulating cell behavior in tissue engineering. *Biomater. Res.* **2019**, *23*, 25. [CrossRef]
45. Papalazarou, V.; Maddocks, O.D.K. Supply and demand: Cellular nutrient uptake and exchange in cancer. *Mol. Cell* **2021**, *81*, 3731–3748. [CrossRef]
46. Windhorst, U.; Lalley, P.M. Action Potential. In *Encyclopedia of Neuroscience*; Springer: Berlin/Heidelberg, Germany, 2008; pp. 22–29.
47. Napotnik, T.B.; Polajžer, T.; Miklavčič, D. Cell death due to electroporation—A review. *Bioelectrochemistry* **2021**, *141*, 107871.
48. Mitchell, R.N.; Schoen, F.J. Functional tissue architecture, homeostasis, and responses to injury. In *Biomaterials Science*; Elsevier: Amsterdam, The Netherlands, 2020; pp. 683–700.
49. Zhu, C.; Liu, F.; Moser, M.A.J.; Zhang, W.; Fang, Z.; Zhang, B. Rapid prediction of ablation zones of irreversible electroporation with electrochemical impedance spectroscopy and artificial neural network in a heterogeneous model. *IEEE Trans. Instrum. Meas.* **2024**, *73*, 2512510. [CrossRef]
50. Bougandoura, O.; Achour, Y.; Zaoui, A. Electroporation in cancer therapy: A simplified model derived from the Hodgkin–Huxley model. *Bioelectricity* **2024**, *6*, 181–195. [CrossRef]
51. Kim, S.H.; Kang, J.M.; Park, Y.; Kim, Y.; Lim, B.; Park, J.-H. Effects of bipolar irreversible electroporation with different pulse durations in a prostate cancer mouse model. *Sci. Rep.* **2024**, *14*, 9902. [CrossRef] [PubMed]
52. Purnama, C.A.; Meiliana, A.; Barliana, M.I.; Lestari, K. Update of cellular responses to the efferocytosis of necroptosis and pyroptosis. *Cell Div.* **2023**, *18*, 5. [CrossRef]
53. Song, P.; Gao, H.; Gao, Z.; Liu, J.; Zhang, R.; Hong-Yuan, K.C. Heat transfer and thermoregulation within single cells revealed by transient plasmonic imaging. *Chem* **2021**, *7*, 1569–1587. [CrossRef]

54. Lam, C.K.; de Groot, B.L. Ion conduction mechanisms in potassium channels revealed by permeation cycles. *J. Chem. Theory Comput.* **2023**, *19*, 2574–2589. [CrossRef]
55. Pan, J.; Chiang, C.-L.; Wang, X.; Bertani, P.; Ma, Y.; Lu, W. Cell membrane damage and cargo delivery in nano-electroporation. *Nanoscale* **2023**, *15*, 4080–4089. [CrossRef] [PubMed]
56. Frias, M.A.; Disalvo, E.A. Breakdown of classical paradigms in relation to membrane structure and functions. *Biochim. Biophys. Acta Biomembr.* **2021**, *1863*, 183512. [CrossRef]
57. Schink, S.; Polk, M.; Athaide, E.; Mukherjee, A.; Ammar, C.; Basan, M. Survival dynamics of starving bacteria are determined by ion homeostasis that maintains plasmolysis. *Nat. Phys.* **2024**, *20*, 1332–1338. [CrossRef]
58. Zmerli, O.; Bellali, S.; Haddad, G.; Hisada, A.; Ominami, Y.; Khalil, J.B. Rapid microbial viability assay using scanning electron microscopy: A proof-of-concept using Phosphotungstic acid staining. *Comput. Struct. Biotechnol. J.* **2023**, *21*, 3627–3638. [CrossRef] [PubMed]
59. Ding, H.-Z. Electrodamage mechanics of dielectric ageing. In Proceedings of the 7th International Conference on Properties and Applications of Dielectric Materials (Cat. No. 03CH37417), Nagoya, Japan, 1–5 June 2003.

fractal and fractional

MDPI

Article

Scale-Free Dynamics of Resting-State fMRI Microstates †

Nurhan Erbil *,‡ and Gopikrishna Deshpande

AU MRI Research Center, Department of Electrical and Computer Engineering, Auburn University, 560 Devall Dr, Suite 266D, Auburn, AL 36849, USA

* Correspondence: nurhaner@hacettepe.edu.tr

† This article is a revised and expanded version of the paper entitled [Erbil, N., Deshpande, G. Microstate Analysis of Spontaneous BOLD signal], which was presented at [18th Organization for Human Brain Mapping, in Beijing, China, 10–14 June 2012] and [Erbil, N., Deshpande, G. Temporally quasi-stable spatial configurations in fMRI reveal scale-free dynamics similar to that of EEG microstates], which was presented at [ISMRM 21st Annual Meeting and Exhibition, in Salt Lake City, UT, USA, 20–26 April 2013].

‡ Current address: Department of Biophysics, Faculty of Medicine, Hacettepe University, Sihhiye, Ankara 06230, Turkey.

Abstract: The functional significance of RSNs is examined via simultaneous EEG-fMRI studies on the basis of the relation of RSNs with different frequency bands of EEG and EEG-based microstate analysis. In this study, we try to identify RSNs from microstates of cortical surface maps of the BOLD signal. In addition, the scale-free dynamics of these map sequences were also examined. The structural and resting state functional MRI images were acquired on a 3T scanner with three different fMRI acquisition protocols from seven subjects. Microstate segmentations from EEG, fMRI, and simulated data were evaluated. Wavelet-based fractal analysis was performed on map sequence time series and the Hurst exponent (H) was calculated. By using HRF-deconvolved fMRI time series, the effect of the HRF (hemodynamic response function) on fMRI-derived microstates was tested. The fMRI map sequence has a system with a memory system smaller than 16 s. When the HRF was deconvolved, the duration of the memory of the system was reduced to 4 s. On the other hand, the results of simulation data indicated that these systems are specific to the resting state BOLD signal. Similar to EEG microstates, fMRI also has microstates and both of them have scale-free dynamics. fMRI microstate dynamics have two different components, one is related to the HRF and the other is independent of the HRF. The significance of fMRI microstates and their relation with RSNs need to be further studied.

Keywords: resting-state networks; simultaneous EEG-fMRI; microstates; Hurst exponent; fMRI microstates

1. Introduction

Resting-state networks (RSNs) in the human brain are defined as coherent fluctuations in slow components (<0.1 Hz) of blood oxygenation level-dependent (BOLD) functional magnetic resonance imaging (fMRI) signals [1,2]. Microstates are clusters of the scalp electrical topography of EEGs (electroencephalograms) across time and are defined as "atoms of thoughts" underlying spontaneous conscious cognitive activity [3–6]. It was shown that rapidly changing EEG microstates are correlated with fMRI RSNs and have scale-free dynamics over scales covering the 256 ms to 16 s range [7,8]. In another study, the combined ICA of EEG and fMRI data was used in order to examine EEG microstates and fMRI RSN networks [9]. It was shown that each RSN was characterized further by a specific electrophysiological signature involving one to a combination of several microstates.

While these studies have informed us a great deal about RSNs that might underlie EEG microstates, they suffer from certain shortcomings that we enumerate below. First, very little is known about the microstate dynamics of fMRI itself and how it compares with that of EEG. Second, fMRI is a hemodynamically smoothed version of underlying neural activity and hence the effect of the hemodynamic response on fMRI microstate dynamics is not clearly understood. In this study, we address these issues by examining the existence of fMRI microstates and testing for the scale-free dynamics of both EEG and fMRI by using simultaneous EEG-fMRI data, as well as investigating the effect of hemodynamic smoothing on fMRI microstates.

It was argued that scale-free dynamics arise only when neuronal systems reach a critical point [10,11]. As a result, they became a focus of interest in the field of neuroscience. The existence of scale-free dynamics was argued as an organizing mechanism that is capable of processing continuously flowing information from multiple sources and producing related responses [12]. The existence of scale-free dynamics of the BOLD time series has been demonstrated previously [13–18]. Task-induced voxel-level fluctuations in fMRI were also examined and it was found that in addition to stimulus-induced signal changes, physiologically based anatomical differences in fMRI time series can be detected and quantified by multifractal parameters [18], indicating scale-free dynamics.

The Hurst exponent (power law exponent), as a measure of long-range dependency, is commonly used for the identification of the scale-invariant structure of a signal. In another study using fMRI time series during task and rest conditions, it was shown that the Hurst exponent was high during rest and reduced during the task, suggesting that the signal contains more long-range memory during rest [9,16]. It is critical to note that scale invariance in time and the scale-free dynamics of brain topology are different from each other [19]. These authors investigated both RSN and non-RSN dynamics on the basis of the Hurst exponent [19]. The group-level RSNs were segmented by a multivariate decomposition approach. It was shown that long memory in functional networks decreased during tasks. The researchers used a multifractal approach and concluded that it can be used as a marker for distinguishing functional networks. The examination of fractal scaling was performed for different groups and patients and it was suggested that fractal properties might be a sensitive measure for the discrimination of conditions [20].

In another resting-state fMRI study, temporal switching of the occurrence of RSNs as well as switching between RSNs across time were examined. It was stated that the network transitions are non-random and hierarchically organized, i.e., the brain is cycling within 'metastates' [21]. Different from our study, these networks were derived from ICA-dependent methods and Hidden Markov Modeling.

The temporal complexity of the fMRI time series has been examined by using multiscale entropy and the Hurst exponent and it was concluded that both the monofractal Hurst exponent and multiscale entropy can be used for analysis of temporal complexity of task-based and resting-state fMRI signals [22].

Several reports have indicated that the monofractal Hurst exponent has been shown to change in relation to both spatial (brain tissue type and functional networks) and temporal (activation and cognition) dynamics [23].

The importance of the development of multimodal measures to be applied as biomarkers and the effect of using them were discussed previously [24,25]. In this study, we focused on the brain topology-related dynamics of resting-state fMRI as a possible multimodal biomarker candidate. We tested the existence of fMRI microstates and their scale-free properties, i.e., spatio-temporal dynamics of fMRI microstates [26,27]. We used the microstate segmentation method to obtain topological maps and issued the same analysis used in the

EEG time series [8]. We also examined the effect of the HRF by using HRF deconvolved data and simulation data.

2. Materials and Methods

2.1. Data Acquisition

This simultaneous EEG-fMRI study was approved by the Institutional Review Board of Auburn University and the study was carried out in agreement with the Code of Ethics of The World Medicinal Association (Declaration of Helsinki). All subjects had no history of neurological or psychiatric disorders and gave their written informed consents before the experiments. Functional and structural magnetic resonance imaging data were acquired on a 3T Siemens Verio scanner with a 12-channel matrix head coil. Simultaneous resting-state EEG-fMRI data were acquired with three different fMRI acquisition protocols.

In the first protocol, functional images were acquired by using the echo-planar imaging (EPI) sequence with 30 ms TE, 1000 ms TR, 90° flip angle, 5 mm slice thickness, and $64 \times 64 \times 18$ acquisition matrix, for 1000 volumes (16.67 min) from 7 subjects (aged 21–28, mean $\pm$ SD = 23 $\pm$ 2.4 years; 2 female, 5 male).

In the second and third protocols, a multiband gradient echo-planar imaging sequence [28] was used with the following parameters:

- MB_600: TR/TE = 600/30 ms, flip angle = 55 degrees, 5 mm slice thickness, $64 \times 64 \times 16$ acquisition matrix for 1000 volumes (10 min);
- MB_200: TR/TE = 200/40 ms, flip angle = 50 degrees, 5 mm slice thickness, $64 \times 64 \times 16$ acquisition matrix for 3000 volumes (10 min).

We acquired fMRI data using these three protocols in order to investigate the effect of increasing temporal sampling resolution (i.e., decreasing TR). In the second and third experiments, data were collected from 7 subjects (aged 24–36, mean $\pm$ SD = 26 $\pm$ 4.8 years; 2 female, 5 male). In all protocols, 'eyes open' and 'eyes closed' conditions were acquired separately. In order to minimize the SAR (Specific Absorption Rate) during multiband acquisition, flip angles were reduced. The details of simultaneous MB-EPI and EEG acquisition were discussed in a previously published paper with the same data set [29]. In all three experiments, T1-weighted structural images were acquired by using a 3D anatomic (MPRAGE) sequence with the following parameters: 176 sagittal slices of 1 mm thickness with 2.52 ms TE, 1900 ms TR, 9° flip angle, and $256 \times 256 \times 176$ acquisition matrix.

Simultaneous EEG data were acquired by using an MR-compatible 64-channel EEG amplifier (Brain Products, Gilching, Germany) and an MR-compatible EEG cap with 63 10–20 system-distributed scalp electrodes and an ECG electrode. The EEG data acquisition clock was synchronized with the MRI scanner clock using Brain Product's SyncBox, resulting in exactly 10,000 data points per TR interval. EEG data were digitized with a sampling frequency of 5 kHz and 0.5 μV resolution, within a DC-250 Hz frequency range and with reference to FCz. The impedance at all recording electrodes was less than 20 kΩ.

2.2. Data Pre-Processing

Image pre-processing analyses were performed using SPM12 software (Wellcome Department of Imaging Neuroscience, London, UK). After slice-timing correction and motion correction (including censoring), images were spatially realigned and normalized to MNI space (Montreal Neurological Institute, resampled voxel size: $2 \times 2 \times 2$ mm^3). Nuisance covariates (white matter and CSF signals and motion parameters) were regressed out. In order to reduce dimensionality, mean time series were calculated for functional regions defined in the CC200 parcellation atlas obtained from spectral clustering of resting-state data [30]. This atlas provides functionally homogeneous regions of interest (ROIs) determined in a data-driven way.

BOLD time series are an indirect measure of neural activity, i.e., they are a convolution of latent neural activity (which is not measured) and the hemodynamic response function (HRF, which is the impulse response of the system representing neurovascular coupling). It has been shown that the HRF varies across brain regions and individuals and this variability is at least partly non-neural in origin [31,32]. The HRF variability has been shown to impact inferences such as functional connectivity obtained from fMRI time series [33,34]. Therefore, we deconvolved the HRF from the fMRI time series using the HRF Estimation MATLAB R2011.a Toolbox [35] and used the resulting latent neural time series in further analyses.

2.2.1. Simulated Data

In order to obtain the simulation data, Gaussian noise (mean = 0, std = 1) matrices were generated with CC200xtime dimensions identical to the experimental fMRI data, using the same EEG sampling frequency (100 Hz). Resulting data were convolved with a canonical hemodynamic response function (HRF) and downsampled according to each TR separately to match each fMRI sampling resolution separately.

2.2.2. Microstate Analysis

Microstate segmentations for EEG, fMRI, and simulation data microstate segmentations were performed for each subject separately using Cartool software by Denis Brunet (brainmapping.unige.ch/cartool). For mean ROI fMRI time series, data obtained from the CC200 atlas mean time series as well as simulation data were recorded and converted to EDF (European Data Format) files for further processing in the Cartool Toolbox. Four template maps for each subject and modality were obtained (illustrated in Figures 1 and 2 for a representative subject).

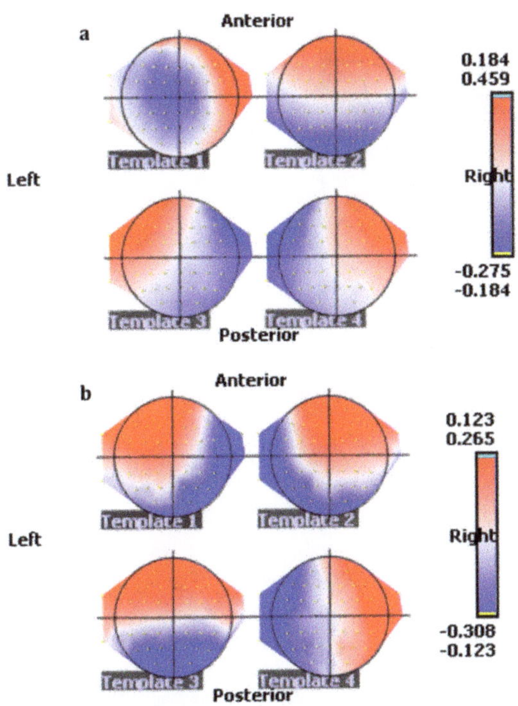

Figure 1. EEG microstate maps of a representative subject for 'eyes closed' (**a**) and 'eyes open' (**b**) conditions.

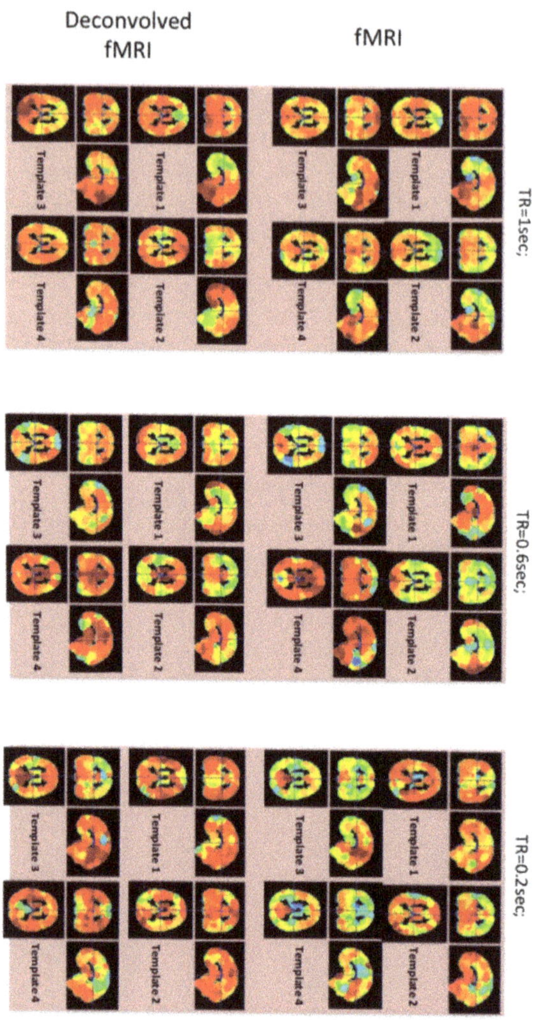

Figure 2. fMRI microstate maps of a representative subject for TR = 1 s, TR = 0.6 s, and TR = 0.2 s for the 'eyes open' condition.

Microstate segmentation is based on both the time and the topographic maps. In the case of EEG, in order to define these quasi-stable maps, the maxima of GFP (Global Field Power), as the standard deviation of data across all electrodes, were determined. GFP is defined as

$$GFP = \sqrt{\frac{\sum_{i=1}^{N}\left(v_i - \overline{v}\right)^2}{N}} \tag{1}$$

where N is the number of electrodes, vi is the voltage at the electrode i, and $\overline{v}$ is the average voltage of all electrodes [5,36]. GFP is a one-number measure of the map at each moment in time. It was shown that a limited number of scalp potential maps remain stable for a certain period of time (60–120 ms) [4]. The maps related to the maxima of GFP are used as templates and the microstate segmentation is performed by using modified k-means cluster analysis [3,37]. The details related to microstate segmentation are given in the prior literature [6,38,39].

2.2.3. Fractal Analysis

The long-range dependency or scaling property represents the memory or self-similarity of a system and is characterized by the Hurst exponent. This analysis concept was introduced by Hurst in 1951 and expanded by Mandelbrot [40–43]. A Hurst exponent (H) smaller than 0.5 means that the system has a short-range temporal dependency. H > 0.5 represents systems with a long-range dependency and H = 0.5 indicates an uncorrelated system [44].

For fractal analysis, the microstates were bipartitioned by associating them with a positive and a negative step, respectively (as described in [8,45]). The cumulative sum of the resulting microstate sequence over time was used for random walk embedding and analyzed using the continuous 'Haar' orthogonal wavelet (Equation (2)) transform by dividing time series with length L into subseries of length 2n, where n = 1, . . ., and m represents the maximum scale (Figure 3) [46].

$$\Psi(t) \equiv \begin{cases} 1 & 0 \le t \le \frac{1}{2} \\ -1 & \frac{1}{2} \le t \le 1 \\ 0 & otherwise \end{cases} \tag{2}$$

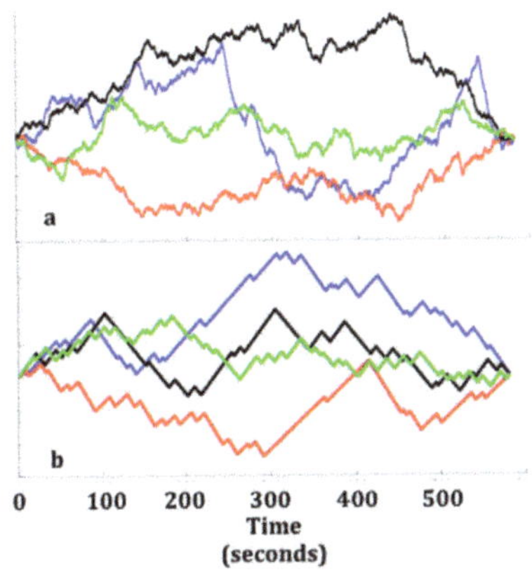

Figure 3. Random walk embedding curves of EEG (**a**) and fMRI (TR = 1) (**b**) microstate sequences of a representative subject. X-axis represents time in seconds. Each colored line represents a different bipartioning combination.

The slope of the scaling diagram is used for the calculation of H (Equation (3)), (Figure 4) [47]. According to limits defined in Table 1, H was calculated for all possible, that is, 3, bipartitionings of microstate sequences for each subject and modality [47].

$$\text{logH\_n} = \text{logc} + \text{Hlogn} \tag{3}$$

Table 1. Relation between the slope of the scaling factor and H [47].

	Differenced Gaussian	**Gaussian**	**Brownian**	**Summed Brownian**
Slope of scaling diagram	(−3, −1)	(−1, 1)	(1, 3)	(3, 5)
Formula Used for H	(H + 3)/2	(H + 1)/2	(H − 1)/2	(H − 3)/2

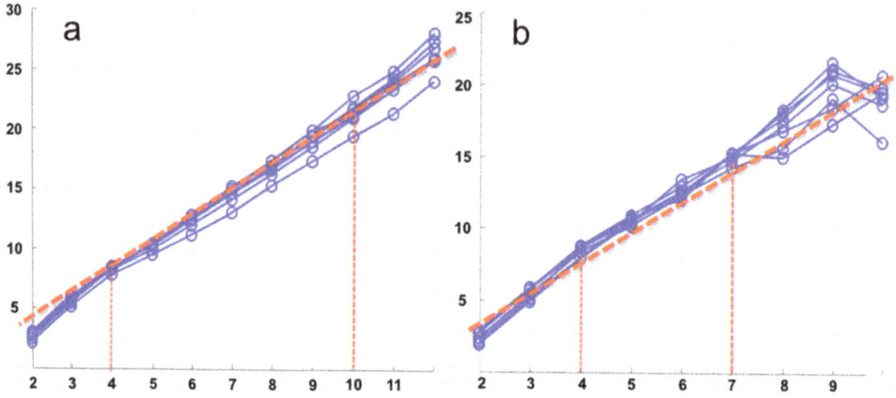

Figure 4. The scaling diagram (scale versus wavelet coefficients in log scale) of EEG (**a**) and fMRI (**b**) time series. The different lines represent different subjects. The red line represents the fitted line representing the group. The slope of the red line represents the Hurst exponent of the corresponding data set at the group level.

3. Results

3.1. Results from Simulated Data

A Hurst exponent value larger than 0.5 is interpreted to imply long-range dependency in the system. The scales with both confidence limits higher than 0.5 are accepted within the long-range dependency limits. Hurst exponents of simulated fMRI data (i.e., Gaussian noise convolved with HRF) were greater than 0.5 for the scales shorter than 4 s for TR = 1 s, 19.2 s for TR = 0.6 s, and longer than 12.8 s for TR = 0.2 s. On the other hand, deconvolved time series did not show the same behavior (Figure 5). H was greater than 0.5 for TR = 1 s, 1.2 s for TR = 0.6 s, and finally 3.2 s for TR = 0.2 s. Simulated data indicated a system with long-duration memory for simulated fMRI, and the duration decreased appreciably for deconvolved simulated fMRI data.

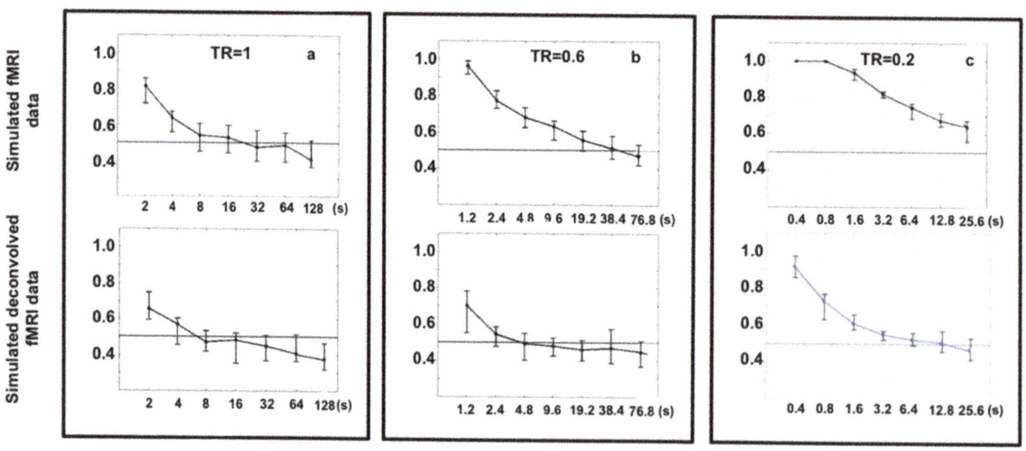

Figure 5. Scale (in seconds) versus H curves of Gaussian noise convolved and deconvolved with HRF. Each point represents the median of H (calculated across subjects) at any given scale whereas vertical lines (error bars) show the upper and the lower 5th percentiles for TR = 1 s (**a**), TR = 0.6 s (**b**) and TR = 0.2 s (**c**).

We have shown that long-range dependency, defined by an H of deconvolved time series, was specific to fMRI and indicated the existence of scale-free dynamics in fMRI time series. Gaussian noise convolved with HRF showed a longer duration memory system compared to the BOLD signal. Another important result related to simulation data is that TR = 0.6 s data have shown longer durations for scale-free dynamics.

3.2. Results from Experimental Data

By using Wilcoxon Signed Rank Tests, Hurst exponents (H) of 'eyes open' and 'eyes closed' conditions were compared. There was no statistically significant difference between calculated H values for deconvolved ($p < 0.647$), raw BOLD ($p < 0.634$) fMRI, and EEG ($p < 0.353$) time series.

The scale-free dynamics range for EEG was around 40 ms. There is no statistically significant difference for the scale-free dynamic range of EEG in relation to fMRI acquisition protocol according to the Chi-square test ($p > 0.339$). For the fMRI time series, it can be seen that deconvolved time series have their own dynamics that are different from the BOLD time series (Figure 6). The scale-free dynamics range is around 4 s for deconvolved time series, while it is larger than 16 s for fMRI time series. On the basis of these results, it can be said that resting state fMRI data represent two different dynamics. The BOLD signal is evidenced in a system with a longer duration memory system (<16 s). On the other hand, the HRF deconvolved time series indicates a system with shorter duration repetition (<4 s).

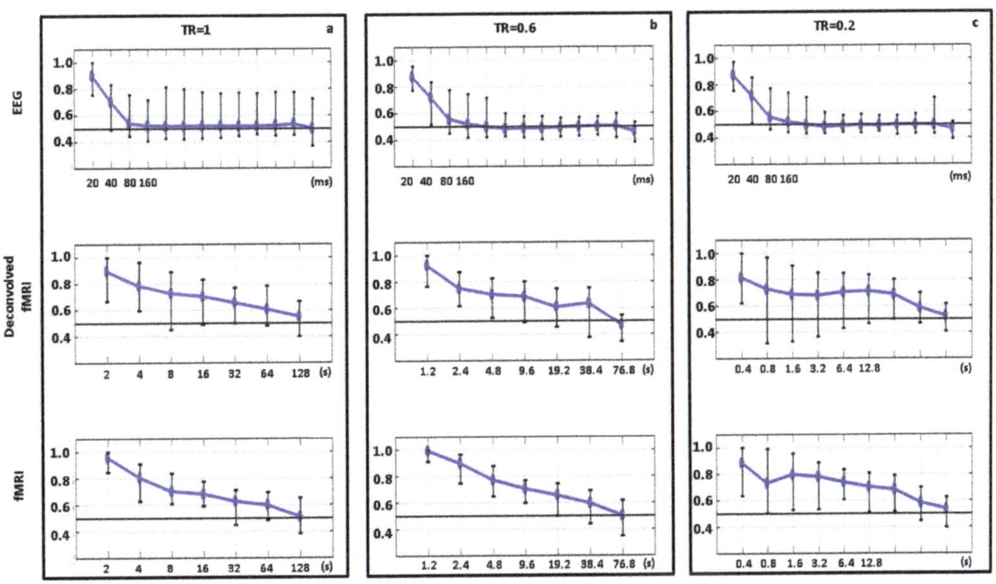

Figure 6. Scale versus H curves of EEG (millisecond), deconvolved fMRI, and fMRI data (seconds). The results shown were estimated by combining data from eyes open and closed conditions. Each point represents the median of H (calculated across subjects) at any given scale, whereas vertical lines (error bars) show the upper and the lower 5th percentiles for TR = 1 s (**a**), TR = 0.6 s (**b**), and TR = 0.2 s (**c**).

4. Discussion

In this study, we have shown that fMRI map series obtained from 'microstate segmentation' also have self-similar dynamics for longer durations (H > 0.5, $p < 0.05$), i.e., the existence of scale-free behavior of both EEG and fMRI microstate sequences from simultaneous acquisitions (Figure 5). We applied the same method used for EEG and found that, similar to EEG, fMRI also has 'microstates' and the duration-based sequence of these microstates indicated a long-range dependent dynamic system [8].

For EEG, as expected, independent from which TR was acquired, scale-free dynamics contain two scales (<40 ms) for fMRI, and four, five, and six scales (<32 s) for each TR (Figure 6), in accordance with the previous findings in the literature [8]. In addition, our results indicated the existence of scale-free dynamics for fMRI microstate time series. On the other hand, as far as the deconvolved time series are concerned, it can be seen that the range of scale-free dynamics decreases to 9.6 s for TR = 1 s and TR = 0.6 s. As a result, it can be concluded that hemodynamic response introduces longer duration scale-free dynamics.

On the basis of our HRF convolved Gaussian noise simulation results, we also showed that scale-free dynamics of fMRI 'microstates' were specific to fMRI (Figure 6) and independent from the TR used in the acquisition. We also tested the effect of the HRF by analyzing HRF-deconvolved fMRI microstates. The duration of scale-free dynamics was decreased to 4 s from 16 s. This result was also in accordance with our simulation data, indicating the existence of approximately 20 s long scale-free dynamics for the HRF convolved Gaussian noise.

Ciuciu et al. focused on the examination of scale-free dynamics of RSNs during rest and task conditions [19]. At that study group level, RSNs were segmented by a multivariate decomposition approach and the time series of ICA-based segmented maps were analyzed. It was shown that long memory in functional networks decreased during tasks, but it was shown that change was not specific to activation areas. They also argued that as far as the topological dynamics of fMRI were concerned, multifractality should be taken into consideration since the HRF cannot be assumed as linear or time-invariant. We have shown that HRF-deconvolved map change dynamics also have a long-memory system; as a result, it can be hypothesized that in addition to the HRF, there were additional systems showing scale-free dynamics. The relation of these fMRI microstates and RSNs needs further investigation and is beyond the scope of this study. In addition, recent work relating RSNs observed by magnetoencephalography (MEG) and BOLD fMRI suggested the coexistence of nonstationary (MEG) and stationary (fMRI) processes on similar anatomical substrates [48].

The results of our data acquired with TR = 200 ms had higher variance that became more prominent after deconvolution. We used a 12-channel head coil. It was shown that parallel imaging can help to increase the total SNR of 2D acquisitions by a factor $\sqrt{MB}$ (multiband) and that the amount of parallel noise amplification depends on the employed MB factor and in-plane acceleration factor if relaxation effects and parallel noise amplification are not taken into consideration [49]. It can be said that the resulting SNR of parallel imaging in TR = 0.2 s was lower compared to other protocols for this coil. On the other hand, it was shown that thermal noise dominated the EPI time series for medium to large voxel sizes for single-channel and 12-channel head coil configurations, but physiological noise dominated the 32-channel array acquisition [50]. The increased variance in TR = 200 ms data set also might result from decreased SNR in relation to physiological noise, which is nonlinear and also depends on the flip angle.

Another possible explanation for increased variance in the TR = 200 ms protocol might be related to the length of step size used in Hurst exponent calculations. The scales indicated by TR = 200 ms were the multiples of 0.2 s. Even though BOLD time series with different TRs have shown similar durations for scale-free dynamics, deconvolved time series were varied in relation to TR. According to the results of the TR = 200 ms protocol, the duration of scale-free dynamics of HRF-deconvolved fMRI time series was shorter than 0.8 s. In this study, different TEs, flip angles, and voxel sizes were used in order to optimize the sequence for a minimum TR. This discrepancy might be related to this difference. In a study using pICA for the analysis of RNSs on simultaneous EEG-fMRI acquisition, it was shown that fast fMRI sampling represents better high-frequency electrical substrates of RSNs [29]. The authors argued that ICA was robust to differences in SNR. But, the differences in the step size and changes in the acquisition protocol might be the source of the difference in the duration of scale-free dynamics indicated with different TRs.

In general, wavelet-based methods were recommended for Hurst exponent analysis and in the literature, most of the studies used this method. In a study, it was shown that for fMRI data sets, the poorest-performing measures were wavelet, detrended fluctuation analysis, aggregated variance, and rescaled range [51]. In this study, we used map sequence dynamics, not fMRI time series. As discussed by Van De Ville et al., wavelet transform analyses are insensitive to low-frequency trends and appropriate for the microstate map sequence analysis [8].

5. Conclusions

Similar to EEG microstates, fMRI also has microstates and both of them have scale-free dynamics. fMRI microstate dynamics have two different components: one is related to the HRF and the other is independent of the HRF. The significance of fMRI microstates and their relation with RSNs needs to be further studied.

6. Limitations

One of the aims of this study is to examine the methods that can be used for the determination of fMRI microstates and investigate whether their temporal dynamics have a fractal structure similar to EEG microstates. However, it was not possible to determine RSN microstates because the number of participants was insufficient [52,53]. In addition to TR, different values of TE and the flip angle might affect the spatiotemporal properties of resting-state fMRI microstates. It was shown that lowering the flip angle can improve the SNR related to the physiological artifacts and that the relation between the time series SNR (tSNR) and physiological noise is nonlinear [50]. The effect of the differing TE and flip angle on fMRI microstates should also be examined.

Author Contributions: Conceptualization, G.D. and N.E.; methodology, G.D. and N.E.; software, N.E.; validation, N.E. and G.D.; formal analysis, N.E.; investigation, N.E. and G.D.; data curation/acquisition, N.E.; writing, N.E.; writing—review and editing, G.D.; visualization, N.E. and G.D.; supervision, G.D. All authors have read and agreed to the published version of the manuscript.

Funding: This research received no external funding.

Institutional Review Board Statement: This study was approved by the Institutional Review Board of Auburn University (#11-372) and was in agreement with the Code of Ethics of The World Medicinal Association (Declaration of Helsinki).

Informed Consent Statement: All participants gave their written informed consent before the experiments.

Data Availability Statement: The data that support the findings of this study are available on request from the authors.

Acknowledgments: The Cartool software (https://denisbrunet.github.io/Cartool/index.html, accessed on 12 December 2024) has been programmed by Denis Brunet from the Functional Brain Mapping Laboratory (FBMLab), Geneva, Switzerland, and is supported by the Center for Biomedical Imaging (CIBM) of Geneva and Lausanne.

Conflicts of Interest: The authors declare no conflicts of interest.

References

1. De Luca, M.; Beckmann, C.F.; De Stefano, N.; Matthews, P.M.; Smith, S.M. fMRI resting state networks define distinct modes of long-distance interactions in the human brain. *NeuroImage* **2006**, *29*, 1359–1367. [CrossRef] [PubMed]
2. Fox, M.D.; Snyder, A.Z.; Vincent, J.L.; Corbetta, M.; Van Essen, D.C.; Raichle, M.E. The human brain is intrinsically organized into dynamic, anticorrelated functional networks. *Proc. Natl. Acad. Sci. USA* **2005**, *102*, 9673–9678. [CrossRef] [PubMed]
3. Lehman, D. Brain Electric Fields and Brain Functional States. In *Evolution of Dynamical Structures in Complex Systems*; Friedrich, R., Wunderlin, A., Eds.; Springer: Berlin/Heidelberg, Germany, 1992; pp. 235–248.
4. Lehmann, D.; Ozaki, H.; Pal, I. EEG alpha map series: Brain micro-states by space-oriented adaptive segmentation. *Electroencephalogr. Clin. Neurophysiol.* **1987**, *67*, 271–288. [CrossRef]
5. Lehmann, D.; Strik, W.K.; Henggeler, B.; Koenig, T.; Koukkou, M. Brain electric microstates and momentary conscious mind states as building blocks of spontaneous thinking: I. Visual imagery and abstract thoughts. *Int. J. Psychophysiol. Off. J. Int. Organ. Psychophysiol.* **1998**, *29*, 1–11. [CrossRef]
6. Michel, C.M.; Koenig, T. EEG microstates as a tool for studying the temporal dynamics of whole-brain neuronal networks: A review. *NeuroImage* **2018**, *180*, 577–593. [CrossRef]
7. Britz, J.; Van De Ville, D.; Michel, C.M. BOLD correlates of EEG topography reveal rapid resting-state network dynamics. *NeuroImage* **2010**, *52*, 1162–1170. [CrossRef]
8. Van de Ville, D.; Britz, J.; Michel, C.M. EEG microstate sequences in healthy humans at rest reveal scale-free dynamics. *Proc. Natl. Acad. Sci. USA* **2010**, *107*, 18179–18184. [CrossRef]
9. Yuan, H.; Zotev, V.; Phillips, R.; Drevets, W.C.; Bodurka, J. Spatiotemporal dynamics of the brain at rest—Exploring EEG microstates as electrophysiological signatures of BOLD resting state networks. *NeuroImage* **2012**, *60*, 2062–2072. [CrossRef]
10. Breakspear, M.; Stam, C.J. Dynamics of a neural system with a multiscale architecture. *Philos. Trans. R. Soc. London. Ser. B Biol. Sci.* **2005**, *360*, 1051–1074. [CrossRef]
11. Werner, G. Brain dynamics across levels of organization. *J. Physiol. Paris* **2007**, *101*, 273–279. [CrossRef]
12. Peng, C.K.; Hausdorff, J.M.; Goldberger, A.L. Fractal mechanisms in neuronal control: Human heartbeat and gait dynamics in health and disease. In *Self-Organized Biological Dynamics and Nonlinear Control*; Walleczek, J., Ed.; Cambridge University Press: Cambridge, UK, 2000; pp. 66–96. [CrossRef]
13. Aguirre, G.K.; Zarahn, E.; D'Esposito, M. Empirical analyses of BOLD fMRI statistics. II. Spatially smoothed data collected under null-hypothesis and experimental conditions. *NeuroImage* **1997**, *5*, 199–212. [CrossRef] [PubMed]
14. Bullmore, E.; Long, C.; Suckling, J.; Fadili, J.; Calvert, G.; Zelaya, F.; Carpenter, T.A.; Brammer, M. Colored noise and computational inference in neurophysiological (fMRI) time series analysis: Resampling methods in time and wavelet domains. *Hum. Brain Mapp.* **2001**, *12*, 61–78. [CrossRef] [PubMed]
15. Bullock, T.H.; McClune, M.C.; Enright, J.T. Are the electroencephalograms mainly rhythmic? Assessment of periodicity in wide-band time series. *Neuroscience* **2003**, *121*, 233–252. [CrossRef] [PubMed]
16. He, B.J. Scale-free properties of the functional magnetic resonance imaging signal during rest and task. *J. Neurosci. Off. J. Soc. Neurosci.* **2011**, *31*, 13786–13795. [CrossRef]
17. He, B.J.; Zempel, J.M.; Snyder, A.Z.; Raichle, M.E. The temporal structures and functional significance of scale-free brain activity. *Neuron* **2010**, *66*, 353–369. [CrossRef]
18. Shimizu, Y.; Barth, M.; Windischberger, C.; Moser, E.; Thurner, S. Wavelet-based multifractal analysis of fMRI time series. *NeuroImage* **2004**, *22*, 1195–1202. [CrossRef]
19. Ciuciu, P.; Varoquaux, G.; Abry, P.; Sadaghiani, S.; Kleinschmidt, A. Scale-Free and Multifractal Time Dynamics of fMRI Signals during Rest and Task. *Front. Physiol.* **2012**, *3*, 186. [CrossRef]
20. Churchill, N.W.; Spring, R.; Grady, C.; Cimprich, B.; Askren, M.K.; Reuter-Lorenz, P.A.; Jung, M.S.; Peltier, S.; Strother, S.C.; Berman, M.G. The suppression of scale-free fMRI brain dynamics across three different sources of effort: Aging, task novelty and task difficulty. *Sci. Rep.* **2016**, *6*, 30895. [CrossRef]
21. Vidaurre, D.; Smith, S.M.; Woolrich, M.W. Brain network dynamics are hierarchically organized in time. *Proc. Natl. Acad. Sci. USA* **2017**, *114*, 12827–12832. [CrossRef]
22. Omidvarnia, A.; Liégeois, R.; Amico, E.; Preti, M.G.; Zalesky, A.; Van De Ville, D. On the Spatial Distribution of Temporal Complexity in Resting State and Task Functional MRI. *Entropy* **2022**, *24*, 1148. [CrossRef]
23. Campbell, O.L.; Weber, A.M. Monofractal analysis of functional magnetic resonance imaging: An introductory review. *Hum. Brain Mapp.* **2022**, *43*, 2693–2706. [CrossRef] [PubMed]
24. Rajkumar, R.; Farrher, E.; Mauler, J.; Sripad, P.; Régio Brambilla, C.; Rota Kops, E.; Scheins, J.; Dammers, J.; Lerche, C.; Langen, K.J.; et al. Comparison of EEG microstates with resting state fMRI and FDG-PET measures in the default mode network via simultaneously recorded trimodal (PET/MR/EEG) data. *Hum. Brain Mapp.* **2021**, *42*, 4122–4133. [CrossRef]

25. Scherr, M.; Utz, L.; Tahmasian, M.; Pasquini, L.; Grothe, M.J.; Rauschecker, J.P.; Grimmer, T.; Drzezga, A.; Sorg, C.; Riedl, V. Effective connectivity in the default mode network is distinctively disrupted in Alzheimer's disease-A simultaneous resting-state FDG-PET/fMRI study. *Hum. Brain Mapp.* **2021**, *42*, 4134–4143. [CrossRef]
26. Erbil, N.; Deshpande, G. Microstate Analysis of Spontaneous BOLD signal. In Proceedings of the18th Organization for Human Brain Mapping, Beijing, China, 10–14 June 2012.
27. Erbil, N.; Deshpande, G. Temporally quasi-stable spatial configurations in fMRI reveal scale-free dynamics similar to that of EEG microstates. In Proceedings of the ISMRM 21st Annual Meeting and Exhibition, Salt Lake City, UT, USA, 20–26 April 2013.
28. Feinberg, D.A.; Moeller, S.; Smith, S.M.; Auerbach, E.; Ramanna, S.; Gunther, M.; Glasser, M.F.; Miller, K.L.; Ugurbil, K.; Yacoub, E. Multiplexed echo planar imaging for sub-second whole brain FMRI and fast diffusion imaging. *PLoS ONE* **2010**, *5*, e15710. [CrossRef]
29. Kyathanahally, S.P.; Wang, Y.; Calhoun, V.D.; Deshpande, G. Investigation of True High Frequency Electrical Substrates of fMRI-Based Resting State Networks Using Parallel Independent Component Analysis of Simultaneous EEG/fMRI Data. *Front. Neuroinformatics* **2017**, *11*, 74. [CrossRef]
30. Craddock, R.C.; James, G.A.; Holtzheimer, P.E., 3rd; Hu, X.P.; Mayberg, H.S. A whole brain fMRI atlas generated via spatially constrained spectral clustering. *Hum. Brain Mapp.* **2012**, *33*, 1914–1928. [CrossRef]
31. Aguirre, G.K.; Zarahn, E.; D'Esposito, M. The variability of human, BOLD hemodynamic responses. *NeuroImage* **1998**, *8*, 360–369. [CrossRef]
32. Handwerker, D.A.; Ollinger, J.M.; D'Esposito, M. Variation of BOLD hemodynamic responses across subjects and brain regions and their effects on statistical analyses. *NeuroImage* **2004**, *21*, 1639–1651. [CrossRef]
33. Rangaprakash, D.; Dretsch, M.N.; Yan, W.; Katz, J.S.; Denney, T.S., Jr.; Deshpande, G. Hemodynamic variability in soldiers with trauma: Implications for functional MRI connectivity studies. *NeuroImage Clin.* **2017**, *16*, 409–417. [CrossRef]
34. Rangaprakash, D.; Wu, G.R.; Marinazzo, D.; Hu, X.; Deshpande, G. Hemodynamic response function (HRF) variability confounds resting-state fMRI functional connectivity. *Magn. Reson. Med.* **2018**, *80*, 1697–1713. [CrossRef]
35. Wu, G.R.; Liao, W.; Stramaglia, S.; Ding, J.R.; Chen, H.; Marinazzo, D. A blind deconvolution approach to recover effective connectivity brain networks from resting state fMRI data. *Med. Image Anal.* **2013**, *17*, 365–374. [CrossRef]
36. Brunet, D.; Murray, M.M.; Michel, C.M. Spatiotemporal Analysis of Multichannel EEG: CARTOOL. *Comput. Intell. Neurosci.* **2011**, *2011*, 813870. [CrossRef]
37. Pascual-Marqui, R.D.; Michel, C.M.; Lehmann, D. Segmentation of brain electrical activity into microstates: Model estimation and validation. *IEEE Trans. Biomed. Eng.* **1995**, *42*, 658–665. [CrossRef]
38. Brodbeck, V.; Kuhn, A.; von Wegner, F.; Morzelewski, A.; Tagliazucchi, E.; Borisov, S.; Michel, C.M.; Laufs, H. EEG microstates of wakefulness and NREM sleep. *Neuroimage* **2012**, *62*, 2129–2139. [CrossRef]
39. Koenig, T.; Lehmann, D.; Merlo, M.C.; Kochi, K.; Hell, D.; Koukkou, M. A deviant EEG brain microstate in acute, neuroleptic-naive schizophrenics at rest. *Eur. Arch. Psychiatry Clin. Neurosci.* **1999**, *249*, 205–211. [CrossRef]
40. Hurst, H.E. Long-Term Storage Capacity of Reservoirs. *Trans. Am. Soc. Civ. Eng.* **1951**, *116*, 770–799. [CrossRef]
41. Mandelbrot, B.B. When Can Price be Arbitraged Efficiently? A Limit to the Validity of the Random Walk and Martingale Models. *Rev. Econ. Stat.* **1971**, *53*, 225–236. [CrossRef]
42. Mandelbrot, B.B. Statistical Methodology for Nonperiodic Cycles: From the Covariance To R/S Analysis. In *Annals of Economic and Social Measurement*; Berg, S.V., Ed.; NBER: Cambridge, MA, USA, 1972; Volume 1, pp. 259–290.
43. Mandelbrot, B.B.; Wallis, J.R. Robustness of the rescaled range R/S in the measurement of noncyclic long run statistical dependence. *Water Resour. Res.* **1969**, *5*, 967–988. [CrossRef]
44. Ihlen, E.A. Introduction to multifractal detrended fluctuation analysis in matlab. *Front. Physiol.* **2012**, *3*, 141. [CrossRef]
45. Von Wegner, F.; Tagliazucchi, E.; Brodbeck, V.; Laufs, H. Analytical and empirical fluctuation functions of the EEG microstate random walk—Short-range vs. long-range correlations. *Neuroimage* **2016**, *141*, 442–445. [CrossRef]
46. Jones, C.L.; Lonergan, G.T.; Mainwaring, D.E. Wavelet packet computation of the Hurst exponent. *J. Phys. A Math. Gen.* **1996**, *29*, 2509–2527. [CrossRef]
47. Serinaldi, F. Use and misuse of some Hurst parameter estimators applied to stationary and non-stationary financial time series. *Phys. A Stat. Mech. Its Appl.* **2010**, *389*, 2770–2781. [CrossRef]
48. De Pasquale, F.; Della Penna, S.; Snyder, A.Z.; Lewis, C.; Mantini, D.; Marzetti, L.; Belardinelli, P.; Ciancetta, L.; Pizzella, V.; Romani, G.L.; et al. Temporal dynamics of spontaneous MEG activity in brain networks. *Proc. Natl. Acad. Sci. USA* **2010**, *107*, 6040–6045. [CrossRef] [PubMed]
49. Preibisch, C.; Castrillon, G.J.; Buhrer, M.; Riedl, V. Evaluation of Multiband EPI Acquisitions for Resting State fMRI. *PLoS ONE* **2015**, *10*, e0136961. [CrossRef] [PubMed]
50. Triantafyllou, C.; Polimeni, J.R.; Wald, L.L. Physiological noise and signal-to-noise ratio in fMRI with multi-channel array coils. *NeuroImage* **2011**, *55*, 597–606. [CrossRef]

51. Rubin, D.; Fekete, T.; Mujica-Parodi, L.R. Optimizing complexity measures for FMRI data: Algorithm, artifact, and sensitivity. *PLoS ONE* **2013**, *8*, e63448. [CrossRef]
52. Krüger, G.; Glover, G.H. Physiological noise in oxygenation-sensitive magnetic resonance imaging. *Magn. Reson. Med.* **2001**, *46*, 631–637. [CrossRef]
53. Gonzalez-Castillo, J.; Roopchansingh, V.; Bandettini, P.A.; Bodurka, J. Physiological noise effects on the flip angle selection in BOLD fMRI. *NeuroImage* **2011**, *54*, 2764–2778. [CrossRef]

fractal and fractional

MDPI

Article

ϑ-Fractional Stochastic Models for Simulating Tumor Growth and Chemical Diffusion in Biological Tissues

Ahmed Ghezal [1] and Najmeddine Attia [2,*]

1 Department of Mathematics, University Center of Mila, Mila 43000, Algeria; a.ghezal@centre-univ-mila.dz
2 Department of Mathematics and Statistics, College of Science, King Faisal University, Al-Ahsa 31982, Saudi Arabia
* Correspondence: nattia@kfu.edu.sa

Abstract: This paper presents an advanced simulation-based investigation of tumor growth and chemical diffusion in biological tissues, using ϑ-fractional stochastic integral equations. Based on the theoretical framework developed in [Fractal Fract. 2025, 9(1), 7], we develop an innovative computational model to explore the practical applications of these equations in the biological field. The model focuses on providing new insights into the dynamic interaction between stochastic effects of a fractional nature and complex biological tissue environments, contributing to a deeper understanding of the mechanisms of chemical diffusion within tissues and tumor growth under different conditions. The paper details the numerical techniques used to solve the ϑ-fractional stochastic integral equations, focusing on the stability and accuracy of the solutions, while demonstrating their ability to accurately and effectively capture key biological phenomena. Through extensive computational experiments, the model demonstrates its ability to replicate realistic tumor growth patterns and complex chemical transport dynamics, providing a powerful and flexible tool for understanding tumor behavior and interaction with potential therapies. These results represent an important step toward improving biological models and enhancing biomedical applications, particularly in the areas of targeted drug design and analysis of tumor dynamics under chemotherapeutic influence.

Keywords: ϑ-fractional stochastic integral equations; stochastic calculus; Ulam–Hyers stability; tumor growth; chemical diffusion in biological tissues

1. Introduction

Fractional calculus, which deals with fractional-order differentiation and integration, has emerged as a pivotal mathematical framework for modeling and analyzing complex systems across various scientific and engineering disciplines. This advanced branch of mathematics goes beyond the traditional limitations of integer-order calculus, providing precise tools for understanding nonlinear, nonlocal, and memory-dependent phenomena that are a fundamental feature of many natural and artificial systems. Applications of fractional calculus extend to diverse fields including electrical engineering, where it is used to improve the efficiency of power systems and filter design, control theory, with a focus on improving the stability of dynamical systems, thermal systems, through the analysis of complex heat conduction, signal processing, where it contributes to the analysis of nonlinear and time-dependent signals, and biological systems, where it is employed to model history-dependent physiological processes such as the transport of biomaterials or cell dynamics. Fractional calculus enables scientists and engineers to address multiple research and application challenges such as asymptotic stability analysis [1,2], which studies the long-term stability of systems, and finite-time stability [3,4], which focuses on the stability of systems over a specific time. It also plays a fundamental role in controller design, which helps improve the control of dynamical systems, and error estimation, which enhances mathematical models' accuracy in predicting complex systems' behavior. With these unique capabilities, fractional calculus provides a comprehensive and flexible framework for modeling multidisciplinary systems, making it an indispensable tool in addressing modern scientific and engineering challenges.

The introduction of fractional ϑ derivatives (ϑ-FDs) and fractional ϑ integrals (ϑ-FIs) is a notable development in fractional calculus, providing additional flexibility in describing systems exhibiting complex diffusion dynamics including subdiffusion and superdiffusion [5]. These tools can reconcile the transitional properties of dynamical systems, allowing for more accurate modeling of phenomena combining slow (constrained) and fast (unconstrained) diffusion in various real applications. Recent studies have investigated the theoretical properties of equations involving ϑ-FDs and ϑ-FIs, focusing on crucial aspects such as the existence, uniqueness, and stability [6,7]. Furthermore, the researchers in [5] proposed an innovative ϑ-subdiffusion equation formulation, specifically designed to model complex transitions between classical subdiffusion and superdiffusion. This application trend reflects the increasing importance of ϑ-fractional derivatives and integrals in addressing the challenges of mathematical modeling of nonlinear and memory-dependent phenomena, such as particle transport in porous media or chemical diffusion in biological tissues. This development highlights the profound potential of ϑ-FDs and ϑ-FIs in achieving significant advances in both theory and application, enhancing the status of fractional calculus as an essential mathematical tool in the study of complex systems.

In the field of stochastic processes, fractional stochastic integral equations (FSIEs) have become a vital mathematical tool due to their unique ability to incorporate the effects of randomness and long memory into mathematical models. These equations provide a flexible framework for describing systems that are affected by stochastic factors and exhibit memory-dependent dynamics, making them of particular interest in various fields such as statistical physics, biological systems, and financial markets. One of the fundamental concepts studied in this context is Ulam–Hayers stability (UHS), which addresses the sensitivity of solutions to perturbations in initial conditions or parameters. This type of stability is of particular importance in practical applications, where models are susceptible to small perturbations due to experimental errors or numerical approximations. UHS has been extensively studied for various types of fractional stochastic equations, with studies [8–10] showing that robust stability can be achieved even in systems with complex dynamical behavior. However, research on the Ulam–Hayer stability of ϑ-FSIEs remains limited. This class of equations is a natural and important extension of conventional FSIEs, offering an additional degree of flexibility in describing transitional phenomena between subdiffusion and superdiffusion. The investigation of UHS for ϑ-FSIEs represents an important step towards improving our understanding of complex multi-effect systems and holds broad potential for practical applications in modeling stochastic phenomena with memory-dependent dynamics, such as chemical diffusion in biological tissues or particle motion in random media.

The theoretical basis of our study is based on the pioneering work of Alsharari et al. [11], where the existence, uniqueness, and stability of UHS solutions of ϑ-FSIEs were analyzed with high precision. In this work, the authors relied on advanced techniques of stochastic calculus and Banach Fixed Point Theory (BFPT) to prove their theoretical results. The equation studied takes the following form:

$$\begin{aligned}\alpha(\omega) = \eta + \int_a^\omega \Psi_1(\varsigma, \alpha(\varsigma))d\varsigma + \sum_{i=2}^{n} \int_a^\omega \vartheta_i'(\varsigma)(\vartheta_i(\omega) - \vartheta_i(\varsigma))^{\gamma_i - 1}\Psi_i(\varsigma, \alpha(\varsigma))d\varsigma \\ + \int_a^\omega F(\varsigma, \alpha(\varsigma))dW(\varsigma),\end{aligned} \tag{1}$$

with $\eta \in \mathbb{R}$, $\gamma_i \in (0,1)$ for $2 \leq i \leq n$, $\omega \in [a, T]$ and specific conditions were imposed on the functions F and Ψ_i to ensure Lipschitz continuity and bounds, which ensures the stability and accuracy of the solutions [11]. Despite the theoretical power of this analysis, the practical applications of these equations, especially ϑ-FSIEs, in modeling realistic phenomena such as tumor growth and chemical diffusion in biological tissues remain insufficiently explored. This study seeks to fill this gap by developing an integrated computational framework that aims to test and apply ϑ-FSIEs in such biological contexts. This framework is based on combining stochastic and fractional properties with biological tissue dynamics, enabling more accurate simulation of complex phenomena involving cell–chemical interactions. The numerical simulation involves the use of advanced numerical techniques to solve ϑ-FSIEs, with an emphasis on the stability and accuracy of the solutions to ensure that the behaviors of biological systems are reliably captured. Through this work, we aim to provide new insights into the applicability of these equations in areas such as the design of targeted therapies and the analysis of the diffusion of chemicals in injured tissues, contributing to the development of more effective mathematical models for biomedical research. Equation (1) was selected as a mathematical model for tumor growth and chemical diffusion due to its ability to represent the complex dynamics of these biological phenomena. This equation relies on three key components that reflect the multiscale nature of the system under study: (1) the kernel-dependent integral terms ϑ, which incorporate the historical effects of interactions between tumor cells and their environment, allowing for the description of delayed chemical diffusion in biological tissues and memory-dependent diffusion; (2) the stochastic terms $dW(\varsigma)$, which represent environmental fluctuations such as random changes in nutrient supply and genetic mutations in cancer cells; (3) the γ_i, which provides an accurate description of anomalous diffusion patterns, describing slow diffusion (subdiffusion) in dense tumor environments and rapid diffusion in areas of high vascular density. This mathematical structure enables the simulation of transitions between different diffusion patterns documented in experimental studies and aids in analyzing tumor responses to environmental changes. The proposed model is based on mathematical principles designed to capture key aspects of tumor growth and diffusion processes. It provides a robust theoretical framework for studying tumor dynamics and serves as a foundation for future research. To strengthen the clinical relevance of this framework, our next steps involve collaborating with oncologists and experimental biologists to integrate tissue-specific data (e.g., MRI tumor measurements or in vitro diffusion rates). This collaboration will enable direct model calibration and validation, bridging the gap between theoretical predictions and real-world biomedical challenges, and ultimately enhancing the model's predictive power and applicability to real-world tumor dynamics.

The main contribution of this paper is to present an advanced numerical simulation of tumor growth and chemical diffusion using ϑ-FSIEs. Through this work, we highlight the dual role of fractional and stochastic dynamics in shaping complex biological patterns, providing a deeper understanding of the interaction of physical and biological factors in biological tissue environments. These simulations provide a detailed insight into the influence of fractional time and stochastic perturbations in controlling tumor growth dynamics and chemical diffusion. In particular, ϑ-FSIEs allow an accurate representation of the transitions between subdiffusion and superdiffusion, reflecting the multi-scale nature of these biological processes. By combining a robust theoretical framework with accurate numerical simulations, this study opens up new avenues for employing ϑ-FSIEs in modeling complex biological systems, further enhancing our contribution to the fields of biomedicine and mathematical computation.

The rest of this paper is organized as follows: Section 2 reviews the main theoretical results obtained. Section 3 presents the numerical results, focusing on the simulation of tumor growth and the diffusion of chemicals in biological tissues. This section demonstrates how ϑ-FSIEs can be applied to realistic models, reviewing the numerical strategies used and their performance in terms of accuracy and stability. The results are analyzed in detail to illustrate the influence of randomness and fractional dynamics on biological processes. Section 4 concludes by providing basic insights into the significance of the study and the results achieved, and discussing the future potential of ϑ-FSIEs in biological modeling. New research directions are proposed, including improving the numerical models and exploring other applications in biophysics and complex stochastic systems.

2. Existence, Uniqueness, and Stability Analysis of ϑ-FSIEs

The seminal work by Alsharari et al. (2025, [11]) focuses on establishing accurate results for a class of ϑ-FSIEs, representing an important advance in analyzing complex systems that combine stochastic effects and fractional dynamics. The primary motivation for this work stems from the need for more accurate and flexible mathematical models capable of describing systems that exhibit memory-dependent behaviors and nonlinear diffusive effects, properties that traditional methods often fail to capture adequately. By adopting a robust mathematical framework that combines fractional calculus and stochastic analysis, the authors address fundamental questions regarding the existence and uniqueness of solutions to ϑ-FSIEs. These results are essential for understanding whether complex systems can be accurately modeled using this class of equations. Furthermore, the work focuses on the stability of solutions, including UHS, which ensures that systems respond to small perturbations in the initial conditions, making the models more robust and applicable in real-world contexts. These results provide a solid foundation for future research into applying ϑ-FSIEs in new fields and more complex real-world problems. By providing this in-depth analysis, Alsharari et al. contribute to the theoretical understanding of ϑ-FSIEs, opening up broad prospects for their application in a variety of complex dynamical systems.

The paper [11] provides important theoretical progress expressed through three main theories. Together, these theories represent an integrated framework for analyzing and studying ϑ-FSIEs, opening new horizons for their application in various fields, which we summarize and analyze below.

Lemma 1 **(Operator definition).** *The following assumptions are made:*

A1. ***Lipschitz condition:***
The functions F, Ψ_l for $1 \leq l \leq n$ satisfy the Lipschitz condition:

$$|F(\omega,u_1) - F(\omega,u_2)| \vee |\Psi_l(\omega,u_1) - \Psi_l(\omega,u_2)| \leq K|u_1 - u_2|,$$

for all $\omega \in [a,T]$, $u_1, u_2 \in \mathbb{R}^2$, with $K > 0$.

A2. ***Boundedness condition:***
The functions F, Ψ_l for $1 \leq l \leq n$ satisfy:

$$\operatorname*{ess\,sup}_{\omega\in[a,T]}|F(\omega,0)| \vee \operatorname*{ess\,sup}_{\omega\in[a,T]}|\Psi_l(\omega,0)| \leq d,$$

for some $d > 0$, where $1 \leq l \leq n$.

Then the operator N_η is well-defined for every $\eta \in \mathbb{R}$, where the operator N_η is defined on the space of stochastic processes $S_m([a,T])$, which represents the set of all measurable and $\mathcal{M}$-adapted processes satisfying

$$\sup_{\omega \in [a,T]} \| \alpha(\omega) \|_m < \infty.$$

More precisely, this space is a Banach space equipped with the norm:

$$\| \alpha \|_{S_m([a,T])} = \sup_{\omega \in [a,T]} \| \alpha(\omega) \|_m.$$

The operator N_η is explicitly defined as

$$\begin{aligned}(N_\eta \alpha)(\omega) = \eta &+ \int_a^\omega \Psi_1(\varsigma, \alpha(\varsigma)) d\varsigma \\ &+ \sum_{i=2}^{n} \int_a^\omega \vartheta_i'(\varsigma)(\vartheta_i(\omega) - \vartheta_i(\varsigma))^{\gamma_i - 1} \Psi_i(\varsigma, \alpha(\varsigma)) d\varsigma \\ &+ \int_a^\omega F(\varsigma, \alpha(\varsigma)) dW(\varsigma).\end{aligned}$$

This preliminary lemma ensures the mathematical soundness of the operator central to the analysis.

The first theorem ensures that the model is mathematically consistent and able to predict accurately, a property essential for applications in engineering and science. This consistency is an indication that the equations used in the model have unique, existing solutions under the assumed conditions, removing any mathematical ambiguity that might lead to unreliable results. On a practical level, this assurance enhances the reliability of the model when used to simulate complex physical and biological systems. For example, in the biological sciences, proving the existence and uniqueness of solutions is essential for modeling biological processes such as tumor growth and the diffusion of chemicals in tissues, where these applications require accurate decisions based on robust mathematical models. Furthermore, this predictive consistency enhances the model's ability to explore unfamiliar scenarios, enabling it to be used as a tool for exploring nonlinear phenomena in fields such as biophysics and environmental modeling. This theoretical foundation paves the way for improving the model and extending it to other, more complex applications, enhancing its value in scientific and engineering research.

Theorem 1 (Existence and uniqueness). *Under the assumptions* **A1** *and* **A2**, *the ϑ-FSIE (1) is guaranteed to have a unique solution.*

The second theorem proves that ϑ-FSIE (1) solutions exhibit a continuous dependence on initial conditions, meaning that small changes in the initial conditions lead to small and proportional changes in the solutions. This property is pivotal in mathematical modeling, as it reflects the stability and predictability of the system. This property enhances the stability and robustness of the solutions under small perturbations in the initial conditions. In biological applications, such as modeling chemical diffusion or tumor dynamics, this property means that model-based predictions are reliable even when there is a small uncertainty in the initial values, such as the initial chemical concentration or the distribution of cancer cells. Furthermore, this property is a fundamental step towards UHS analysis, which provides deeper insights into the long-term dynamic behavior of the system, making the model more suitable for practical applications that require accurate and consistent responses under small environmental or cognitive changes.

Theorem 2 (Continuous dependence on initial conditions [11]). *For two initial values $\eta_1, \eta_2 \in \mathbb{R}$, the difference between their respective solutions $\alpha_1(\varsigma)$ and $\alpha_2(\varsigma)$ of (1) vanishes as $\eta_1 \longrightarrow \eta_2$:*

$$\lim_{\eta_1 \longrightarrow \eta_2} \sup_{\varsigma \in [a,T]} \| \alpha_1(\varsigma) - \alpha_2(\varsigma) \|_{ms} = 0.$$

The latter theorem proves that the ϑ-FSIE (1) is stable according to the UHS criterion. This property indicates that the approximate solutions, resulting from small disturbances or errors in the initial data, remain close to the exact solutions. This stability is an important indicator of the robustness and reliability of the model, especially in practical applications where errors and approximations are inevitable. This property plays a crucial role in ensuring that the model can tolerate small deviations without significantly affecting the accuracy of its predictions. For example, in numerical simulations of biological or physical processes, such as tumor growth or chemical diffusion, UHS stability ensures that errors due to numerical slicing, computational approximations, or experimental measurements do not lead to significant deviations in the results. Furthermore, UHS stability provides a solid basis for the design of efficient numerical algorithms, as it ensures that the approximations resulting from numerical solutions will not deviate significantly from the theoretical solutions. This is of great importance in complex systems where fractional dynamics interact with stochastic effects, posing a challenge for accurate modeling and reliable simulation. The applications of UHS also extend to dynamical systems, optimal control problems, and model-based decision-making, where this stability lends confidence in the reliability of predictions and their relevance to real behaviors. Thus, the UHS stability of the ϑ-FSIE (1) equation enhances the mathematical framework of the model and improves its practical applicability in various scientific and engineering fields.

Theorem 3 (Ulam–Hyers stability). *If A1 and A2 are satisfied, then the ϑ-FSIE (1) is UHS.*

The results presented by Alsharari et al. [11] represent a major step forward in the theory of fractional stochastic systems. By taking advantage of continuity conditions and Lipschitz boundary, the authors provide a powerful mathematical framework for studying ϑ-FSIEs. The theorems presented ensure that these equations not only have unique and well-behaved solutions but also have desirable stability properties, such as UHS. These results are pivotal for the practical application of fractional stochastic models, as they provide accurate and reliable tools for analyzing complex systems that combine fractional and stochastic effects. This is particularly evident in areas such as control theory, where control of fine-grained dynamical systems is required, signal processing, where non-local dynamics play a major role in signal optimization, and biological systems, where these models enable a deeper understanding of biological interactions involving diffusion and stochastic processes. Furthermore, these results provide insights into how to balance accurate modeling and numerical considerations in practical applications. The ability to prove the existence and uniqueness of solutions, along with stability properties, makes it possible to build models that can deal with the actual challenges associated with volatility and uncertainty in systems.

3. Numerical Simulation and Analysis of Tumor Growth Dynamics

Understanding tumor growth and the dynamics of chemical diffusion within biological tissues requires advanced simulation techniques and powerful analytical frameworks. In this context, simulations are built based on Equation (1). Through this complex model, how the tumor evolves and how environmental and therapeutic factors affect this growth are determined. This model uses numerical integration techniques to simulate the complex interactions between tumor cells and their surrounding chemicals, and the effects of chemotherapies and radiation. The process begins by simulating tumor evolution using this equation, and subsequently progresses to evaluate the different effects of treatments by simulating chemical interactions with therapeutics and using neural networks to recognize patterns and predict future tumor evolution. We also use predictive modeling techniques to enhance our understanding of how the tumor responds to the environment and treatment, which contributes to providing deeper insights into its behavior under multiple conditions. These numerical simulations provide powerful tools to support therapeutic decision-making and guide future research in oncology.

Figure 1 illustrates the natural growth trajectory of a tumor in the absence of any treatment, revealing a typical exponential growth pattern characterized by a steady increase in tumor size over time. This exponential growth reflects the process of accelerated tumor cell proliferation, where the tumor continues to expand at an increasing rate when there are no therapeutic interventions to stop it. This pattern is a critical parameter in studying the behavior of untreated tumors, highlighting the aggressive nature of the tumor and its ability to spread rapidly and widely into neighboring tissues. These data do not emphasize the importance of early detection of tumors and initiating appropriate therapeutic interventions as soon as possible to prevent this uncontrolled increase in tumor size. Although this exponential growth indicates a relatively early stage of tumor development, tumor development in the absence of treatment remains an essential starting point for understanding tumor dynamics and how biological factors influence its response to treatment.

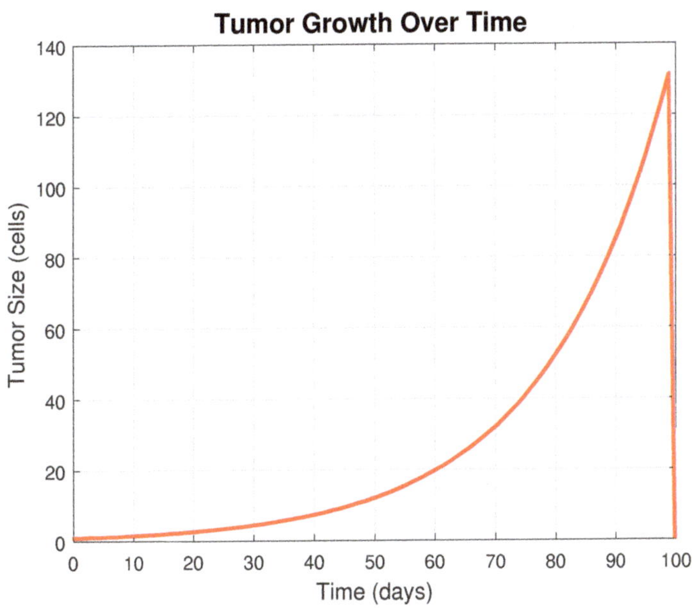

Figure 1. Baseline tumor growth over time.

Figure 2 compares tumor growth under three different treatment conditions: no treatment, chemotherapy, and placebo. The "no treatment" curve replicates the baseline from Figure 1, reflecting the steady exponential growth pattern that characterizes an untreated tumor. This pattern shows a continuous increase in tumor size over time without intervention, reflecting the aggressive and rapid growth nature of malignant tumors in the absence of treatment. This condition serves as an important reference for evaluating the effectiveness of different treatments. In contrast, the "chemotherapy" curve shows a significant decrease in growth rate, indicating that chemotherapy has succeeded in significantly slowing tumor growth. Although chemotherapy reduces tumor growth, this decrease is not always sufficient to completely stop tumor progression, highlighting the limitations of some chemotherapies in controlling growth in the long term. Nevertheless, chemotherapy remains an effective treatment option in many cases requiring a rapid response. The "placebo" curve shows a more pronounced suppression of tumor growth than chemotherapy, suggesting that a placebo may provide superior benefits in managing tumor dynamics. Alternative treatment may include the use of innovative therapeutic techniques or therapeutic combinations specifically developed to attack the tumor in different ways than conventional treatments. This treatment shows a strong effect in reducing tumor size in the long term, which opens the door to research into its potential as a more effective alternative to some chemotherapies, especially in cases that do not respond to conventional drugs. This comparison contributes to shedding light on the relative effectiveness of different interventions in managing tumor dynamics, providing deeper insights into optimal treatment strategies. Through this analysis, the most effective treatments can be identified based on their different effects in reducing tumor growth, thus improving future treatment strategies. This comparison also provides a basis for developing personalized therapeutic frameworks based on tumor type and response to treatment, which could enhance the improvement of patient care.

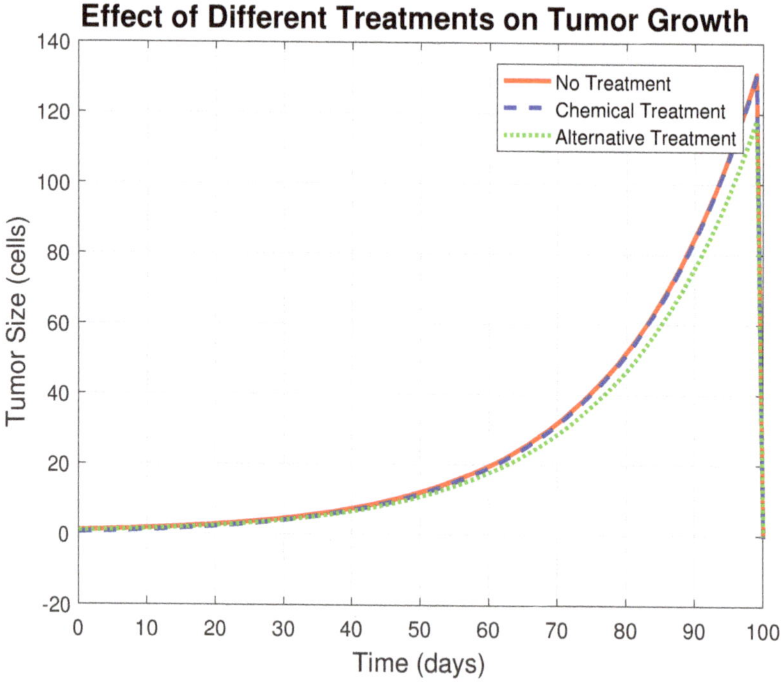

Figure 2. Comparative analysis of treatment strategies.

Figure 3 illustrates the ability of the neural network model to recognize and replicate observed tumor growth patterns. By comparing the observed data with the model's predictions, it is clear that the neural network accurately captures the underlying dynamics of tumor growth, including exponential patterns and changes in tumor size over time. The model has a high ability to predict tumor progression under different conditions, whether untreated or multi-treatment, enhancing the accuracy of predictive understanding of tumor behavior. The strength of neural networks is their ability to learn from large and complex data sets, making them an ideal tool for analyzing biological patterns that may be hidden or complex to traditional methods. The network's ability to adapt to observed data and generate accurate results makes it a reliable tool for understanding tumor growth processes and their interactions with different treatments. Validation of the model by comparing predictions with actual data shows that the neural network captures not only general trends in tumor growth but also subtle responses to changes in therapeutic parameters. This reliability strengthens the position of neural networks as powerful analytical tools for understanding complex, multidimensional biological processes. Not only does this analysis provide deeper insights into tumor behavior under different influences, it also paves the way for the use of neural networks in predictive modeling, allowing researchers and clinicians to predict future tumor evolution based on current data. These networks can then be used to guide advanced treatment strategies, providing accurate predictions that support better, scientifically informed treatment decisions.

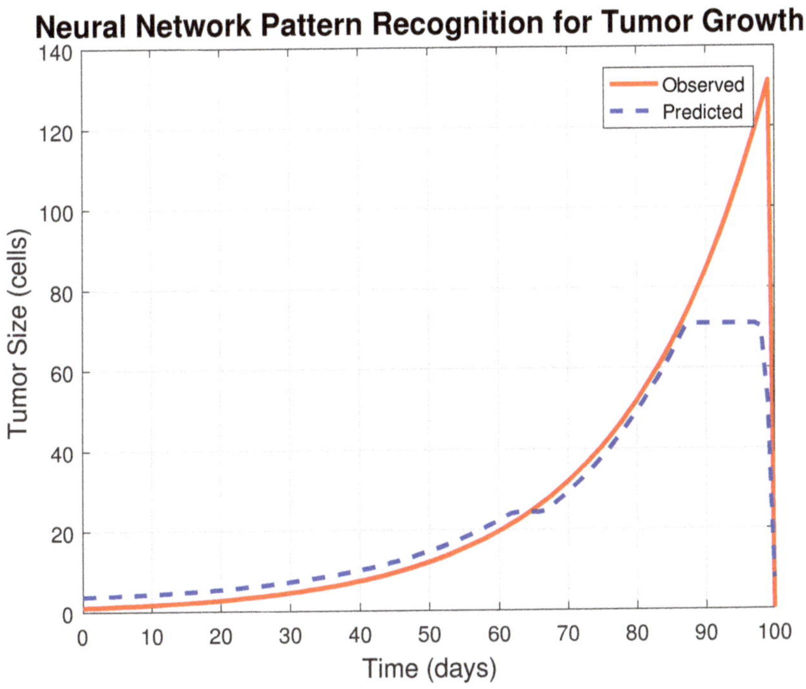

Figure 3. Neural network-based pattern recognition for tumor growth.

Figure 4 illustrates the ability of the neural network to predict future tumor growth, expanding the focus to predict long-term tumor evolution dynamics. The neural network allows growth trends to be extrapolated from observed data and accurately predicted over extended periods. The predicted values generated by the network closely match the actual data, highlighting the power of the model in simulating and identifying potential tumor growth trajectories under a variety of conditions. The results show that the neural network is not limited to processing current data, but can also provide accurate estimates of the future based on past patterns, providing an invaluable tool in estimating future tumor evolution. These predictive capabilities are invaluable in clinical decision-making, as clinicians and researchers can use them to proactively identify potential tumor growth trends. With this predictive ability, personalized treatment plans that take into account potential tumor evolution can be designed, contributing to more personalized and effective treatments for each patient. In addition, this ability allows changes in tumor status to be anticipated, enabling early therapeutic interventions to prevent progression or improve treatment efficacy at different stages of growth. Overall, the importance of neural networks lies in providing data-driven prediction solutions, which contribute to dynamically guiding treatment based on a deep understanding of the biological behavior of tumors. The ability of these networks to predict tumor growth opens a new horizon in data-driven medical treatment, which enhances the effectiveness of clinical procedures and directs them toward the most positive outcomes.

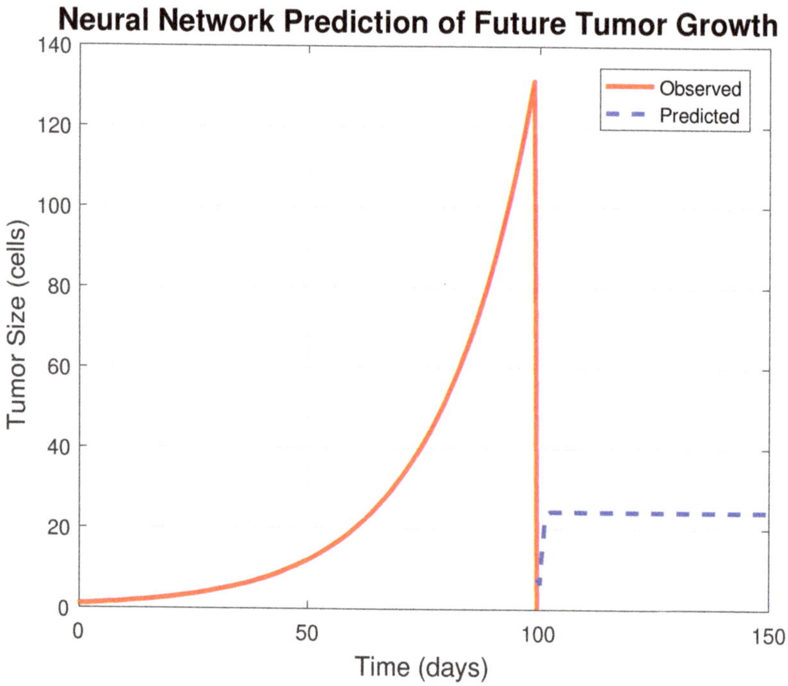

Figure 4. Predictive modeling of tumor growth using neural networks.

Remark 1. *In this paper, we performed numerical simulations using the following schemes: (1) a fixed-time-step Euler forward method ($\Delta t = 1$) for the logistic tumor growth model, (2) adaptive numerical integration using the integral() function in MATLAB (https://www.mathworks.com/products/matlab.html) to model chemical diffusion, and (3) a prediction model using support vector machines (SVMs) for long-term prediction. To ensure the accuracy of the results, we performed a sensitivity analysis by varying the growth parameters (0.03–0.07) and diffusion parameters (0.6–1.0), and verified the stability of the solutions as the grid resolution changed (n = 100 to n = 1000). The results demonstrated numerical stability with a less than 5% relative change in the main variables, while the prediction model achieved an accuracy with a mean squared error of 0.05. This methodology strikes a balance between computational accuracy and computational efficiency over the studied parameter range.*

Remark 2. *The ϑ-FSIEs-based model offers clear competitive advantages over traditional models used to simulate tumor growth and chemical diffusion in biological tissues. First, the incorporation of stochasticity and fractional effects allows for a more accurate representation of nonlinear biological* *phenomena, which is critical for the study of complex biological systems. Second, simulations have shown that the model offers high numerical stability, with the relative error reduced to less than 5%when varying growth and chemical diffusion parameters, enhancing the reliability of the results. Furthermore, the model is flexible in incorporating different biological parameters and can be easily adjusted to simulate multiple scenarios, including the effects of chemotherapy and tumor–environment interactions. Finally, this approach offers improved computational efficiency. This modeling framework not only contributes to a better theoretical understanding of tumor progression mechanisms but can also serve as a practical tool for clinical decision-making by providing more accurate predictions of tumor response to various treatments.*

4. Conclusions

This paper presents an advanced framework for simulating tumor growth and chemical diffusion in biological tissues using ϑ-FSIEs. By combining theoretical analysis and numerical simulation, we explored the dynamic interactions between fractional and stochastic effects in complex biological environments. The results highlight the importance of fractional time and stochastic perturbations in shaping tumor growth dynamics and chemical transport processes, providing new insights into the applicability of ϑ-FSIEs in modeling biological phenomena such as tumor progression and therapeutic interventions. Incorporating fractional effects into biological modeling provides an additional layer of accuracy in simulating biological systems characterized by random and nonlinear behavior, a common feature in tumor progression and chemical diffusion. This model allows the study of the effects of small perturbations on the system, helping to understand how small changes in parameters affect complex biological dynamics. Simulations demonstrated the ability of the ϑ-FSIE model to replicate realistic tumor growth patterns and model the diffusion of chemicals in biological tissues with high accuracy. This framework also provided valuable insights into the effects of different treatment strategies, especially chemotherapy. Through comparative analyses, we observed the potential of alternative therapies to suppress tumor growth over long periods, opening new avenues for research into therapeutic strategies. Furthermore, by incorporating neural network-based predictive modeling, we enhanced our understanding of tumor growth under different conditions, demonstrating the power of these networks to accurately predict tumor progression. The ability of neural networks to recognize complex patterns and predict future growth trajectories adds a crucial layer to the modeling framework, providing valuable support in decision-making about treatment strategies. These networks may also provide support in evaluating the efficacy of future therapies by simulating various treatment scenarios. Additionally, simulations of tumor growth under various conditions, including untreated scenarios and treatment-based interventions, provide an application case that validates the model's predictive capabilities. The primary tumor growth (Figure 1) is consistent with the observed exponential growth patterns, supporting the model's accuracy in simulating real-world tumor dynamics. Furthermore, a comparative analysis of chemotherapy and alternative therapies (Figure 2) highlights the model's ability to assess treatment efficacy, making it a valuable tool for evaluating therapeutic strategies. Predictive modeling using neural networks (Figures 3 and 4) enhances the model's potential for clinical decision-making, demonstrating its ability to predict tumor progression under various treatment regimens.

In conclusion, the combination of stochastic and fractional dynamics enables a more comprehensive understanding of tumor behavior and chemokinesis, contributing to the development of more effective mathematical models for biomedical applications. The use of this model could enhance the accuracy of predictions about tumor progression and guide research efforts toward personalized therapeutic approaches. Next steps will prioritize improving numerical methods and exploring their potential in other areas of biophysics and complex systems, particularly in targeted therapy design and chemotherapy-driven tumor dynamics. The model's flexibility also allows extensions to scenarios like tumor–vascular interactions or environmental–genetic effects.

To strengthen clinical relevance, we plan to collaborate with experimental biologists for tissue-specific data (e.g., MRI tumor measurements or in vitro diffusion rates), enabling direct model calibration and validation. This will bridge the gap between theoretical predictions and real-world biomedical challenges.

Author Contributions: Conceptualization, N.A.; methodology, A.G.; formal analysis, N.A. and A.G.; writing—original draft preparation, A.G.; writing—review and editing, N.A. and A.G. All authors have read and agreed to the published version of the manuscript.

Funding: This work was supported by the Deanship of Scientific Research, Vice Presidency for Graduate Studies and Scientific Research, King Faisal University, Saudi Arabia [KFU251420].

Data Availability Statement: No new data were created or analyzed in this study. Data sharing is not applicable to this article.

Conflicts of Interest: The authors declare that there are no conflicts of interest.

References

1. Monje, C.A.; Chen, Y.; Vinagre, B.M.; Xue, D.; Feliu-Batlle, V. *Fractional-Order Systems and Controls: Fundamentals and Applications*; Springer: Berlin/Heidelberg, Germany, 2010; ISBN 9781849963350.
2. Wu, Z. Multiple asymptotic stability of fractional-order quaternion-valued neural networks with time-varying delays. *Neurocomputing* **2021**, *448*, 301–312. [CrossRef]
3. Ben Makhlouf, A. A novel finite time stability analysis of nonlinear fractional-order time delay systems: A fixed point approach. *Asian J. Control* **2022**, *24*, 3580–3587. [CrossRef]
4. Ben Makhlouf, A.; Mchiri, L.; Rhaima, M. Stability analysis of finite time for a class of nonlinear time-delay fractional-order systems. *Fractal Fract.* **2024**, *8*, 4. [CrossRef]
5. Kosztoowicz, T. Subdiffusion equation with fractional Caputo time derivative with respect to another function in modeling transition from ordinary subdiffusion to superdiffusion. *Phys. Rev. E* **2023**, *107*, 064103. [CrossRef] [PubMed]
6. Derbazi, C.; Baitiche, Z.; Zada, A. Existence and uniqueness of positive solutions for fractional relaxation equation in terms of Ψ-Caputo fractional derivative. *Int. J. Nonlinear Sci. Numer. Simul.* **2023**, *24*, 633–643. [CrossRef]
7. Derbazi, C.; Baitiche, Z.; Benchohra, M. Coupled system of Ψ-Caputo fractional differential equations without and with delay in generalized Banach spaces. *Results Nonlinear Anal.* **2022**, *5*, 42–61. [CrossRef]
8. Derbazi, C.; Baitiche, Z. Uniqueness and Ulam-Hyers-Mittag-Leffler stability results for the delayed fractional multiterm differential equation involving the Φ-Caputo fractional derivative. *Rocky Mt. J. Math.* **2022**, *52*, 887–897. [CrossRef]
9. Ahmadova, A.; Mahmudov, N.I. Ulam-Hyers stability of Caputo type fractional stochastic neutral differential equations. *Stat. Probab. Lett.* **2021**, *168*, 108949. [CrossRef]
10. Mchiri, L. Ulam-Hyers stability of fractional Itô-Doob stochastic differential equations. *Math. Methods Appl. Sci.* **2023**, *46*, 13731–13740. [CrossRef]
11. Alsharari, F.; Fakhfakh, R.; Kahouli, O.; Ben Makhlouf, A. Some existence, uniqueness, and stability results for a class of ϑ-fractional stochastic integral equations. *Fractal Fract.* **2025**, *9*, 7. [CrossRef]

fractal and fractional

MDPI

Article

Application of Fractional Fourier Transform and BP Neural Network in Prediction of Tumor Benignity and Malignancy

Xuanyu Liu †, Nan Gao †, Shuoran He † and Lizhen Wang *

School of Mathematics, Northwest University, Xi'an 710127, China; liuxuanyu@stumail.nwu.edu.cn (X.L.); gaonan@stumail.nwu.edu.cn (N.G.); heshuoran@stumail.nwu.edu.cn (S.H.)

* Correspondence: wanglizhen@nwu.edu.cn

† These authors contributed equally to this work.

Abstract: To address the limitations of traditional tumor diagnostic methods in image feature extraction and model generalization, this study innovatively proposes a synergistic diagnostic model that integrates fractional Fourier transform (FrFT) and error back-propagation (BP) neural networks. The model leverages the time–frequency analysis capability of FrFT and incorporates the fractal characteristics observed during tumor proliferation, effectively enhancing multi-scale feature extraction and representation. Experimental results show that the proposed model achieves an accuracy of 93.177% in classifying benign and malignant tumors, outperforming the support vector machine (SVM) method. The integration of FrFT improves feature distinguishability and reduces dependence on manual extraction. This study not only represents a breakthrough in tumor diagnostic technology but also paves new avenues for the application of fractional calculus and fractal geometry in medical image analysis. The findings show great potential for clinical application and future development.

Keywords: tumor diagnosis; fractional calculus; fractal feature; fractional Fourier transform; BP neural network

1. Introduction

1.1. Background

Tumors, especially malignant ones, remain among the major global health threats. According to the World Health Organization, in 2022, approximately 19.96 million new malignant tumor cases were reported worldwide, resulting in 9.73 million deaths [1]. Accurate prediction of tumor benignity or malignancy plays a crucial role in early detection and improving patient outcomes.

Conventional diagnostic methods such as medical imaging and biopsy are often invasive, inefficient, and prone to false positives, limiting their suitability for early screening. Computer-aided diagnosis (CAD) technologies have emerged as promising tools in medical image analysis, enhancing diagnostic efficiency and objectivity through machine learning. However, existing CAD systems still struggle to extract informative features and achieve robust classification, especially when dealing with complex, non-stationary medical signals.

Tumor images often exhibit fractal-like patterns and complex time–frequency structures that are challenging to capture using traditional Fourier transforms. The fractional Fourier transform (FrFT), by introducing a fractional-order parameter, extends classical Fourier analysis and enables more flexible and effective multi-scale feature extraction. Meanwhile, backpropagation (BP) neural networks are widely used for classification due to their powerful nonlinear modeling capability, but they are sensitive to input features and susceptible to overfitting.

https://doi.org/10.3390/fractalfract9050267

To address these challenges, this study proposes an FrFT-BP hybrid model. FrFT is used to preprocess tumor images and extract fractional time–frequency features, which are then fed into a BP neural network for classification, aiming to improve both feature representation and classification performance.

1.2. *Status of Research*

FrFT breaks through the limitation of traditional Fourier transform in time–frequency resolution by introducing the fractional-order parameter, which is especially suitable for feature extraction of non-smooth signals. In 1980, Namias first proposed the mathematical theory of FrFT, which laid the theoretical foundation for its use in the field of signal processing [2]. In 1994, Almeida verified the advantages of FrFT in the time–frequency analysis of biological signals [3]; in 2019, Zhan Hongfeng et al. extended the feature domain with FrFT to extract as much valid information as possible from different dimensions, which significantly improved the correct recognition rate of classification results [4]. However, most of the existing studies focus on the processing of single-modal data and lack an efficient synergy mechanism with deep learning models.

BP neural networks are widely used in medical classification tasks due to their powerful nonlinear fitting ability. In 1986, the backpropagation algorithm proposed by Rumelhart et al. laid the foundation for the development of BP networks [5]. In 2023, Ge Mengfei et al. combined a neural network with the Adaboost method to increase the accuracy of predictive classification of breast cancer to 95.55% [6]. However, the high sensitivity of traditional BP neural networks to input features and their reliance on manually designed feature extraction methods limit their performance in complex medical imaging.

1.3. *Research Objectives, Hypotheses, and Innovativeness*

The rationale of this study lies in combining FrFT with BP neural networks for tumor classification. FrFT enables the extraction of fine-grained, non-stationary features from tumor images, improving the quality of inputs. The BP network enhances classification with its nonlinear learning capability. The synergy reduces reliance on manual feature design, enhances generalization, and improves accuracy [7].

The innovation of this study lies in the integration of the FrFT as a preprocessing tool for input features into the BP neural network, thereby constructing a novel framework of fractional neural networks. The FrFT possesses enhanced time–frequency resolution, enabling it to capture non-stationary and complex signal characteristics that traditional Fourier transforms struggle to extract. This addresses key limitations of existing approaches, such as low feature utilization and high dependency on manual feature engineering. In particular, FrFT effectively enhances the representation of tumor-specific fractal features, leading to higher-quality inputs for the neural network. When combined with the powerful nonlinear fitting capabilities of the BP neural network, the model achieves improved generalization and stability, especially in small-sample medical data scenarios where traditional networks are prone to overfitting. This synergy not only reduces reliance on handcrafted features but also paves the way for building accurate and low-invasive intelligent diagnostic tools for tumor prediction, demonstrating both structural innovation and practical relevance.

Based on this, the research objective of this paper is to construct and validate a benign and malignant tumor prediction model integrating FrFT and a BP neural network and to improve its classification performance and generalization ability when dealing with complex medical data. Considering that medical data are characterized by high dimensionality, nonlinearity, and noise sensitivity, this paper further proposes the hypothesis that if the input data have a high signal-to-noise ratio and feature integrity after FrFT preprocessing, the constructed FrFT-BP model will significantly outperform the traditional methods in terms of classification accuracy and robustness.

1.4. Structure of the Paper

This paper adopts the research path of "theory construction–method design–experimental verification" and is organized as follows:

Section 2 systematically elaborates on the theoretical foundation of FrFT and neural networks. It includes the mathematical definition, basic properties, and unique advantages of FrFT in signal processing and analyzes the core algorithm and architectural features of BP neural networks.

Section 3 constructs the FrFT-BP collaborative diagnostic model. The composition of the experimental dataset, the FrFT preprocessing process, and the network parameter optimization strategy are explained in detail, and a hybrid training method based on the L-M algorithm is proposed.

Section 4 conducts the analysis of benign and malignant tumor prediction results and carries out comparative experimental research. Through multi-dimensional visualization tools such as a performance chart, training status chart, and regression chart, the model's prediction performance on clinical data is analyzed and compared with traditional SVM methods.

Section 5 summarizes the research results, argues for the theoretical contribution of FrFT in enhancing feature differentiability, and explores the prospect of the application of the fusion technique of fractional calculus and deep learning in the field of smart healthcare.

2. Theoretical Foundation

2.1. Fractional Fourier Transform

2.1.1. Definition of FrFT

The FrFT is a tool for transforming a signal from the time (or spatial) domain to the frequency domain. Unlike the classical Fourier transform, the FrFT not only involves the frequency domain, but also allows the "order" of the transform angle to be adjusted α in order to realize different levels of signal transformation. This gives the FrFT a unique advantage in signal processing applications, especially in non-local characterization, where the FrFT is able to retain more information about the signal [8].

For a one-dimensional signal $x(t)$, FrFT is defined as follows [9]:

$$X_p(\mu) = F_p[X(t)] = \int_{-\infty}^{+\infty} K_p(\mu,t)x(t)\,dt, \tag{1}$$

where $K_p(\mu,t) = A_p e^{i\mu^2 \cot\alpha - it^2 \csc^2\alpha}$ is called the kernel function of the fractional Fourier. $A_p = \sqrt{1-j\cot\alpha}$, α is the counterclockwise rotation angle of the fractional-order Fourier domain with respect to the time domain, and the corresponding fractional order is $P = 2\alpha/\pi$. When $p = 4n$, $K_p(\mu,t) = \delta(\mu - t)$; when $p = 4n+2$, $K_p(\mu,t) = \delta(\mu+t)$. The fractional Fourier transform kernel is denoted as follows.

$$K_p(\mu,t) = \begin{cases} \sqrt{\frac{1-j\cot\alpha}{2\pi}} \exp\left(j\frac{\mu^2+t^2}{2}\cot\alpha - j\frac{\mu t}{\sin\alpha}\right), \alpha \neq n\pi, \\ \delta(\mu - t), \alpha = 2n\pi, \\ \delta(\mu + t), \alpha = (2n+1)\pi. \end{cases} \tag{2}$$

The inverse of the fractional order Fourier is

$$x(t) = \int_{-\infty}^{+\infty} K_p(\mu,t)X_p(\mu)d\mu. \tag{3}$$

When the FrFT of the transform of $p = 1$ and when $\alpha = \pi/2$, from Equation (1),

$$x_1(u) = \int_{-\infty}^{+\infty} e^{-j2\pi ut}x(t)dt. \tag{4}$$

From Equation (4), the FrFT is the ordinary Fourier transform when $p = 1$. Therefore, the FrFT can also be seen as an extension of the conventional Fourier transform [10].

2.1.2. Basic Properties

- **Linear properties:** FrFTs have the characteristics of linear transforms and can be combined—that is,

$$F^p\left[\sum_n c_n f_n(u)\right] = \sum_n c_n[F^p f_n(u)].$$

- **Order additivity (rotational additivity):**

$$F^{p_1}F^{p_2} = F^{p_1+p_2}.$$

- **Reversible nature**

$$(F^p)^{-1} = F^{-p}.$$

According to the rotational additivity, it is known that after performing an FrFT with the transformed angle $\alpha = p\pi/2$, its inverse transformation is equivalent to performing an FrFT with the angle $-\alpha$. This property implies that if a signal's time–frequency domain has been rotated by a specific angle through the FrFT, the restoration of the signal's original state can be easily achieved by performing an FrFT with the corresponding negative angle on the signal [11].

- **Nature of exchange**

$$F^{p_1}F^{p_2} = F^{p_2}F^{p_1}.$$

- **Combining properties**

$$(F^{p_1}F^{p_2})F^{p_3} = F^{p_1}(F^{p_2}F^{p_3}).$$

- **Time shift characteristic**

$$F^p[x(t-v)] = X_p(\mu - v\cos\alpha)\exp\left(j\frac{v^2}{2}\sin\alpha\cos\alpha - jv\mu\sin\alpha\right).$$

indicates the frequency shift of the signal.

- **Frequency shift characteristics**

$$F^p\left[x(t)e^{j\sigma t}\right] = X_p(\mu - \sigma\cos\alpha)\exp\left(-i\frac{\sigma^2}{2}\sin\alpha\cos\alpha - i\mu\sigma\sin\alpha\right),$$

σ indicates the frequency shift of the signal.

2.1.3. Application of FrFT in Data Processing

Fractional neural networks can be categorized into two types in terms of structural form: the first type combines FrFT with feedforward neural networks, where the activation function of the nodes in the hidden layer is replaced by the fractional-order kernel function, and the weight from the input layer to the hidden layer is replaced by the fractional-order parameter. This method searches for the optimal order parameter through network training and gradient correction iterations, and performs data prediction at that optimal order. The second category is the use of FrFT as a preprocessing tool for neural network inputs, which is suitable for data characterized by Chirp-like signals. The Chirp-like signals are analyzed by fractional Fourier Transform to extract their unique time–frequency features, and the neural network performs prediction, function approximation, or classification identification based on these feature parameters. The optimal fractional neural network proposed in this paper belongs to this category. In this paper, FrFT is used as a data preprocessing tool, aiming to improve the non-local characteristics of the data and thus enhance the learning ability of the neural network on the data. By adjusting the value of the order parameter α of FrFT, the input features can be optimized so that the neural network can better extract the key information from the data, and thus improve the accuracy of benign and malignant tumor prediction [12].

2.2. *Neural Network Theory*

2.2.1. Overview of Neural Networks

Neural networks are a kind of machine learning model inspired by biological nervous systems, which consist of a large number of artificial neurons, and realize complex function approximation through multi-layer nonlinear transformations, which makes them show their unique value in medical pattern recognition tasks, especially in the problem of tumor benignity and malignancy discrimination, which is characterized by high dimensionality, nonlinearities, and small samples.

2.2.2. The BP Neural Network

The BP neural network is a typical multilayer feedforward neural network composed of input, hidden, and output layers, which is trained through four steps: forward propagation, computation of error, back-propagation, and iterative training. The BP neural network has a strong nonlinear fitting capability [13]. In this study, the BP neural network is selected as the baseline model due to its adaptability to medical prediction problems, particularly in capturing complex nonlinear relationships in structured, non-sequential data and in offering stable gradient-based optimization [14].

Compared with other neural network architectures such as Convolutional Neural Networks (CNNs) and Recurrent Neural Networks (RNNs), the BP network presents several advantages in the context of this research. CNNs are primarily designed for image-related tasks and rely on local spatial features for convolution operations. However, the input features in this study are extracted numerical descriptors of tumors with no inherent spatial correlation, making CNNs structurally mismatched. RNNs, on the other hand, are designed for sequential or temporal data modeling, such as speech or text. Since the input data in this study consist of independent samples without temporal dependency, RNNs are not suitable for this scenario either.

In contrast, BP neural networks impose minimal assumptions on input data structure and are capable of learning high-order nonlinear mappings through multilayer nonlinear transformations in the hidden layers. Their universal approximation capability has been theoretically validated by the Universal Approximation Theorem. Furthermore, BP networks leverage the chain rule for efficient gradient computation and can be optimized using second-order algorithms such as the Levenberg–Marquardt method, ensuring rapid convergence. In this study, although the FrFT-based preprocessing significantly increases the dimensionality of the input features, the BP network maintains efficient training and convergence performance, with computational complexity remaining within clinically acceptable limits. Therefore, considering structural compatibility, computational efficiency, and generalization performance, the BP neural network is a rational and effective model choice for this specific application.

3. Application of Fractional-Order Calculus Theory to Neural Networks

3.1. *Experimental Data*

The data for this study were obtained from a clinical dataset publicly released by the Northwest University Mathematical Modeling Competiton Organizing Committee in

2023, which consisted of data with nine characteristics, with each cancer case assigned one tumor benign and malignant label provided by a hospital. The dataset contains a total of 608 case samples, including 389 benign and 219 malignant cases, and the image data are anonymized.

3.2. Experimental Methodology

In this paper, we propose a fusion prediction model based on FrFT and the BP neural network, aiming to enhance the neural network's ability to characterize the tumor data through the non-local characteristics of fractional-order calculus [15]. The method uses FrFT to preprocess the original tumor data with a time–frequency domain transform and realizes multi-dimensional signal analysis by adjusting the order in the FrFT, which effectively overcomes the problem of limited generalization performance of traditional neural networks due to local feature extraction [16].

Specifically, we first preprocess the tumor data using FrFT, which effectively enhances the non-local characteristics of the data and extracts unique time–frequency features by adjusting the transform order. The preprocessed data are converted into real-valued features, which are used as inputs to the BP neural network. The output layer of the BP neural network is responsible for predicting the benignness or malignancy of the tumor. During the training process, we use the Levenberg–Marquardt algorithm to optimize the weights and biases of the network to minimize the prediction error. The L-M algorithm is a second-order optimization method that improves the speed of convergence during the learning process by combining the advantages of the gradient descent method and the Newton method [17]. Its update formula is $\Delta\omega = \left(J^T J + \mu I\right)^{-1} J^T e$, where J is the Jacobi matrix of error pair weights, μ is the damping factor, and e is the error vector. The L-M algorithm balances convergence speed and stability by dynamically adjusting μ.

In order to validate the prediction performance of the model, we used a comprehensive assessment of the sum of squared errors (SSE), mean square error (MSE), and root mean square error (RMSE).

The Figure 1 shows the structure of a fractional BP neural network, which is detailed as follows:

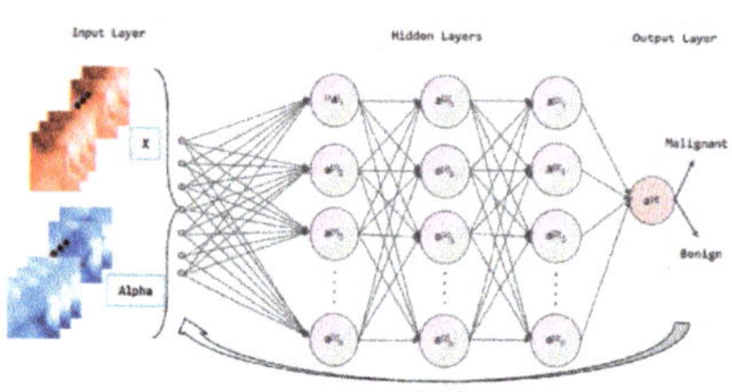

Figure 1. Structure of fractional BP neural network.

(A) Input Layer: The annotation X represents medical instance data input, and the annotation α represents the FrFT parameters.

(B) Hidden Layers: Multiple fully connected layers with node notation $a_i^{[l]}$ (l: layer index, i: node index).

(C) Output Layer: Binary classification (Malignant/Benign) with MSE optimization target.

3.3. Experimental Design

(1) Data processing and FrFT preprocessing

First, this paper uses a dataset in Excel table format containing nine features and a label for tumor benignity and malignancy. The data are transformed by FrFT and the output is a complex-valued result, and we take its magnitude as the final feature data and keep it as a real value. With this treatment, the non-local characteristics of the signal are preserved [18].

(2) Data normalization and training set and test set division

In order to eliminate the scale differences between features and ensure that the training of the model is not affected by the data magnitude, the input data are normalized in [19].

In terms of dataset division, random assignment was used to divide the dataset into training and test sets, where the training set accounted for 80% of the total data and the test set accounted for 20%.

(3) Selection of optimal hidden layer nodes

Too few nodes in the hidden layer will limit the network's ability to learn complex nonlinear relationships, leading to underfitting, while too many nodes will easily trigger the phenomenon of overfitting, reducing the model's ability to generalize on new samples. In order to ensure the training effect of a BP neural network, this study adopts the method of cross-validation to select the optimal number of nodes in the hidden layer. The specific steps are as follows:

Step 1: Set different number of implicit layer nodes (10, 20, 30, 40) for experimentation.

Step 2: Train the network 10 times for each hidden layer node and record the test set mean square error (MSE), that is,

$$MSE = \frac{1}{N}\sum_{i=1}^{N}(y_i - \hat{y}_i)^2,$$

where y_i is the true value, $\hat{y}_i$ is the predicted value, and N is the sample size.

Step 3: Select the number of hidden layer nodes with minimum MSE as the final network structure.

(4) Network training and prediction

Network training is optimized using the Levenberg–Marquardt (L-M) algorithm. The specific process is as follows:

Step 1: Initialize the weights ω and bias b, and set the initial damping factor $\mu = 0.01$ and the maximum number of iterations $T = 2000$.

Step 2: Forward propagation calculates the output error e and constructs the Jacobian matrix J.

Step 3: Solve the linear equation, that is,

$$\Delta\omega = \left(J^T J + \mu I\right)^T J^T e,$$

and update the weights, that is,

$$\omega_{k+1} = \omega_k + \Delta\omega.$$

Step 4: If the error decreases after the update, accept the update and set $\mu = \mu/10$; otherwise, reject the update and order $\mu = \mu \times 10$.

Termination condition: The maximum number of iterations is reached or the error is less than the threshold $\varepsilon = 10^{-7}$.

After the training is completed, predictions are made using the test set data and compared with the actual labels to evaluate the performance of the model.

Remark 1. *If μ is too small, the training MSE will converge fast but the test MSE will be elevated, causing the algorithm to fall into local minima. If μ is too large, the training convergence speed* *will be significantly reduced and the test MSE will be elevated, leading to over-regularization and damaging the model capacity. Therefore, it is important to calculate the appropriate initial μ value, set the initial value of μ as [0.001, 0.01, 0.1, 1, 10], and record the training MSE convergence curve with the test MSE (as shown in Figure 2). Based on the convergence curve analysis, taking into account MSE and number of rounds, we chose μ = 0.01 as it presents the optimal balance between training efficiency and stability, satisfying the dual constraints of medical AI models on training efficiency and computing resources.*

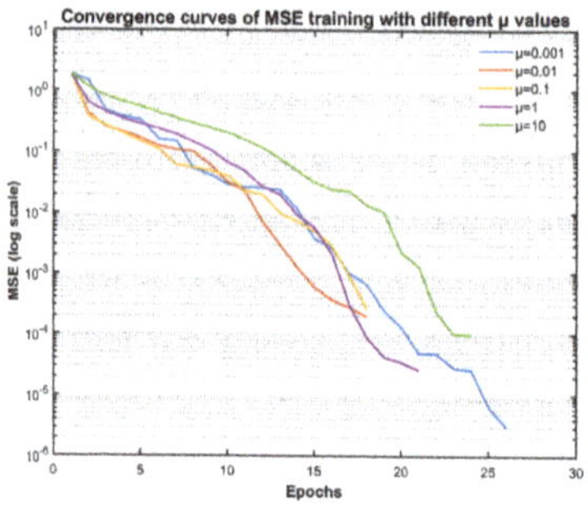

Figure 2. Convergence curves of MSE training with different μ values.

(5) Error analysis and performance evaluation

After the model prediction results are obtained, this paper provides a comprehensive assessment of the model's prediction performance using a variety of error metrics, including the sum of squared errors (SSE), mean absolute error (MAE), mean square error (MSE), root mean square error (RMSE), and mean absolute percentage error (MAPE).

SSE and MSE measure the sum of the squares of the deviations of the predicted values from the true values, which can reflect the overall error level; MAE provides an average assessment of the absolute values of the errors, which is a more intuitive description of the average prediction bias; RMSE places more emphasis on the large error values based on the MAE, which is more sensitive to the fluctuation of the errors; and MAPE is used to assess the relative percentage of the errors, which facilitates the comparison of the data with different scales.

Although the above metrics provide a multifaceted perspective for performance evaluation, there are some limitations in each metric: SSE and MSE are extremely sensitive to outliers, which may lead to underestimation of the overall performance due to a few extreme error values; MAPE produces abnormally large values when the target value is close to zero, which affects the interpretability; and RMSE magnifies the effect of large errors, which may hide the fact that the model performs well in most of the samples. Therefore, relying on a single metric may lead to a misjudgment of model performance.

To compensate for the limitations of these error metrics, this study further combines graphical analysis tools, such as a Regression Chart and a Comparison Chart of Predicted Results, to assess the model's fitting ability and prediction stability. In addition, group comparative analysis of the performance metrics of the training set, validation set, and test set are conducted in this study (i.e., Performance Chart), so as to verify the generalization ability and robustness of the model at different stages. The combination of multiple means makes the model assessment more comprehensive and reliable, ensuring the objectivity and credibility of the conclusions.

This flowchart (Figure 3) presents the key implementation steps of the FrFT-BP hybrid model:

(1) Perform multi-scale time–frequency decomposition on the original tumor features using FrFT ($\alpha = 0.7$) (Step 1).
(2) Using normalization to process the training set data (Step 2).
(3) Determine the optimal number of hidden layer nodes through cross validation (Step 3).
(4) Apply Levenberg–Marquardt second-order optimization algorithm for network training, including forward propagation → error backpropagation → Hessian matrix update (Step 4).
(5) Evaluate the performance of the model based on seven indicators including SSE, MAE, MAPE, etc. (Step 5).

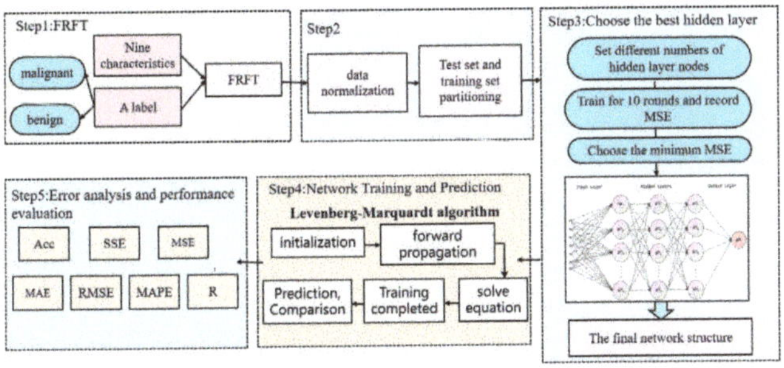

Figure 3. Flowchart of experimental design.

4. Analysis of Outcomes of Tumor Benignity and Malignancy Prediction

4.1. Implementation Details

The experiments were implemented in MATLAB R2022b using a customized function to perform the FrFT on the input data. The FrFT kernel was designed based on the time-domain definition with adjustable fractional order α. Each sample's real and imaginary parts were extracted and concatenated to form the new input features.

The BP neural network was constructed using MATLAB's `newff` function from the Neural Network Toolbox. The input data were normalized to [0, 1], and the output labels were normalized using `mapminmax`. The training was conducted using the Levenberg–Marquardt algorithm (`trainlm`), with the following parameters:

- Learning rate: 0.001.
- Maximum epochs: 2000.
- Performance goal (MSE): 10^{-7}.
- Transfer functions: `tansig` for hidden layer and `purelin` for output layer.

The optimal number of hidden neurons was determined through empirical testing, starting from $\sqrt{n+m}+1$ to $\sqrt{n+m}+10$, where n and m denote the number of input and output neurons, respectively. The best architecture was selected based on the lowest mean squared error (MSE) on the training set.

All experiments were conducted on a personal computer with the following specifications:

- CPU: R7-5825U
- RAM: 16 GB
- Operating System: Windows 11

4.2. Evaluation of the Neural Network Training Outcomes

This paper uses three charts, the performance chart, the training state chart, and the regression chart, to demonstrate the neural network's training effect and prediction ability while training. These figures thoroughly highlight the key indicators used during the training process as well as the model's effect after training.

- **Performance Chart**

The performance chart (as shown in Figure 4) shows how the mean square error (MSE) varies with the number of iterations during the BP neural network's training process. The chart shows how well the network fits the training data in each cycle. The performance chart shows gradually decreasing inaccuracy, which often suggests that the network is constantly improving its fit to the training data. As the training develops, the error stabilizes, indicating that the network is close to optimal and the training process converges.

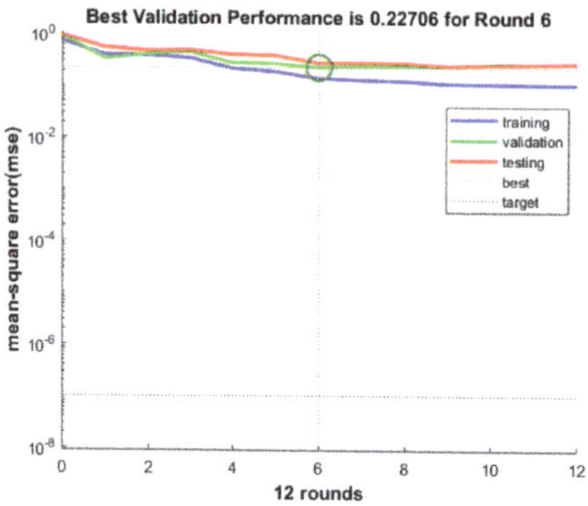

Figure 4. Performance chart.

The model's training quality can be visualized by observing the chart, where the error decreases faster and more smoothly, indicating better training results.

- **Training Status Chart**

The training status chart usually shows the network training state at various stages of the training process. The figure (as shown in Figure 5) shows the training dynamics of the neural network model in 10 rounds of iterations; the gradient continues to decrease, the μ exponential level decreases, and the validation check reaches the early stopping condition within a reasonable number of rounds, all of which indicate that the neural network has effectively completed the learning of the data features and successfully avoided the occurrence of the overfitting phenomenon.

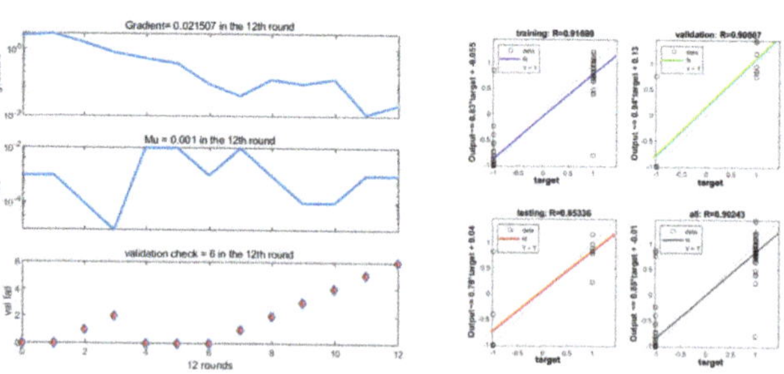

Figure 5. Training status chart (**left**) and regression chart (**right**).

- **Regression Chart**

The regression graph shows the relationship between the predicted values and the true values. The graph illustrates the relationship for the four processes: Training, Validation, Testing, and All.

(1) Training set regression performance (Training: R = 0.9806)

The blue fitted line in the figure is very close to the ideal line (Y = T), with a correlation coefficient R of 0.9806. This indicates that the neural network has an extremely strong fit on the training data. The regression equation is as follows:

$$\text{Output} \approx 0.95 \times \text{target} - 0.018$$

The slope is close to 1 and the intercept is close to 0, further indicating that the deviation between the predicted values and the true values is small, and the fitting is excellent.

(2) Validation set regression performance (Validation: R = 0.86481)

The green fitted line deviates slightly from the ideal line, with an R value of 0.86481. Although slightly lower than the training set, it still shows a strong correlation. The regression equation is

$$\text{Output} \approx 0.8 \times \text{Target} - 0.07$$

This shows that the model still has some generalization ability on data not involved in training and does not show serious overfitting.

(3) Regression performance on the test set (Testing: R = 0.91254)

The fitting performance in the test set is good, with an R value of 0.91254, a slope of 0.83, and an intercept of −0.14. This indicates that the model predicts unknown data more accurately and has good robustness.

(4) Overall regression performance (All: R = 0.95612)

The regression plot of the integrated dataset shows an overall correlation coefficient R of 0.95612, indicating strong overall prediction ability. The regression equation is

$$\text{Output} \approx 0.92 \times \text{Target} - 0.037$$

This is also close to the ideal line, further validating the model's good learning ability across the sample space.

All four regression plots demonstrate a high correlation between the predicted output and the actual target. The R-values of the training and overall datasets are particularly close to 1, indicating that the model accurately captures the nonlinear relationship between inputs and targets, showing strong potential for practical application.

Further comparison of the prediction results is shown in Figure 6. The left figure verifies the discriminative ability of the BP neural network in benign and malignant tumor prediction. The network output is highly consistent with the real labels on the whole, indicating that the model has good generalization ability and robustness in the binary classification task. The right panel reveals the predictive stability and robustness of the BP neural network in tumor benign and malignant classification. The model predicts the vast majority of test samples accurately with high error concentration and no systematic bias in the overall error.

With a prediction accuracy of 93.177%, the experimental results show that the model based on the combination of the FrFT and BP neural network makes more accurate predictions on the test set. The model accurately predicts whether a tumor is benign or malignant, as evidenced by the small gap between the predicted and true values in the chart of true and predicted values.

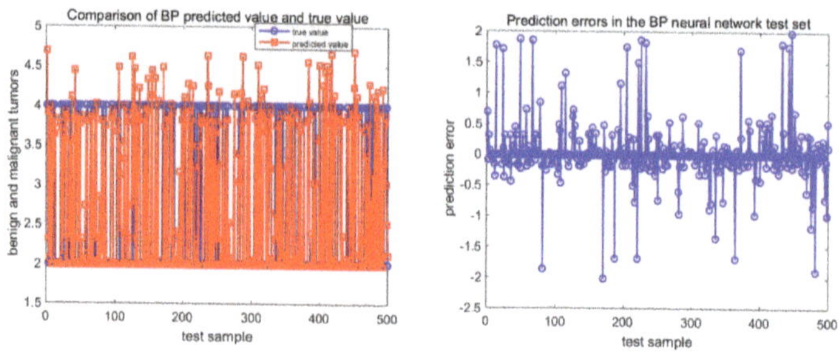

Figure 6. Comparison chart of predicted results.

4.3. Prediction Accuracy Under Different Orders

The figure (as shown in Figure 7) shows the variation in prediction accuracy of the neural network model under different orders α. The accuracy peaks at $\alpha = 0.7$ (93.177%), indicating the importance of selecting an appropriate order for optimal model performance.

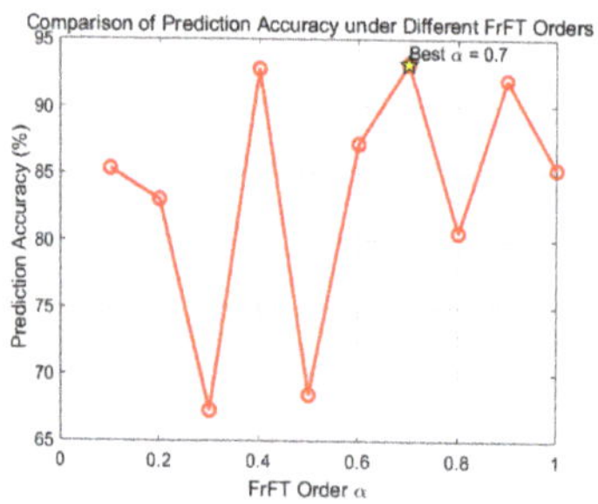

Figure 7. Comparison of prediction accuracy under different FrFT orders.

4.4. Comparative Experimental Design

Since the support vector machine (SVM) method is suitable for processing high-dimensional medical data and can classify nonlinear data through the kernel function, this paper uses it as a comparison model and conducts comparative experiments based on the same preprocessed dataset to evaluate the performance of the two methods under several evaluation metrics such as accuracy, sum of squares of errors (SSE), mean absolute error (MAE), mean square error (MSE), root mean square error (RMSE), mean percentage error (MAPE) and correlation coefficient (R) under several evaluation indexes.

The following (Table 1) are the results:

Table 1. Comparison of the results of the indicators of the two models.

INDEX	Acc	SSE	MAE	MSE	RMSE	MAPE	*R*
BP	93.177	83.789	0.193	0.178	0.421	6.823	0.901
SVM	64.130	132	0.717	1.435	1.198	17.935	−0.560

The experimental results show that the model based on FrFT combined with the BP neural network proposed in this paper outperforms the SVM model in all the metrics in the benign–malignant tumor prediction task.

Specifically, the model has smaller SSE and MSE, which indicates that it fits the sample data better during the training process; the MAE and RMSE are also lower, which show stronger predictive stability and robustness; the correlation coefficient R value is close to

1, which further verifies that the model prediction results are highly consistent with the real values.

In contrast, despite its good generalization ability, the performance of the SVM method is highly dependent on the selection of the kernel function and the accurate tuning of parameters when facing the complex nonlinear structure of tumor data. If the kernel function is not properly set, the model may not be able to fully explore the implicit associations between higher-order features. In contrast, the BP neural network used in this paper constructs the higher-order feature interaction structure through multi-layer nested nonlinear activation functions and combines with the frequency domain feature enhancement provided by FrFT, which enables the model to adaptively capture the multi-scale information, thus improving the ability to recognize the benignness and malignancy of tumors.

In addition, under the premise of moderate sample size, high feature dimensions, and complex nonlinear relationships among variables, BP neural networks have more modeling flexibility and expressive ability than SVMs. Therefore, the method in this paper shows better performance and adaptability in such medical prediction scenarios.

4.5. Discussion on Computational Complexity

In terms of computational complexity, the proposed FrFT-BP neural network includes a preprocessing step where the fractional Fourier transform is applied to each input sample. This step has a complexity of $O(N \cdot d)$ for N samples and d features. While this introduces additional computation compared to traditional BP or SVM models, it significantly enhances the feature representation, leading to improved learning efficiency and accuracy.

Compared with SVMs, especially those using nonlinear kernels, which typically require solving quadratic programming problems with complexity ranging from $O(N^2)$ to $O(N^3)$, our model is computationally more efficient and scalable. Additionally, SVMs often require parameter tuning and kernel selection, which further adds to the computation burden.

Overall, the FrFT-BP method achieves a favorable balance between accuracy and computational cost, making it a practical choice for large-scale classification problems.

4.6. Error Sources and Research Limitations

Although the FrFT-BP model proposed in this paper shows high classification accuracy on the current dataset, there are still some non-negligible sources of error and research limitations. First, the input data have certain fractal characteristics and non-stationarity, and although the feature extraction stage improves the signal characterization ability with the help of FrFT, the selection of fractional order is still dependent on experiments and lacks the theoretical optimality guarantee; second, there is a certain category imbalance and labeling subjectivity in the training data, which may lead to unstable prediction of the model on the boundary samples. In addition, although the overall accuracy of SVM is lower than that of the present method, it shows better generalization ability in the case of high-dimensional features, which suggests that we should pay attention to the adaptability of different models to the data structure in model selection.

From a system perspective, the model has not yet been validated cross-platform in different imaging devices and clinical scenarios, and its ability to process high-resolution images (e.g., 4K pathology slices) and computational efficiency still need to be further optimized. Meanwhile, due to the sensitivity of medical data, the regulatory constraints on data access and sharing are also a realistic bottleneck for future large-scale deployment. Therefore, despite the superior performance of the model in experiments, its generalized application still needs to be continuously improved in terms of model interpretability, real-time reasoning capability, and system integration.

5. Conclusions and Outlook

5.1. Conclusions

In this paper, a benign–malignant tumor prediction model combining FrFT and BP neural networks is proposed. The experimental results show that the FrFT can effectively enhance the non-local characteristics of the data and improve the prediction accuracy of the BP neural network. The model not only has high prediction accuracy, but also performs well in error analysis, proving its potential application in tumor prediction.

5.2. Impact on Field of Medical Image Analysis and Tumor Diagnosis

(1) Enhanced characterization of medical image features

The FrFT-BP neural network fusion model proposed in this study achieves the enhanced characterization of tumor morphological features through the time–frequency rotational property of FrFT. Experiments show that the model improves the prediction accuracy while improving its classification performance compared with the traditional integer-order Fourier transform. This method provides a new mathematical tool for mining the deep time–frequency features of tumors.

(2) Promoting real-time aided diagnosis

The FrFT-BP neural network fusion model proposed in this study effectively improves the model efficiency by reducing the number of training iterations through the second-order convergence property of the Levenberg–Marquardt algorithm. It provides a technical prototype for outpatient real-time screening and helps the intelligent transformation of domestic medical equipment.

(3) Optimization of clinical decision support system

The FrFT-BP neural network fusion model proposed in this study can be used to assist doctors in diagnosis, and at the same time, doctors can be reminded to make follow-up consultations in time for complicated cases, in order to prevent patients from missing the golden stage of early cancer treatment.

5.3. Future Prospects

- **Expand the application of medical data:** Apply existing mathematical frameworks to the analysis of pathological sections, genomic data, etc., and explore how to combine different types of medical data through fractional-order methods. At the same time, develop new mathematical tools to more accurately identify the features of tumor edges.
- **Interdisciplinary research:** Combining mathematics and artificial intelligence technology to predict the development trend of tumors is promising direction of research. By using fractional time series analysis and recurrent neural networks, a model can be constructed to predict the probability of tumor deterioration, which could help with early detection and treatment. Meanwhile, studying the efficacy of drugs in cancer treatment and exploring the relationship between tumor characteristics and drug metabolism are important directions of study.
- **Exploration of clinical application:** It is important to conduct actual testing on a certain type of tumor case to verify the stability of the model under different devices and scanning methods, ensuring its wide applicability in clinical practice. Simultaneously optimizing the algorithm to meet the fast processing requirements of 4K medical images should also be explored.

5.4. Potential Challenges in Clinical Application

While the proposed method shows promising results in classification accuracy and generalization, several challenges remain for its clinical deployment. These include the following:

- **Data Privacy:** Medical data are sensitive and subject to strict regulations, making data access and sharing a potential barrier.
- **Model Interpretability:** Deep learning models, including BP neural networks, are often criticized for their "black box" nature, which limits clinicians' trust.
- **Scalability:** Real-time application in clinical workflows requires integration with hospital systems and optimization for inference speed.
- **Patient Rights:** The model is designed to assist physicians in decision-making or prompt follow-up examinations, rather than replacing clinical diagnoses, thereby potentially reducing the risk of misdiagnosis. Furthermore, the diagnostic report will clearly indicate that it is an "AI-assisted result", and patients can access the model version and performance metrics through the hospital information system.

Future work will focus on addressing these issues through interpretable model designs, federated learning frameworks, and collaborations with clinical institutions.

5.5. Ethical Statement

This study is based on publicly available datasets that do not involve any personally identifiable patient information. No clinical trials or patient interventions were conducted. Any future clinical application of the proposed method will be subject to formal ethical review and institutional approval to ensure compliance with data protection and research ethics guidelines.

Author Contributions: Writing—original draft, X.L., N.G. and S.H.; Writing—review & editing, X.L., N.G. and S.H.; Project administration, L.W. All authors have read and agreed to the published version of the manuscript.

Funding: This work is supported by the National Natural Science Foundation of China (Grant No. 12271433).

Data Availability Statement: The raw data supporting the conclusions of this article will be made available by the authors on request. The dataset utilized in this study originates from the Northwest University Mathematical Modeling Competition Organizing Committee, which has made the data publicly available through competition problems. Although the specific location of the database has not been disclosed, the relevant data can be obtained by contacting the relevant Committee. In this research, we have rigorously filtered the published dataset, excluding any unknown or ambiguous data points to ensure the accuracy and reliability of our study. This data processing procedure not only enhances the quality of the data but also provides a solid foundation for subsequent analysis.

Conflicts of Interest: The authors declare that they have no conflicts of interest.

References

1. Bray, F.; Laversanne, M.; Sung, H.; Ferlay, J.; Siegel, R.L.; Soerjomataram, I.; Jemal, A. Global Cancer Statistics 2022: GLOBOCAN estimates of incidence and mortality worldwide for 36 cancers in 185 countries. *CA Cancer J. Clin.* **2024**, *74*, 205–249. [CrossRef] [PubMed]
2. Namias, V. The Fractional Order Fourier Transform and its Application to Quantum Mechanics. *Geoderma* **1980**, *25*, 241–265. [CrossRef]
3. Almeida, L.B. The fractional Fourier transform and time-frequency representations. *IEEE Trans. Signal Process.* **1994**, *42*, 3084–3091. [CrossRef]
4. Zhan, H. Classification method of motor imagery eeg signals based on FrFT and RVM. *Comput. Appl. Softw.* **2020**, *37*, 146–153.
5. Rumelhart, D.E.; Hinton, G.E.; Williams, R.J. Learning representations by back-propagating errors. *Nature* **1986**, *323*, 533–536. [CrossRef]
6. Ge, M.; Li, Z.; Liu, J.; Wang, H.; Wang, J. Diagnosis and prediction of breast cancer based on BP_Adaboost model. *J. Terahertz Sci. Electron. Inf. Technol.* **2023**, *21*, 1014–1021.
7. Chen, Y. An Improved Quantum Genetic Algorithm Optimized BP neural network for Malignant Tumor Diagnosis. *Inf. Comput.* **2022**, *34*, 179–181.

8. Zheng, J. Time-Frequency Scattering Convolutional Network Based on Short-time Fractional Fourier Transform. Ph.D. Dissertation, Harbin Institute of Technology, Harbin, China, 2021.
9. Tao, R.; Deng, B.; Wang, Y. *Fractional Fourier Transform and Its Applications*; Tsinghua University Press: Beijing, China, 2009; pp. 10–13.
10. Li, S. Research and Hardware Implementation of Fractional Fourier Transform Algorithm Based on FPGA. Ph.D. Dissertation, Guizhou University, Guiyang, China, 2024.
11. Shao, Y. The Application of Fractional Fourier Transform in Signal Analysis. Master's Thesis, Chinese Master's Theses Full-Text Database, Harbin University of Science and Technology, Harbin, China, 2016.
12. Li, X.; Xing, L. Traffic flow forecast based on optimal order fractional neural network. *Comput. Eng. Appl.* **2012**, *48*, 226–230.
13. Liu, T. Improvement Research and Application of BP Neural Network. Ph.D. Dissertation, Northeast Agricultural University, Harbin, China, 2011.
14. Ping, L.; Lingke, Z.; Anze, T. Design of BP neural network prediction system based on MATLAB. *Comput. Appl. Softw.* **2008**, *25*, 149–150+184.
15. Li, Y.; Xin, M. Fault detection of industrial processes based on fractional order Fourier transform and convolutional neural network. *Electron. Meas. Technol.* **2024**, *47*, 1–8.
16. Xiang, P.; Li, H.; Song, J.; Hou, S.; Zhou, H. Hyperspectral anomaly detection with local correlation fractional Fourier transform and vector pulse coupled neural network. *Infrared Phys. Technol.* **2022**, *127*, 104430. [CrossRef]
17. Zhao, H.; Zhou, R.; Lin, T. Neural network Supervised Control Based on Levenberg-Marquardt Algorithm. *J. Xi'An Jiaotong Univ.* **2002**, *36*, 523–527.
18. Lu, X.; Song, L.; Xu, H.; Su, D. Single sample electromagnetic spectrum recognition utilizing fractional Fourier transform. *Chin. J. Aeronaut.* **2024**, *37*, 435–446. [CrossRef]
19. Liu, X. Study on Data Normalization in BP neural network. *Mech. Eng. Autom.* **2010**, *3*, 122–123+126.

MDPI AG
Grosspeteranlage 5
4052 Basel
Switzerland
Tel.: +41 61 683 77 34

Fractal and Fractional Editorial Office
E-mail: fractalfract@mdpi.com
www.mdpi.com/journal/fractalfract

www.ingramcontent.com/pod-product-compliance
Lightning Source LLC
Chambersburg PA
CBHW061618210926
51850CB00009B/2369
* 9 7 8 3 7 2 5 8 4 8 4 7 8 *